Copyright 2020 by Linda Wegner -All rights reserved.

No part of this book may be reproduced or transmitted in any form or by any means, electronic or mechanical, including photocopying and recording, or by any information storage and retrieval system, without permission in writing from the publisher. This is a work of fiction. Names, places, characters and incidents are either the product of the author's imagination or are used fictitiously, and any resemblance to any actual persons, living or dead, organizations, events or locales is entirely coincidental. The unauthorized reproduction or distribution of this copyrighted work is ilegal.

Disclaimer Notice:

Please note the information contained within this document is for educational and entertainment purposes only. All effort has been executed to present accurate, up to date, reliable, complete information. No warranties of any kind are declared or implied. Readers acknowledge that the author is not engaged in the rendering of legal, financial, medical, or professional advice. The content within this book has been derived from various sources. Please consult a licensed professional before attempting any techniques outlined in this book.

By reading this document, the reader agrees that under no circumstances is the author responsible for any losses, direct or indirect, that are incurred as a result of the use of the information contained within this document, including, but not limited to, errors, omissions, or inaccuracies.

CONTENTS

- INTRODUCTION 8
- 2-WEEKS MEAL PLAN 9
  - Day 1 9
    - Breakfast Egg Crepes With Avocados 9
    - Easy Keto Pepperoni Meatballs 9
    - Keto Curried Tomato Soup 9
    - Keto Guacamole Burgers 9
  - Day 2 10
    - Keto Cloud Bread 10
    - Garlic Bacon Wrapped Chicken Bites Recipe 10
    - Cream Of Celery Soup 10
    - Keto Broccoli Beef Stir-Fry Recipe 10
  - Day 3 11
    - Healthy Chocolate Peanut Butter Low Carb Smoothie 11
    - Easy Pan-Fried Lemon Chicken 11
    - Keto Broccoli Soup Recipe 11
    - Kale Keto Tofu Stir Fry 11
  - Day 4 12
    - Keto Roasted Brussels Sprouts With Garlic 12
    - Keto Chicken Hearts Recipe 12
    - Fresh Tomato Basil Soup 12
    - Bacon-Wrapped Meatloaf 12
  - Day 5 13
    - Keto "Everything" Avocado Breakfast 13
    - Paleo Guacamole Burger Recipe 13
    - Baked Sausage With Creamy Basil Sauce 13
    - Turkey Meatloaf 13
  - Day 6 14
    - Keto Boosted Coffee Recipe 14
    - Keto Almond Butter Cookie Dough 14
    - Keto Baked Bacon Omelet 14
    - Keto Electrolyte Drink 14
  - Day 7 15
    - Keto Brunch Spread 15
    - Keto 5-Ingredient Coconut Flour Cookies 15
    - Keto Fried Chicken With Broccoli 15
    - Rosemary Mint Soda 15
  - Day 8 16
    - Keto 3-Ingredient Muffins Recipe 16
    - Keto Madeleine Cookies 16
    - Keto Smoked Salmon Plate 16
    - Keto Chocolate Coconut Cups 16
  - Day 9 17
    - Crispy Keto Chicken Thighs Recipe 17
    - Keto 4-Ingredient Almond Flour Cookies 17
    - Keto Smoked Salmon And Avocado Plate 17
    - Low Carb Keto Chocolate Bar 17
  - Day 10 18
    - Three Ingredient Keto Steak Sauté 18
    - Keto Shortbread Cookies 18
    - Keto Fried Cabbage With Crispy Bacon 18
    - Frozen Blueberry Fat Bombs 18
  - Day 11 19
    - Keto Breakfast Pizza 19
    - Keto "Peanut Butter" Cookies 19
    - Keto Smoked Salmon Plate 19
    - Coconut Fat Bombs 19
  - Day 12 20
    - Keto Lemon Baked Salmon Recipe 20
    - Keto Pecan Crisps Recipe 20
    - Keto Smoked Salmon And Avocado Plate 20
    - Cheese Meatloaf 20
  - Day 13 21
    - Herb Roasted Bone Marrow 21
    - Low Carb Onion Rings 21
    - Keto Salmon-Filled Avocados 21
    - Keto Pizza Casserole 21
  - Day 14 22
    - Grilled Beef Liver 22
    - Farmhouse Beans & Sausage 22
    - Keto Fried Salmon With Green Beans 22
    - 4-Ingredient Pancakes 22
- Smoothies & BREAKFASTs Recipes 23
  - Perfect Keto Avocado Breakfast Bowl 23
  - Sheet Pan Brussels Sprouts With Bacon 23
  - Kale And Chives Egg Muffins 23
  - 3-Ingredient Bacon And Egg Breakfast Muffins 23
  - Keto Mushroom Omelet 23
  - Coconut Macadamia Bars – Breakfast In Five 24
  - 10-Minute Keto Toast Recipe 24
  - Keto Smoothie - Blueberry 24
  - Perfect Keto Peaches And Cream Fat Bombs 24
  - Creamy Triple Chocolate Keto Shake 24
  - Frozen Keto Berry Shake 25
  - Minty Green Protein Smoothie Shake 25
  - Keto Beetroot Shake For Athletes 25
  - Healthy Chocolate Peanut Butter Low Carb Smoothie 25
  - Mckee Strawberry Keto Milkshake 25
  - Coconut Milk Strawberry Smoothie 25
  - Blueberry Coconut Yogurt Smoothie Recipe 25
  - Keto Chocolate Smoothie 26
  - Strawberry Avocado Keto Smoothie With Almond Milk 26
  - Low Carb Blueberry Protein Power Smoothie 26
  - Strawberry Protein Smoothie 26
  - Low-Carb Blueberry Vanilla Smoothie 26
  - Dairy-Free Peanut Butter And Jelly Smoothie 26
  - Keto Organic Peanut Smoothie 26
  - Energizing Keto Smoothie 27
  - Keto Blueberry Ginger Smoothie 27
  - Refreshing Cucumber Celery Lime Smoothie 27
  - Sleep In" Smoothie 27
  - Keto Chocolate Peppermint Smoothie Recipe 27
  - Keto Raspberry Avocado Smoothie 27
  - Easy Keto Avocado Toast Recipe 27
  - Chocolate Protein Waffles 27
  - Keto Lemon Ginger Green Juice Shots Recipe 28
  - Keto Red Velvet Smoothie Recipe 28
  - Keto Spinach Avocado Green Smoothie 28
  - Strawberry Avocado Coconut Smoothie 28
  - Cinnamon Chocolate Breakfast Smoothie Recipe 28
  - Strawberry & Mint Smoothie 28
  - Keto Chocolate Raspberry Spinach Green Smoothie 29
  - Keto Ginger Cilantro Smoothie 29

- Keto Smoothie Recipe {With Chocolate & Chia Seeds} 29
- Low-Carb 5 Minute Mocha Smoothie 29
- Salted Caramel Keto Smoothie 29
- Buttery Coconut Flour Waffles 29
- Vegan Keto Porridge 30
- Cinnamon Faux-St Crunch Cereal 30
- Coconut Flour Crepes 30
- Keto Four-Ingredient Pancake With Almond Flour Recipe 30
- Keto Bacon Asparagus Mini Frittata Recipe ... 30
- Paleo Egg Frittata Muffins Recipe [Keto, Dairy-Free] 31
- Keto Oatmeal: 5-Minute Low-Carb Oatmeal ... 31
- Meat-Lover Pizza Cups 31
- Cold Brew Protein Shake Smoothie 31
- Coco-Nutty Grain-Free Granola 31
- Keto Sausage And Egg Breakfast Sandwich ... 32
- Easy Low Carb Keto Breakfast Casserole 32
- Low Carb Orange Dreamlike Smoothie 32
- Holley's Ham And Swiss Breakfast Muffins ... 32
- Cheesy Egg White Veggie Breakfast Muffins .. 32
- Cinnamon "Rice" Breakfast Pudding 33
- High Protein Low Carb Breakfast Casserole ... 33
- Everything But The Bagel 33

Poultry Recipes 34
- Baked Pesto Chicken 34
- Simple Bone Broth 34
- Spring Soup With Poached Egg 34
- Boiled Eggs With Butter And Thyme 34
- Keto Dijon Smothered Chicken Drumsticks ... 34
- Keto Crispy Rosemary Chicken Drumsticks ... 35
- Chicken Breast With Olive Tapenade 35
- Pan-Seared Beef Tongue 35
- Beef Tongue Into Delicious Crispy Beef 35
- Keto Crockpot Shredded Chicken 35
- Keto Buffalo Cauliflower Wings 36
- Smoked Paprika Chicken 36
- Slow Cooker Paleo Chicken Broth 36
- Lemon Parsley Chicken 36
- Bbq Chicken Livers And Heart 36
- Keto Crockpot Garlic Chicken 37
- Slow Cooker Chicken Adobo Keto 37
- Slow Cook Chicken Curry 37
- Split Chicken Breast With Onions And Mushrooms 37
- Crock Pot Chicken Stock 37
- Crockpot Chicken Stock 38
- Bbq Chicken Livers And Hearts 38
- Healthy Buffalo Chicken Dip 38
- 2 Ingredient Paleo Crockpot Chicken 38
- Lemon Pepper Chicken 38
- Juicy Ranch Chicken 39
- World's Moistest Chicken 39
- Avocado Chicken Salad 39
- Chicken Liver With Raw Garlic And Thyme ... 39
- Bacon-Wrapped Tahini And Sun-Dried Tomato Stuffed Chicken Breasts 39
- Paleo Crispy Garlic Curry Chicken Drumsticks Recipe 40
- Pomegranate Chicken Salad Recipe 40
- Chicken Pepper Poppers For Bbqs And Potlucks 40
- Paleo Garlic Chicken Nuggets 40
- Keto Lemon Pepper Roast Chicken 41
- Chicken Caesar 41
- Chicken, Bacon, And Apple Mini Meatloaves Recipe 41
- Garlic Lemon Chicken Breast 41
- Easy 5 Ingredient Paleo Roast Chicken 42
- Simple Marinated Chicken Hearts 42
- Keto Almond Butter Chicken Saute 42
- Homemade Thai Chicken Broth 42
- Garlic Ghee Baked Chicken Breast 42
- Grilled Chicken Drumsticks With Garlic Marinade 43
- Baked Chicken Meatballs - Habanero & Green Chili 43
- Grilled Chicken With Chimichurri Sauce 43
- Balsamic, Garlic, And Basil Marinated Chicken Breasts 43
- Keto Golden Chicken Bacon Fritter Balls Recipe 44
- Easy Paleo Chicken Pepper Stir-Fry 44
- Keto Macadamia Crusted Chicken Breast 44
- Keto Crockpot Garlic Chicken 44
- Bacon Avocado Ranch Chicken Burger And Tabasco Sauce 44
- Stuffed Chicken With Asparagus & Bacon 45
- Easy Mozzarella & Pesto Chicken Casserole .. 45
- Bacon-Wrapped Chicken Tenders With Ranch Dip 45
- Chili Roasted Chicken Thighs 45
- Super Easy Spicy Baked Chicken 45
- Chicken Al Forno With Vodka Sauce & Two Kinds Of Cheese 46
- Easy Mexican Chicken Casserole With Chipotle 46
- Ranch Chicken 46
- Chicken Bacon Ranch Casserole 46
- 5 Ingredient Bacon Wrapped Chicken Breast .. 46
- Parmesan Chicken Tenders 47
- Broiled Chicken Thighs With Artichokes And Garlic 47
- Rosemary Garlic Chicken Kabobs 47
- Keto Honey Mustard Chicken 47
- Crockpot Green Chile Chicken 47
- Blackened Dijon Chicken 48
- Blackened Ranch Pan-Fried Chicken Thighs .. 48
- Keto Slow Cooker Greek Chicken 48
- Instant Pot Keto Crack Chicken 48
- Creamy Mexican Slow Cooker Keto Chicken .. 49
- Basil Stuffed Chicken Breasts 49
- Low Carb Chicken Nuggets Keto 49
- Keto Honey Mustard Chicken 49

Pork, Beef & Lamb Recipes 50
- Vegged Up Paleo Beef Burgers 50
- Slow Cooker Pork 50
- Paleo Slow Cooker Pork Recipe 50
- World's Easiest Crockpot Pork Roast 50
- Keto Roasted Bone Marrow Recipe 50

- Easy Slow Cooker Keto Pot Roast 50
- Rosemary Liver Burgers 50
- Keto Oven-Baked Steak With Garlic Thyme Portabella Mushrooms 51
- Low-Carb Stuffed Poblano Peppers 51
- Mini Zucchini Avocado Burgers 51
- Keto Instant Pot Roasted Bone Broth Recipe ... 51
- Paleo Crock Pot Oxtail With Mustard Gravy 52
- Cowboy Burgers (Keto) 52
- Lamb & Leek Burgers 52
- Easy Broiled Table Seasoned Mini Beef Patties 52
- Corned Beef Hash 52
- Slow-Cooked Keto Corned Beef Brisket 53
- Keto Steak Au Poivre 53
- Hidden Liver Meatballs 53
- Keto Spicy Beef Avocado Cups 53
- Simple Beef Tenderloin Filet Mignon 53
- Keto Skirt Steak 54
- Three Ingredient Keto Steak Sauté 54
- Easy Marinated Grilled Steak Tacos 54
- Paleo-Italian Carpaccio 54
- Butter Coffee Rubbed Tri-Tip Steak 54
- Paleo Rib Eye Steak 55
- Keto Spicy Beef Avocado Cups 55
- Keto Rosemary Roast Beef And White Radishes 55
- Keto Broccoli Beef Stir-Fry 55
- Cube Steak 55
- Beef (Heart) Steak 56
- Keto Corned Beef And Hash Recipe 56
- Keto Sous-Vide Fillet Steak Recipe 56
- Keto Beef Liver With Asian Dip 56
- Pan Seared Duck Breast 57
- Keto Steak Au Poivre 57
- Keto Oven-Baked Steak With Garlic Thyme Portabella Mushrooms 57
- Keto Sous-Vide Fillet Steak Recipe 57
- Tuscan-Style Grilled Rib Eye Steak 58
- Corned Beef And Cauliflower Hash 58
- Easy Zucchini Beef Saute, Garlic, And Cilantro. 58
- Easy Paleo Broccoli Beef Recipe 58
- Low Carb Pork Medallions 58
- Stuffed Pork Chops – 5 Ingredients 59
- Chipotle Steak Bowl 59
- Bacon-Wrapped Pork Chops 59
- Slow Cooker Keto Corned Beef Cabbage 59
- Shredded Taco Pork 60
- Kalua Pork 60
- Coffee Barbecue Pork Belly 60
- Low Carb Tortilla Pork Rind Wraps 60
- Keto Chili Dog Pot Pie Casserole 60
- Keto Barbecue Dry Rub Ribs 61
- Easy Keto Instant Pot Chile Verde 61
- Garlic Butter Baked Pork Chops 61
- Stuffed Pork Chops With Bacon And Gouda 61
- Rosemary Garlic Butter Pork Chops 62
- Pecan Crusted Pork Chops 62
- Stuffed Pork Chops – 5 Ingredients 62
- Pot Pork Chops Dinner 62
- Crispy Pork Chops Keto 63
- Caramelized Onion And Bacon Pork Chops 63
- Keto Pork Belly 63
- Lemon Pepper Pork Chops 63
- Boneless Pork Chops Recipe 63
- Slow Cooker Keto Meatballs 64
- Easy Zucchini Beef Saute, Garlic, And Cilantro. 64
- Easy Keto Broccoli Beef Recipe 64
- The Best Bunless Burger Recipe Burgers 64
- Keto Slow Cooker Onions 64
- Lamb Lollipops With Garlic And Rosemary Recipe 65
- Grilled Lamb In Paleo Mint Cream Sauce 65
- Grilled Lamb Chops With Dijon-Basil Butter 65
- Garlic & Rosemary Lamb Chops 65
- Greek Lamb Chop Marinade 66
- Lamb, Red Onion And Herb Koftas 66
- Sausage Kale Soup With Mushroom 66
- Lamb & Leek Burgers With Lemon Cream 66
- Guilt-Free Slow Cooked Shoulder Of Lamb 66
- One-Pot Braised Lamb With Caramelized Onions And Rosemary 67

Side Dishes & SNACKS Recipes 68
- Keto Jalapeno Poppers 68
- Lemon Fruit And Nut Bars 68
- Cauliflower Fried Rice With Bacon Recipe 68
- Spicy Keto Deviled Eggs 68
- Keto Cheese Omelet 68
- Halloumi Cheese With Butter-Fried Eggplant .. 69
- Keto Brunch Spread 69
- Broccoli & Cheddar Keto Bread 69
- White Lasagna Stuffed Peppers 69
- Easy Taco Casserole Recipe 70
- Spicy Keto Cheese Chips 70
- Boiled Eggs With Butter And Thyme 70
- Keto Cookie Dough (With Chocolate Chips) 70
- Lemon Turmeric Roasted Cauliflower Keto 70
- Fluffy Microwave Scrambled Eggs 71
- Pizza Eggs Keto 71
- Caesar Salad Deviled Eggs 71
- Caesar Egg Salad Lettuce Wraps 71
- Sour Cream And Chive Egg Clouds 71
- Low Carb Keto Egg Noodles 72
- Egg Fast Recipe: Egg Puffs 72
- Egg Fast Fried Boiled Eggs With Yum Yum Sauce 72
- Microwave Paleo Bread 72
- Low-Carb Keto Tuna Pickle Boats 72
- Keto-Friendly Baked Cheese Crisps 73
- One-Minute Keto Mug Bread 73
- Keto Cinnamon Chocolate Chia Pudding 73
- Turkey And Cheese Rolls 73
- Low Carb Bacon & Eggs 73
- Portobello Mushroom Mini Keto Pizzas 73
- Best Keto Popcorn Cheese Puffs 74
- Keto Low Carb Tortilla Chips 74
- Cheddar And Everything Seasoning Fat Bombs 74
- Bacon-Wrapped Avocado Fries 74
- Keto Stove-Top Bone Broth 74
- The Ultimate Keto Buns 74
- Crispy Sweet Potato Fries 75

- Keto Pizza Chips 75
- Avocado Baked Eggs 75
- Garlic Dill Baked Cucumber Chips 75
- Baked Eggs And Asparagus With Parmesan 76
- Keto Sausage Balls 76
- Egg & Chorizo Muffins 76
- Egg Muffins With Sausage, Spinach, And Cheese 76
- Spicy Sausage, Cheese, And Egg Muffins 77
- Ghee Aka Clarified Butter 77
- Basic Keto Cheese Crisps 77
- Cheesy Keto Biscuits 77
- Oven-Baked Bacon 77
- Cauliflower-Spinach Side Dish 77
- Low-Carb Keto Cheese Taco Shells 78
- Keto Garlic Cheese 'Bread' 78
- Savory Salmon Fat Bombs 78
- Bacon-Wrapped Mozzarella Sticks 78
- Bacon Onion Butter 78
- Bacon & Egg Fat Bombs 79
- Jalapeno Popper Deviled Eggs With Bacon 79
- Eggplant French Toast 79
- Mock French Toast 79
- Garlic Parmesan Baked Tortilla Chips 80
- Crispy Cheddar Crisps 80
- Grain-Free "Whole Grain" Crackers 80
- Sour Cream And Chive Crackers 80
- Salt And Vinegar Zucchini Chips 80
- Brussels Sprouts Chips 81
- Sesame Mirin Kale Chips 81
- Spicy Cheddar Crisps 81
- Crispy Green Bean Chips 81
- Carrot Chips 81
- Tomato Chips 82
- Keto Curry Candied Bacon Recipe 82
- Parmesan Crisps Baked With Zucchini And Carrots 82
- Pumpkin Spice Apple Chips 82
- Keto Salt And Pepper Crackers 82
- Rosemary And Sea Salt Crackers 83
- Homemade Baked Banana Chips 83
- Rosemary & Sea Salt Flax Crackers 83
- Cauliflower Mac And Cheese In 4 Minutes 83
- Easy Low Carb Cauliflower Pizza Crust Recipe 83
- Keto Deviled Eggs 84
- Spicy Keto Deviled Eggs 84
- Italian Keto Plate 84
- Meat-Lover Pizza Cups 84
- Taco Sauce – Low Carb, Gluten-Free 85
- Fathead Pizza Dough- Keto 85
- Bacon, Braunschweiger, & Pistachio Truffles ... 85
- Coconut Flour Pizza Crust Recipe 85
- Better Than Fat Head Pizza – Pizza Crust 85
- Easy Crockpot Bone Broth 86
- Spinach Pizza Crust 86
- Steamed Artichoke 86
- Fat Head Pizza - The Holy Grail 86
- Asparagus + Goat Cheese Frittata 87
- Fancy Af Egg Clouds Recipe 87
- Egg Nest Recipe With Braised Cabbage 87
- Eggs En Cocotte Recipe 87
- Cloud Eggs 88
- Huevos Pericos Colombian Scrambled Eggs 88
- Caesar Egg Salad Lettuce Wraps 88
- Low Carb Cheese Enchiladas 88
- Keto 2 Minute Avocado Oil Mayo 88
- Taco Sauce 89
- Bacon-Wrapped Scallops 89
- Low Carb Fried Mac & Cheese 89
- Caprese Grilled Eggplant Roll-Ups 89
- Roasted Squash, Pomegranate Seeds And Spiced Walnut Salad 89
- Roasted Butternut Squash Cubes 90
- Wilted Organic Kale & Bacon 90
- 90-Second Keto Bread In a Mug 90
- Grain-Free Butter Bread 90
- Pumpkin Spice Roasted Pecans 90
- Keto Hollandaise 91
- Keto Bacon Wrapped Asparagus With a Secret Sauce 91
- Keto Honey Mustard Dressing 91
- Parmesan Chive And Garlic Keto Crackers 91
- Spinach-Mozzrella Stuffed Burgers 92

DESSERTS 93
- Macadamia Nut Fat Bomb 93
- Sugar-Free Low Carb Dried Cranberries 93
- Strawberry Ice Cream 93
- Malted Milk Ice Cream 93
- Low Carb Chocolate Mason Jar Ice Cream 93
- Sugar-Free Coconut Ice Cream 94
- Chocolate Chip Ice Cream 94
- Keto Crème Brule 94
- Keto Peanut Butter Fudge Fat Bomb 94
- Low Carb Jello Pops 94
- Strawberry Cheesecake Fat Bombs 95
- English Toffee Fat Bombs 95
- Low Carb Rolls 95
- Cinnamon Bun Fat Bomb Bars 95
- Lemon Cheesecake Fat Bombs With Cream Cheese 96
- Fat Bombs 96
- Keto Chocolate Nut Clusters 96
- Happy Almond Bombs – Keto Fat Bombs 96
- Paleo Vegan Coconut Cranberry Crack Bars 97
- No-Bake Keto Butter Cookies 97
- 3-Ingredient Keto No-Bake Coconut Cookies Recipe 97
- 4 Ingredient Chocolate Peanut Butter No-Bake Cookies 97
- 4 Ingredient Low Carb Hot Chocolate Ice Cream 97
- Healthy 3 Ingredients No Bake Paleo Vegan Coconut Crack Bars 98
- Easy Stovetop Sugar-Free Candied Almonds 98
- Healthy No Churn Workout Protein Ice Cream 98
- 4-Ingredient No-Bake Chocolate Coconut Crack Bars 98
- 3-Ingredient Keto Peanut Butter Fudge 98
- Easy Keto Garlic Roasted Bok Choy 99
- 3 Ingredient Flourless Sugar Free Cookies 99

- 4 Ingredient Keto Vegan Chocolate Coconut Cookies 99
- 3 Ingredient Keto Almond Butter Cups 99
- 4 Ingredient Keto Vegan Chocolate Snowball Cookies 100
- No-Bake Keto Vegan Peanut Butter Cookies 100
- Keto Chocolate Peanut Butter Cookies 100
- Keto Vegan Chocolates 100
- Fresh Strawberry Lime Popsicles 100
- Strawberry Low Carb Popsicles Freezer Pops 101
- 3-Ingredient Keto Raspberry Lemon Popsicles 101
- Peanut Butter Chocolate Cookies 101
- Fudgy Macadamia Chocolate Fat Bomb 101
- Jello Cream Cheese Fat Bomb 101
- Low Carb Chocolate Coconut Fat Bombs 101
- Keto Peanut Butter Cookies 102
- Pumpkin Seed Bark And Dark Chocolate & Sea Salt 102
- Low Carb Chocolate Bark 102
- Chocolate Coconut Gummies 102
- 3 Ingredient Keto Chocolate Coconut Cups 102
- Keto Vanilla Almond Fat Bomb 103
- Keto Almond Butter Fat Bomb Sandwiches Recipe 103
- Keto Coconut Fat Bomb Sandwiches Recipe 103
- White Chocolate Fat Bombs 103
- Nutella Fat Bombs 103
- Raspberry Fat Bombs - Cream Heart Jellies 103
- Keto Fat Bombs | Cookies And Cream 104
- Keto Avocado Dessert 104
- Low Carb Pumpkin Cheesecake Mousse 104
- Strawberry Dole Whip Recipe 104
- Easy Keto Ham And Cheese Rolls Recipe 104
- Keto Bagels Recipe With Fathead Dough 105
- Protein Pudding - Chocolate Or Vanilla 105
- Cream Cheese Pancakes – Low Carb & Keto 105
- Kathleen's Cottage Pancakes 105
- Chocolate Protein Pancakes 105
- Low-Carb Waffles 106
- Almond Joy Fruit And Nut Bars 106
- Pumpkin Pie Fruit And Nut Bars 106
- Low Carb Keto Banana Nut Protein Pancakes 106
- Keto Chocolate Mason Jar Ice Cream 106
- Chocolate Peanut Butter Balls 107
- Keto Cheesecake Cupcakes 107
- Easy Keto Fudge Recipe With Cocoa Powder 107
- Keto Muffins 107

Drinks Recipes 108
- Keto Traditional Coffee Recipe 108
- Vanilla Latte Martini 108
- Keto Boosted Coffee Recipe 108
- Keto Coconut Coffee Recipe 108
- Keto Frothy Coffee Recipe 108
- Keto Collagen Boosted Coffee 108
- Keto Iced Lemon Coffee Recipe 108
- Low Carb Blueberry Mojitos 108
- Apple Martini 109
- Blueberry Martini 109
- Cranberry Ginger Mulled Wine 109
- Black Beauty – Low Carb Vodka Drink 109
- Low Carb Strawberry Margarita Gummy Worms 109
- Dairy-Free Boosted Keto Coffee 109
- Cacao Coffee Recipe 110
- Coconut Milk Latte 110
- Chamomile Mint Tea Recipe 110
- Keto Iced Apple Green Tea 110
- Turmeric Ginger Lime Tea Recipe 110
- Zingy Salted Lime Soda 110
- Cucumber Basil Ice Cubes Recipe 111
- Cucumber Lime Water 111
- Honeysuckle Tea 111
- Keto Turmeric Bone Broth 111
- Kamikaze Shot Sugar-Free 111
- Low Carb Pina Colada 111
- Dirty Chai 111
- Low Carb Margaritas 112
- Spiked Root Beer Float 112
- The Splendido 112
- Low Carb Margarita 112
- Low Carb Mojito 112
- Cosmopolitan Cocktail Recipe 112
- Traditional Lime Mojito Recipe With Honey 113
- Pumpkin Spice Boosted Keto Coffee 113
- Almond Coconut Milk Creamer 113
- The Garden Surprise – Keto Gin Cocktail 113
- Keto Blueberry Mojito 113

Seafood & Fish Recipes 114
- Curry-Roasted Shrimp With Oranges 114
- Seared Salmon With Green Peppercorn Sauce 114
- Five-Spice Tilapia 114
- Shrimp Stacks 114
- Express Shrimp & Sausage Jambalaya 114
- Keto Steamed Clams With Basil Garlic Butter 115
- Oyster Broiled With Spicy Sauce 115
- Garlic Lemon Butter Crab Legs 115
- Low Carb Soft Shell Crab 115
- Salmon Roasted In Butter 116
- Salmon Garlicky Black Pepper And Egg Free Lemon Aioli 116
- Keto Bacon Wrapped Salmon With Pesto 116
- Grilled Salmon With Creamy Pesto 116
- Grilled Swordfish Skewers With Pesto Mayo 116
- Schlemmerfilet Bordelaise Herbed Almond And Parmesan Crusted Fish 117
- Baked Lemon Butter Tilapia 117
- Low-Carb Fish Curry With Coconut And Spinach 117
- Low-Carb Almond And Parmesan Baked Fish 117
- Keto Fried Fish 117
- Baked White Fish With Pine Nut, Parmesan With Basil Pesto Crust 118
- Smoky Tuna Pickle Boats – Low Carb & Gluten-Free 118
- Easy Keto Fried Coconut Shrimp 118
- Shrimp Recipe With Garlic Butter Cauliflower Rice 118
- Low Carb Spicy Shrimp Hand Rolls 119

- Chimichurri Shrimp 119
- Zero Carb Fried Shrimp 119
- Baked Butter Garlic Shrimp 119
- Grilled Salmon With Creamy Pesto Sauce 120
- Keto Grilled Lobster Tails With Creole Butter 120
- Smoked Salmon Pinwheels 120
- Keto Tuna Salad 120
- Salmon Florentine 120
- Roasted Salmon With Parmesan Dill Crust 121
- Parmesan Crusted Cod 121
- Baked Butter Garlic Shrimp 121
- Baked Lobster Tails With Garlic Butter 121
- Keto Coconut Shrimp Recipe 121
- Keto Shrimp And Cucumber Appetizer Recipe 122
- Paleo/Gf Popcorn Shrimp Recipe 122
- Keto Lemon Baked Salmon Recipe 122
- Keto Smoked Salmon Salad With Poached Egg 122
- Quick Keto Bacon-Wrapped Salmon 123
- Low Carb Oatmeal With Coconut Flour 123
- Baked Rosemary Salmon 123
- Keto Baked Salmon With Lemon And Butter .. 123
- Keto Fried Salmon With Asparagus 123
- Pink Peppercorn Smoked Salmon Salad Recipe 124
- Five-Minute Keto Curried Tuna Salad Recipe . 124
- Five-Minute Keto Fried Sardines Recipe With Olives 124
- Five-Minute Keto Sardines And Onions Recipe 124
- Easy Sardines Salad Recipe 124
- Fried Mahi Fish Bites 124
- Poached Cod In Tomato Sauce 125
- Keto Baked Salmon With Lemon And Butter .. 125
- Prosciutto-Wrapped Salmon Skewers 125
- Keto Tuna Plate 125

Vegetarian Recipes 126
- Keto Simple Vegan Bok Choy Soup 126
- Zucchini Noodles 126
- Balsamic Marinated Tomatoes 126
- Paprika Roasted Radishes With Onions 126
- Spaghetti Squash With Crispy Sage Garlic Sauce 126
- Cilantro Lime Cauliflower Rice 126
- Oven Roasted Cabbage Wedges 127
- Butter Roasted Radishes 127
- Parmesan-Roasted Cauliflower 127
- Roasted Buffalo Cauliflower 127
- Lemon Parmesan Broccoli Soup 127
- Cold Sesame Cucumber Noodle Salad Recipe 128
- Low-Carb Cauliflower Hash Browns 128
- Roasted Cabbage 128
- No-Cook Refreshing Mint Avocado Chilled Soup 128
- Keto Fried Halloumi Cheese With Mushrooms 128
- Goat Cheese Salad With Balsamico Butter 129
- Roasted Garlic Parmesan Cauliflower 129
- Crunchy & Nutty Cauliflower Salad 129
- Zucchini Noodles With Avocado Sauce 129
- Grain-Free Keto Granola 129
- Cheesy Ranch Roasted Broccoli 130
- Keto Creamy Avocado Pasta With Shirataki ... 130
- Easy Zucchini Noodle Alfredo 130
- Creamy Mushroom And Cauliflower Risotto Recipe 130
- Grilled Halloumi Brochette 130
- Simple Cauliflower Keto Casserole 131
- Stuffed Zucchini With Goat Cheese & Marinara 131
- Simple Greek Salad 131
- Moroccan Roasted Green Beans 131
- Caprese Style Portobello's 131
- Cheesy Garlic Roasted Asparagus 131
- Easy Roasted Broccoli 132
- Three-Step Green Beans Recipe 132
- Hassel Back Caprese Salads 132
- Steamed Artichoke And Garlic Butter 132
- Acorn Squash Slices 133
- Keto Parsley Cauliflower Rice 133
- Sautéed Radishes With Green Beans 133
- Sweet Potato & Bean Quesadillas 133
- Toasted Ravioli Puffs 133
- Tomato & Avocado Sandwiches 134
- Apple, White Cheddar & Arugula Tarts 134
- Risotto Cakes 134

Appendix : Recipes Index 135

INTRODUCTION

The ketogenic eating regimen, or keto for fast, is a very low-carb weight-reduction plan this is high in fats and mild in protein. It's like other sans grain and low-carb counts energy, like paleo and atkins, and calls for eating meats, dairy, eggs, fish, nuts, spreads, oils, and non-dull greens.

Supplanting the greater a part of the frame's sugar consumption with fats makes it's higher at eating fat for power. Typically, cells use glucose which originates from sugars to make energy. Yet, when there are more ketones within the blood than glucose, the frame will devour positioned away fats. This metabolic country is known as ketosis.

The food regimen isn't always new. It's clearly been applied for a vast period of time as a remedy for children with epilepsy whose seizures weren't reacting to the drug. Studiestrusted source has indicated that the keto food regimen is compelling for lessening seizures. Along those strains, specialists believe it might likewise have superb benefits for other neurological conditions, like alzheimer's chemical imbalance, parkinson's, different sclerosis, lousy cerebrum wounds, and thoughts tumors.

In any case, keto is typically regular for its weight-loss advantages. The consuming routine is frequently used to assist manipulate with yearning and lift weight loss in folks who are fat. It may likewise assist with glucose manipulate in individuals with type 2 diabetes.

Regardless of whether you are hoping to strive a keto weight loss plan simply because or add new dishes on your day by day exercise, these plans have you secured.

2-WEEKS MEAL PLAN
DAY 1

Breakfast

BREAKFAST EGG CREPES WITH AVOCADOS

Prep Time: 5mints, Cook Time: 10mints, Total Time: 15mints; Servings: 1

Ingredients
- 1 tsp olive oil
- 2 eggs
- Handful alfalfa sprouts
- 1/4 avocado
- Few slices turkey cold
- 1 tsp mayonnaise

Instructions
1. Heat oil in a little medium measured skillet over medium heat
2. When the container is hot break the eggs into the dish and utilizing your spatula to mix them so they are a similar thickness all around and totally covering the skillet.
3. Cook until crispy, flip over and keep on cooking for one more moment.
4. Remove from skillet, top with ingredients and serve.

Nutrition Fact:: Calories: 454, Fat 31g, Carbs 12g, Sugars 4.4g, Protein 22g

Lunch

EASY KETO PEPPERONI MEATBALLS

Prep Time: 5mints, Cook Time: 15mints, Total Time: 20mints; Serving: 4

Ingredients
- 1 lb ground beef or chicken
- 1/4 lb pepperoni slices
- 1 egg, whisked
- Hot sauce, to taste
- Salt and pepper

Instructions
1. Preheat stove to 400°F.
2. Blend the ground hamburger, ground pepperoni, and egg together.
3. Structure little meatballs from the blend
4. Put on a parchment paper-lined heating plate and cook for 15 minutes, turning over after 10 minutes.
5. Enjoy as a starter or serve with some hot sauce or Keto BBQ sauce as a primary.

Nutrition Fact: Calories: 451, Fat 37g, Carbs 0.6g, Sugar 0.4g, Protein 20g

Dinner

KETO CURRIED TOMATO SOUP

Prep Time: 10mints, Cook Time: 4hrs, Total Time: 4hrs 10mints; Serves: 4-6

Ingredients
- 4 pounds ripened garden tomatoes
- 2 cups full-fat coconut milk
- 1 tsp salt, onion, and 1 cup of water
- 2 Tsp curry powder
- 1 tsp minced garlic

Instructions
1. Mix all the ingredients in a cooker and set it on high.
2. Cook for 3 1/2 to 4 hours, till a hot soup forms.
3. If you want to cook this on low, it will take 5-6 hours. Serve the soup hot, embellished with cut cilantro if you desire.

Nutrition Fact: Calories: 213, Fat 0.1g, Carbs 8g, Sugar 0.4g, Protein 15g

Dessert

KETO GUACAMOLE BURGERS

Prep Time: 10mints, Cook Time: 20mints, Total Time: 30mints; Serving: 2

Ingredients
- 300 g ground beef
- 2 eggs
- 2 Tsp coconut oil
- 1/2 cup guacamole

Instructions
1. With your hands, shape the ground meat into 2 patties.
2. Cook the 2 burger patties, either in a skillet with a touch of coconut oil or on a barbecue.
3. When the burgers are cooked thoroughly, put to the side.
4. Fry the eggs in a skillet.
5. Put 1 seared egg over every burger and afterward top with guacamole.

Nutrition Fact: Calories: 349, Fat 56g, Carbs 4g, Sugar 0.3g, Protein 23g

DAY 2

Breakfast

KETO CLOUD BREAD

Prep Time: 10mints, Cook Time: 30mints, Total Time: 40mints; Serving: 10 pieces

INGREDIENTS
- 3 eggs, room temperature
- 3 tbsp cream cheese, softened
- 1/4 tsp cream of tartar
- 1/4 tsp salt

Instructions
1. Preheat stove to 300°F and line oven trays with fabric paper.
2. Cautiously remote egg whites from yolks, put whites in one bowl and yolks in another.
3. In the bowl of egg yolks, add cream cheese and blend until nicely mixed.
4. In the bowl of egg whites, add cream of tartar and salt. Utilizing a hand blender, mix until evenly blended.
5. Pouring step by step, use a spatula or spoon to add yolk combination to egg whites and carefully overlap till there aren't any white streaks.
6. Spoon blend onto arranged oven tray approximately ½ to ¾ inches tall and around five inches separated
7. Cook in the stove at the center rack for half-hour, till tops, are darker in color.
8. Allow to cool and enjoy.

Nutrition Fact: Calories: 35, Fat 2.8g, Carbs 0.4g, Sugar 1.4g, Protein 8g

Lunch

GARLIC BACON WRAPPED CHICKEN BITES RECIPE

Prep Time: 10mints, Cook Time: 30mints, Total Time: 40mints; Serving: 4

Ingredients
- 1 large chicken breast
- 8–9 thin slices of bacon
- 3 Tsp garlic powder

Instructions
1. Preheat stove to 400°F and line an oven tray with aluminum foil.
2. Put the garlic powder into a bowl and dunk every chicken piece into the garlic powder.
3. Wrap each with bacon strips. Put the bacon-wrapped chicken pieces on the oven tray spacing them out so they're not touching.
4. Heat for 25-30 minutes until the bacon is done. Turn the pieces and cook for another 15 minutes.
5. Serve warm.

Nutrition Fact: Calories: 230, Fat 13g, Carbs 5g, Sugar 2g, Protein 22g

Dinner

CREAM OF CELERY SOUP

Prep Time: 25mints, Total Time: 45mints; Servings: 4

Ingredients
- 1 bunch celery
- 1 sweet yellow onion
- 1 cup of coconut milk
- 2 cups of water and sea salt
- 1/2 tsp dill

Instructions
1. Add all ingredients into an Instant Pot. Seal top, and afterward press the "Soup" button.
2. The "Soup" setting will run for 30 minutes and afterward consequently go into "keep warm mode" for a couple of hours
3. After Instant Pot has depressurized, remove the top, and afterward cautiously mix soup utilizing a drenching blender. Keep blender submerged to avoid hot soup from splattering. Mix until smooth.
4. Serve warm.

Nutrition Fact: Calories: 321, Fat 2.4g, Carbs 5.3g, Sugar 1.6g, Protein 23g

Dessert

KETO BROCCOLI BEEF STIR-FRY RECIPE

Prep Time: 10mints, Cook Time: 10mints, Total Time: 20mints; Serving: 2

Ingredients
- 1/2 lb broccoli florets
- 1/2 lb beef steak
- Onion, Salt and pepper
- 2 Tsp Easy Stir-Fry Sauce
- 4 Tsp avocado oil

Instructions
1. Put 2 Tsp of avocado oil into a skillet or pot on medium heat. Add the broccoli florets into the skillet and sauté until somewhat soft. Remove and put on a plate.
2. Add 2 more Tsp of avocado oil into the skillet and turn the heat to high.
3. Add the chopped onion and beef steaks and sauté until the meat is cooked. Add the broccoli and pan fry food for 2-3 additional minutes. Season with salt and pepper, to taste

Nutrition Fact: Calories: 573, Fat 51g, Carbs 9g, Sugar 3g, Protein 22g

DAY 3

Breakfast

HEALTHY CHOCOLATE PEANUT BUTTER LOW CARB SMOOTHIE

Prep Time: 5mints, Total Time: 5mints; Serving: 3
INGREDIENTS
- 1/4 cup Peanut butter
- 3 tbsp Cocoa powder
- 1 cup Heavy cream
- 1 1/2 cup almond milk
- 6 tbsp Powdered erythritol
- 1/8 tsp Sea salt

Instructions
1. Add all ingredients in a blender.
2. Puree until smooth. Add sugar for taste if desired.

Nutrition Facts: Calories 435, Fat 41g, Carbs 10g, Sugar 3g, Protein 9g

Lunch

EASY PAN-FRIED LEMON CHICKEN

Prep Time: 10mints, Cook Time: 10mints, Total Time: 50mints; Servings: 1
Ingredients
- 1 chicken breast
- Zest and juice of 1 lemon
- 1-2 tsp olive oil or avocado oil
- 1/4 tsp sea salt
- 1/8 tsp black pepper

Instructions
1. In a massive plastic zip top P.C., add the chicken breast, lemon zest and juice, olive oil, salt and pepper.
2. Utilize a meat pounder to even thickness of the chicken breast.
3. Leave the chicken to marinate for a half-hour for better taste but you may prepare immediately.
4. Heat a skillet over medium-high heat and add a greater quantity of your fat of choice, for instance, coconut oil.
5. Cook the chicken until thoroughly done and serve warm.

Nutrition Facts: Calories 298, Fat 10g, Carbs 5g, Sugar 2g, Protein 26g

Dinner

KETO BROCCOLI SOUP RECIPE

Prep Time: 5mints, Cook Time: 25mints, Total Time: 30mints; Serving: 4

Ingredients
- 1 head broccoli
- 4 cups chicken broth or bone broth
- 2 Tsp of pine nuts
- Salt and freshly ground black pepper
- 2 Tsp coconut cream

Instructions
1. Remove the stalks from the florets of the head of broccoli and cut the stalks.
2. Empty the chicken stock into a pot and bring it to a boil. At that point add the cut stalks.
3. Cook for 10 minutes then add the florets and cook for another 10-15 minutes until the broccoli is soft.
4. Meanwhile, in a different hot, dry container, toast the pine nuts until golden.
5. When the broccoli has cooked, remove the dish from the heat and utilize a hand blender to blend into a smooth soup. Season with salt and freshly ground black pepper
6. Separate into two bowls and sprinkle with coconut cream if you wish.
7. Add toasted pine nuts on top and serve.

Nutrition Fact: Calories 134, Fat 5g, Carbs 8g, Sugar 2g, Protein 4g

Dessert

KALE KETO TOFU STIR FRY

Prep Time: 20mints, Cooking Time: 35mints, Total Time: 55mints; Serving: 3

Ingredients:
- 1 block extra-firm tofu
- 6 cups kale
- 1 clove garlic
- 2 Tbsp Bragg's liquid amino
- 1 Tbsp sesame seeds

Instructions
1. Enclose a square of tofu in a paper towel. Give tofu a chance to dry out for around 15-20 minutes.
2. Spray a griddle with a non-stick cooking spray. Add minced garlic and bring to medium-high heat.
3. Add tofu, framing an even layer. Cook for 2 minutes.
4. Add kale and fluid amino, and cook for 8 to 10 minutes, blending occasionally.
5. Top with sesame seeds, and serve and enjoy

Nutrition Fact: Calories: 300, Fat 28g, Carbs 7g, Sugar 1g, Protein 11g

DAY 4

Breakfast

KETO ROASTED BRUSSELS SPROUTS WITH GARLIC

Prep Time: 7mints, Cook Time: 30mints, Total Time: 37mints; Serving: 2

INGREDIENTS
- 2 cups Brussels sprouts
- 3-5 cloves garlic
- 1 tablespoon avocado oil
- salt + pepper

Instructions
1. Preheat stove to 400 degrees F.
2. Wash the Brussels Sprouts and pat dry.
3. Cut them down the middle and remove external leaves that are loose.
4. Put them right onto a heating sheet.
5. Cut cloves of garlic into enormous pieces.
6. Cover the Brussels sprouts and garlic with avocado oil, salt, and pepper.
7. Cook for 15 minutes and afterward give a shake to turn the sprouts and garlic.
8. Cook for another 15 to 20 minutes.
9. Serve warm.

Nutrition Fact: Calories: 106, Fat 7g, Carbs 9g, Sugar 1g, Protein 3g

Lunch

KETO CHICKEN HEARTS RECIPE

Prep Time: 5mints, Cook Time: 30mints, Total Time: 35mints; Servings: 3

Ingredients
- 1 Pound Chicken Hearts
- 1 tsp salt & Pepper
- 1 tsp cayenne pepper
- 1 tsp garlic powder
- 1 tsp onion powder

Instructions
1. Pat dry chicken hearts with a paper towel
2. Mix hearts with flavors to your taste. I like them spicy (Simple organ meat formula for chicken hearts)
3. Put hearts in Copper Chef Crisper plate.
4. Cook for 30 minutes at 350 degrees F.
5. Serve warm

Nutrition Facts: Calories 239, Fat 14g, Carbs 3g, Sugar 1g, Protein 24g

Dinner

FRESH TOMATO BASIL SOUP

Prep Time: 5mints, Cook Time: 10mints, Total Time: 15mints; Serving: 6

Ingredients
- 5 cups of fresh tomato puree
- 1 stick of salted butter
- 8 oz cream cheese
- a handful of fresh basil leaves
- 1 tbsp Healthy Mama Gentle Sweet
- salt and pepper to taste

Instructions
1. Puree enough new tomatoes in a blender to rise to five cups of puree. (You may need about; 4 huge tomatoes and possibly 16 ounces of cherry tomatoes.)
2. Empty the puree into an enormous pot and add the spread and cream cheese. Heat to a stew and cook until the spread and cream cheddar liquefy.
3. Cautiously empty the soup once again into the blender and add the basil or utilize a drenching blender to puree until smooth along with the melted butter and tbsp of Mama Gentle Sweet.

Nutrition Facts: Calories 287, Fat 28g, Carbs 6g, Sugars 4g, and Protein 3g

Dessert

BACON-WRAPPED MEATLOAF

Prep Time: 35mints, Cooking Time: 1hr 15mints, Total Time: 1hrs 50mints; Serving: 6

Ingredients
- 1 lb ground turkey
- 1/4 large onion or one small onion
- 1-2 cloves garlic
- Bacon– 6 to 8 strips

Instructions
1. Chop your onions
2. Blended the onion and the ground turkey together
3. Add two cloves of squashed garlic, salt, and pepper
4. Spread out the pieces of bacon on an oven tray fixed with parchment paper and place portions of meat in the middle in the shape of a loaves.
5. Wrap the loaf with the bacon and use sticks to keep bacon in place.
6. Secured the portions and let them chill in the ice chest for around 30 minutes.
7. When they had chilled, put the meatloaves in the stove to heat at 400 F for 50 to an hour.
8. Remove the sticks and presented with broccoli sautéed with garlic in olive oil.

Nutrition Fact: Calories: 113, Fat 6.9g, Carbs 6.8g, Sugar 4.3g, Protein: 7.9g

DAY 5

Breakfast

KETO "EVERYTHING" AVOCADO BREAKFAST

Prep Time: 5mints, Total Time: 5mints; Serving: 2

INGREDIENTS
- 1 Tsp of garlic powder
- 1 Tsp of onion powder
- Salt and pepper
- 1 large avocado

Instructions
1. To make everything flavorful, join the minced garlic, minced onion, and salt and pepper in a little bowl.
2. Put an equivalent measure of cut avocado on 2 plates. Sprinkle the ideal measure of flavoring on the avocado and serve.

Nutrition Fact: Calories: 160, Fat 15g, Carbs 9g, Sugar 1g, Protein 2g

Lunch

PALEO GUACAMOLE BURGER RECIPE

Prep Time: 15mints, Cooking Time: 15mints, Total Time: 30mints; Serving: 4

Ingredients
- 1 burger/patty
- 1 egg
- 1/4 cup guacamole

Instructions
1. Cook the burger/patty.
2. Fry an egg.
3. Put the seared egg over the burger and top with the guacamole.

Nutrition Fact: Calories: 113, Fat 6.9g, Carbs 6.8g, Sugar 4.3g, Protein 7.9g

Dinner

BAKED SAUSAGE WITH CREAMY BASIL SAUCE

Prep Time: 5mints, Cook Time: 40mints, Total Time: 45mints; Serving: 12

Ingredients
- 3 lb Italian sausage chicken, turkey, or pork
- 8 oz cream cheese
- 1/4 cup basil pesto
- 1/4 cup heavy cream
- 8 oz mozzarella

Instructions
1. Preheat stove to 400 degrees F. Layer a huge meal dish with a cooking spray. Put the sausage in the preparing dish. Heat for 30 minutes
2. In the meantime, mix together the cream cheese, pesto, and heavy cream.
3. Spread the sauce over the wiener. Top with mozzarella. Prepare for an extra 10 minutes or until the wiener is 160 degrees F when checked with a meat thermometer.

Nutrition Facts: Calories 550, Fat 49g, Carbs 2g, Sugars 0.2g, Protein 21g

Dessert

TURKEY MEATLOAF

Prep Time: 15mints, Cooking Time: 25mints, Total Time: 40mints; Serving: 4

Ingredients:
- 2 lbs of lean ground turkey
- 1 egg
- 2 Tsp of coconut amino
- 1 tsp every one of garlic powder, salt, and pepper
- 1/2 cup onion, pepper, and celery

Instructions
1. Preheat stove to 375°.
2. Add all ingredients in a huge blending bowl.
3. Layer a portion dish with coconut oil.
4. Empty ground turkey blend into the portion container
5. Cook for 60 minutes.
6. Remove from the stove and let rest for 10 minutes.
7. Cut, and serve!

Nutrition Fact: Calories: 321, Fat 9g, Carbs 14g, Sugar 4.1g, Protein 24g

DAY 6

Breakfast

KETO BOOSTED COFFEE RECIPE

Prep Time: 2mints, Total Time: 2mints; Serving: 16 ounces

INGREDIENTS
- 2 cups freshly brewed hot coffee
- 2 Tsp grass-fed butter
- 1 scoop Perfect Keto MCT Powder
- 1 tsp Ceylon cinnamon

Instructions
1. Add the entirety of the ingredients in a blender.
2. Utilizing an inundation blender or frothier, mix on low then accelerate to high for 30 seconds or until foamy.
3. Serve and enjoy.

Nutrition Fact: Calories: 280, Fat 31g, Carbs 2.8g, Sugar 2.2g, Protein 1g

Lunch

KETO ALMOND BUTTER COOKIE DOUGH

Prep Time: 5mints, Total Time: 5mints; Serving: 12

Ingredients
- 1 cup almond butter
- 1 Tsp flax meal
- Tsp water
- 1 tsp vanilla extract
- Sweetener and Dash of salt

Instructions
1. Add all of the ingredients in a huge bowl.
2. Smear into little bowls and blend in with a spoon.

Nutrition Fact: Calories: 134, Fat 12g, Carbs 4g, Sugar 1g, Protein 5g

Dinner

KETO BAKED BACON OMELET

Prep Time: 5mints, Cooking Time: 20mints, Total Time: 25mints; Serving: 2

Ingredients
- 4 eggs
- 5 oz. bacon
- 3 oz. butter
- 2 oz. fresh spinach
- salt and pepper

Instructions
1. Preheat the stove to 400°F. Oil an individual serving-sized dish with the butter.
2. Fry bacon and spinach in the rest of the butter.
3. Whisk the eggs until foamy. Blend in the spinach and bacon, including the fat left over.
4. Add some finely chopped chives. Season to taste with salt and pepper
5. Empty the egg blend into preparing dishes and heat for 20 minutes or until set and golden.
6. Let cool for a couple of moments and serve.

Nutrition Fact: Calories 737, Fat 72g, Carbs 2g, Sugar 14g, Protein 21g

Dessert

KETO ELECTROLYTE DRINK

Prep Time: 5mints, Total Time: 5mints; Serving: 3

Ingredients
- 1 gram of Celtic Sea Salt
- 2 fluid Oz. Unsweetened Aloe vera Juice
- 1 tsp fresh lemon juice
- 24 fluid Oz spring water

Instructions
1. Combine all ingredients, and serve and enjoy.
2. You can utilize chilled water or drink over ice for additional refreshment.

Nutrition Facts: Calories 242, Fat 7g, Carbs 3g, Sugar 2.3g, Protein 12g

DAY 7

Breakfast

KETO BRUNCH SPREAD

Prep Time: 10mints, Cook Time: 20mints, Total Time: 30mints; Serving: 4

INGREDIENTS
- 4 large eggs
- 24 asparagus spears
- 12 slices of pastured, sugar-free bacon

Instructions
1. Pre-heat your stove to 400°F
2. Cut your asparagus removing an inch from the bottoms.
3. Two by two, wrap them with one cut of bacon.
4. Put inside the stove set the clock for 20mins.
5. In the meantime, get a little pot of water to a boil. Add four eggs in the bubbling water. Leave for six minutes.
6. Strip away the shell.
7. When the asparagus is ready, serve on a plate or reducing board.
8. If you do not have an egg holder use coffee cups to hold your eggs up.
9. Plunge your asparagus lances into your eggs. Blow to cool and enjoy!

Nutrition Fact: Calories: 426, Fat 38g, Carbs 3g, Sugar 2g, Protein 17g

Lunch

KETO 5-INGREDIENT COCONUT FLOUR COOKIES

Prep Time: 10mints, Cook Time: 15mints, Total Time: 25mints; Serving: 15

Ingredients
- 3/4 cup coconut flour
- 4 eggs
- 1 tsp baking powder
- 1/2 cup ghee
- Sweetener

Instructions
1. Preheat stove to 350°F.
2. Combine every one of the ingredients to shape a batter.
3. Take little wads of batter and level to frame a little treat. Note the batter is somewhat delicate and runny.
4. Put onto a parchment paper lined on a heating plate. Ensure there's space between the treats.
5. Heat for 10-13 minutes until somewhat seared around the edges.
6. Let cool and serve!

Nutrition Fact: Calories: 100, Fat 9g, Carbs 2g, Sugar 0.3g, Protein 2g

Dinner

KETO FRIED CHICKEN WITH BROCCOLI

Prep Time: 5mints, Cooking Time: 15mints, Total time:; Serving: 2

Ingredients
- 9 oz. broccoli
- 3½ oz. butter
- 10 oz. boneless chicken thighs
- Salt and pepper
- ½ cup mayonnaise

Instructions
1. Rinse and trim the broccoli. Cut into little pieces, including the stem.
2. Heat up a touch of margarine in a skillet where you can fit both the chicken and the broccoli
3. Season the chicken and fry over medium heat for around 5 minutes on every side, or until golden in color and cooked thoroughly.
4. Add more spread and put the broccoli in a similar skillet. Fry for another couple of minutes.
5. Season to taste and present with the rest of the spread.

Nutrition Fact: Calories 733, Fat 66g, Carbs 5g, Sugar 22g, Protein 29g

Dessert

ROSEMARY MINT SODA

Prep Time: 7mints, Total Time: 7mints; Serving: 4

Ingredients
- 25 oz. bottle mineral water
- 4 sprigs rosemary
- 4 sprigs mint
- 1 lime cut into 4 wedges
- 2 Tsp maple syrup

Instructions
1. In four enormous glasses crush 1 wedge of lime into the base of each glass. Add ½ tsp of maple syrup if utilizing alongside the lime and mix together.
2. Add the ideal measure of ice, I, as a rule, add about ½ far up the glass. Softly crush the herbs in your grasp. Stick 1 stem of rosemary and 1 stem of mint into each glass.
3. Empty the mineral water into each glass and enable it to sit for around 30 seconds to allow the herbs to soak and serve right away.

Nutrition Facts: Calories 462, Fat 12g, Carbs 4g, Sugar 3g, Protein 21g

DAY 8

Breakfast

KETO 3-INGREDIENT MUFFINS RECIPE

Prep Time: 10mints, Cook Time: 25mints, Total Time: 35mints; Serving: 12

INGREDIENTS
- 2 cups whole nuts
- 5 medium eggs, whisked
- Stevie and spices, to taste

Instructions
1. Preheat stove to 350°F (175°C).
2. Oil a 12-cup biscuit plate.
3. Use Nourishment processes to ground hazelnuts into flour form.
4. In a huge blending bowl, whisk together the eggs and hazelnut flour to make a batter.
5. Add the Stevie and flavors.
6. Fill the biscuit plate.
7. Heat for 25 minutes until a mixed drink stick embedded into the center shows that the dough has been cooked.
8. Let cool totally and serve and enjoy it.

Nutrition Fact: Calories: 117, Fat 10g, Carbs 4g, Sugar 1g, Protein 6g

Lunch

KETO MADELEINE COOKIES

Prep Time: 10mints, Cook Time: 15mints, Total Time: 25mints; Serving: 10 cookies

Ingredients
- cup almond flour
- 1/3 cup flax meal
- 2 Tsp coconut oil
- 2 eggs
- Erythritol or Stevie and Dash of salt

Instructions
1. Preheat stove to 320°F.
2. Combine to form a batter. Fold into 20 little Madeleine-molded pieces and utilize the back of a lubed fork to press into the highest point of the batter scoring lines to make the Madeleine treats look.
3. Cook for 12-15 min until somewhat caramelized.

Nutrition Fact: Calories: 124, Fat 11g, Carbs 4g, Sugar 1g, Protein 5g

Dinner

KETO SMOKED SALMON PLATE

Prep Time: 5mints, Total Time: 5mints; Serving: 2

Ingredients
- ¾ lb smoked salmon
- 1 cup mayonnaise
- 2 oz. baby spinach
- 1 tbsp olive oil
- salt and pepper

Instructions
1. Put salmon, spinach, a slice of lime, and a enough mayonnaise on a plate.
2. Spray olive oil over the spinach and season with salt and pepper.

Nutrition Fact: Calories 403, Fat 65g, Carbs 1g, Sugar 23g, Protein 28g

Dessert

KETO CHOCOLATE COCONUT CUPS

Prep Time: 2mints, Cook Time: 3mints, Total Time: 5mints; Servings: 18 cups

Ingredients
- 1/2 cup coconut butter, melted
- 1/2 cup cocoa powder
- 1/2 cup coconut oil
- 1 serving sweetener of choice

Instructions
1. Line an 18 small biscuit tin with smaller than usual biscuit liners and put aside.
2. In a microwave-safe bowl or stovetop, dissolve your coconut oil. Add your cocoa powder and blend until completely mixed and no clusters remain. In the event that you use alternatives to add sugar, add it here now as well.
3. Moving rapidly, coat the base and sides of the biscuit liners with dissolved chocolate. Guarantee a little is extra to top with water. Put the chocolate-covered biscuit tins in the cooler to solidify.
4. When firm, place the coconut spread into the cups. Top with the rest of the chocolate and cool again until firm.

Nutrition Fact:: Calories: 45, Fat 0.5g, Carbs 1g, Sugar 0.3g, Protein 9g

DAY 9

Breakfast

CRISPY KETO CHICKEN THIGHS RECIPE

Prep Time: 5mints, Cook Time: 40mints, Total Time: 45mints; Serving: 4
INGREDIENTS
- 12 chicken thighs
- 4 Tsp of olive oil
- 2 Tsp salt

Instructions
1. Preheat stove to 450°F (230°C).
2. Add salt on every chicken thigh and put on a lubed heating plate. Ensure the thighs are not touching each other on the plate. Sprinkle the olive oil or avocado oil over the chicken thighs.
3. Cook for 40 minutes until the skin is done.

Nutrition Fact: Calories: 713, Fat 56g, Carbs 0.2g, Sugar 0.3g, Protein 32g

Lunch

KETO 4-INGREDIENT ALMOND FLOUR COOKIES

Prep Time: 10mints, Cook Time: 10mints, Total Time: 20mints; Serving: 15 cookies

Ingredients
- 2 cups almond flour
- 6 Tsp ghee
- 1 egg
- Keto sweetener

Instructions
1. Preheat range to 350°F.
2. Combine each one of the ingredients to form a batter.
3. Take little bundles of batter and shape into cookies.
4. Put onto a cloth paper-lined a preparing plate. Ensure there's space among the treats.
5. Cook for 7-10mins till really cooked and crunchy.

Nutrition Fact: Calories: 125, Fat 12g, Carbs 3g, Sugar 1g, Protein 3g

Dinner

KETO SMOKED SALMON AND AVOCADO PLATE

Prep Time: 5mints, Total Time: 5mints; Serving: 2
Ingredients
- 7 oz. smoked salmon
- 2 avocados
- ½ cup mayonnaise
- salt and pepper

Instructions
1. Split the avocado down the middle, remove the pit, and scoop out avocado pieces with a spoon. Put on a plate.
2. Add salmon and a healthy amount of mayonnaise to the plate.
3. Top with freshly ground black pepper and a sprinkle of sea salt.

Nutrition Fact: Calories 634, Fat 42g, Carbs 4g, Sugar 22g, Protein 35g

Dessert

LOW CARB KETO CHOCOLATE BAR

Prep Time: 5mints, Cook Time: 5mints, Total Time: 10mints; Serving: 8
Ingredients
- 2 tbsp coconut oil
- 2 1/2 oz unsweetened baking chocolate
- 6 tbsp Powdered erythritol
- 2 tbsp Inulin
- 1/4 tsp Liquid sunflower lecithin
- 1/8 tsp Sea salt and 1 tsp Vanilla extract

Instructions
1. Liquefy cocoa margarine and preparing chocolate in a twofold heater over low heat.
2. Mix in the powdered erythritol and inulin a little at a time. Mix in the sunflower lecithin and salt. Heat until everything is smooth and disintegrated.
3. Remove from heat. Mix in vanilla concentrate.
4. Empty the liquefied chocolate blend into molds. Refrigerate for 30 minutes, until firm.

Nutrition Facts: Calories 143, Fat 15g, Total Carbs 4g, Sugar 2g, Protein 1g

DAY 10

Breakfast

THREE INGREDIENT KETO STEAK SAUTÉ

Prep Time: 10mints, Cook Time: 20mints, Total Time: 30mints; Serving: 1

INGREDIENTS
- 1 beef ribeye steak
- 1/2 onion, peeled and sliced
- 2 cloves of garlic
- 2 Tsp avocado oil, to cook with

Instructions
1. Add avocado oil to a skillet and sauté the steak, onion, and garlic.

Nutrition Fact: Calories: 798, Fat 70g, Carbs 7g, Sugar 3g, Protein 25g

Lunch

KETO SHORTBREAD COOKIES

Prep Time: 20mints, Total Time: 30mints; Serving: 10 cookies

Ingredients
- 1 cup almond flour
- 1/4 cup erythritol
- 1 tsp baking powder
- 1 egg
- 2 Tsp ghee

Instructions
1. Preheat the stove to 350 F.
2. Mix the almond flour, erythritol and baking powder in a bowl.
3. In a different bowl whisk the egg with the softened ghee and the vanilla concentrate. Add the egg blend to the almond flour blend utilizing a wooden spoon until it meets up
4. Utilize a tsp to gather up portions roughly 0.9oz in weight and structure into little balls. Put the balls onto a preparing plate fixed with parchment paper.
5. Utilize a fork to tenderly to check whether the treats are done.
6. Remove from stove and permit to cool. Enjoy instantly or store in a sealed shut compartment.

Nutrition Fact: Calories: 85, Fat 8g, Carbs 2g, Sugar 0.1g, Protein 3g

Dinner

KETO FRIED CABBAGE WITH CRISPY BACON

Prep Time: 5mints, Cooking Time: 15mints, Total Time: 20mints; Serving: 2

Ingredients
- 10 oz. bacon
- 1 lb green cabbage
- 2 oz. butter
- salt and pepper

Instructions
1. Chop cabbage and bacon into little pieces.
2. In an enormous skillet, fry the bacon over medium heat until firm.
3. Add cabbage and margarine and fry until delicate. Season with salt and pepper to taste

Nutrition Fact: Calories 850, Fat 79g, Carbs 9g, Sugar 32g, Protein 21g

Dessert

FROZEN BLUEBERRY FAT BOMBS

Prep Time: 5mints, Total Time: 5mints; Serving: 15

Ingredients
- 250 g cream cheese
- 75 g blueberries fresh
- 3 tbsp granulated sweetener

Instructions
1. Put every one of the ingredients inside the blender beat till smooth.
2. Put in the ice chest or cooler till the combination is thick enough to fold into balls.
3. Fold the combo into 15 balls and place them inside the cooler.
4. It may be stored inside the cooler for as long as one month.

Nutrition Facts: Calories 52, Fat 5.6g, Carbs 1.9g, Sugar 1.1g, Protein 1.3g

DAY 11

Breakfast

KETO BREAKFAST PIZZA

Prep Time: 10mints, Cooking time: 25mints, Total Time: 35mints; Serving: 2
INGREDIENTS:
- 2 cups grated cauliflower
- 2 Tsp coconut flour
- 1/2 tsp salt
- 4 eggs
- 1 tsp psyllium husk powder

Instructions:
2. Preheat the stove to 350 degrees F. Line a pizza tray or sheet skillet with the material.
3. In a blending bowl, add all ingredients aside from garnishes and blend until mixed. Put aside for 5 minutes to permit coconut flour and psyllium husk to ingest fluid and thicken up.
4. Cautiously pour the pizza base onto the dish. Utilize your hands to form it into a round, even pizza base.
5. Cook for 15 minutes, or until golden dark colored and completely cooked.
6. Remove from the stove and top breakfast pizza with your picked ingredients. Serve warm.
Nutrition Fact: Calories: 454, Fat 31g, Carbs 15g, Sugars 4.4g, Protein 22g

Lunch

KETO "PEANUT BUTTER" COOKIES

Prep Time: 10mints, Cook Time: 15mints, Total Time: 25mints; Serving: 12
Ingredients
- 1 cup almond butter
- 1 egg
- 1 tsp vanilla extract
- Sweetener and Dash of salt
- 1 tsp baking soda

Instructions
1. Preheat stove to 350 F (175 C).
2. Combine every one of the ingredients in an enormous bowl.
3. Structure 12-15 little treats with your hands and put them on a heating plate fixed with parchment paper. Make a point to leave room between the treats.
4. Heat for 10 minutes
Nutrition Fact: Calories: 136, Fat 12g, Carbs 4g, Sugar 1g, Protein 5g

Dinner

KETO SMOKED SALMON PLATE

Prep Time: 5mints, Total Time: 5mints; Serving: 2
Ingredients
- ¾ lb smoked salmon
- 1 cup mayonnaise
- 2 oz. baby spinach
- 1 tbsp olive oil
- salt and pepper

Instructions
1. Put salmon, spinach, a smidge of lime, and a healthy spoonful of mayonnaise on a plate.
2. Splash olive oil above the spinach and season with salt and pepper.
Nutrition Fact: Calories 534, Fat 45g, Carbs 7g, Sugar 17g, Protein 31g

Dessert

COCONUT FAT BOMBS

Prep Time: 5mints, Total Time: 1hr 5mints; Servings: 30 fat bombs
Ingredients:
- 1 Can Coconut Milk
- 3/4 cup coconut oil
- 1 cup unsweetened coconut flakes
- 20 drops Liquid Stevie

Instructions:
1. Add coconut oil to a blending bowl. Microwave for 20 seconds to dissolve
2. Add Stevie and coconut milk to the coconut oil. Blend.
3. Finally, add coconut chips and blend.
4. Fill fat bomb paperwork and put them inside the cooler for 60mins.
5. These fat bombs are nice saved within the cooler.
Nutrition Facts: Calories 89.1, Fat 9.7g, Carbs 0.87, Sugar 0.4g, Protein 0.33g

DAY 12

Breakfast

KETO LEMON BAKED SALMON RECIPE

Prep Time: 5mints, Cook Time: 20mints, Total Time: 25mints; Serving: 2
INGREDIENTS
- 2 Lemons
- 2 Fillets of salmon, fresh or frozen
- 2 Tsp of olive oil
- Salt and freshly ground black pepper
- Thyme sprigs, to garnish

Instruction
1. Preheat the oven to 350°F (180°C).
2. Put a large portion of the cut lemons on the base of a dish.
3. Lay the salmon fillets over the cut lemons and spread with the rest of the lemon cuts.
4. Sprinkle olive oil over the salmon and heat in the stove for 20 minutes.
5. Season with salt and pepper and embellishment with thyme
6. Present with your decision of keto-accommodating side dishes.

Nutrition Fact: Calories: 571, Fat 44g, Carbs 2g, Sugar 2g, Protein 36g

Lunch

KETO PECAN CRISPS RECIPE

Prep Time: 10mints, Cook Time: 10mints Total Time: 20mints; Serving: 6
Ingredients
- cups pecans
- 12 pecan halves for topping
- ¼ cup erythritol
- 1 egg, whisked
- 1/4 cup flax or chia seed

Instructions
1. Heat stove to 350 F.
2. Use Nourishment processor to ground the 1.5 cups pecanss, erythritol, egg, flax/chia meal to form a batter.
3. Put 12 biscuit liners into a biscuit skillet.
4. Partition the blend into the 12 liners.
5. Heat for 8-10 minutes.
6. Remove from stove and let cool somewhat before putting away in a sealed shut compartment.

Nutrition Fact: Calories: 170, Fat 14g, Carbs 7g, Sugar 1g, Protein 7g

Dinner

KETO SMOKED SALMON AND AVOCADO PLATE

Prep Time: 5mints, Total Time: 5mints; Serving: 2
Ingredients
- 7 oz. smoked salmon
- 2 avocados
- ½ cup mayonnaise
- Salt and pepper

Instructions
1. Split the avocado into equal parts, remove the pit, and scoop out avocado pieces with a spoon. Put on a plate.
2. Add salmon and a generous blob of mayonnaise to the plate.
3. Top with freshly ground black pepper and a sprinkle of sea salt.

Nutrition Fact: Calories 342, Fat 8g, Carbs 2g, Sugar 6g, Protein 34g

Dessert

CHEESE MEATLOAF

Prep Time: 15mints, Cook Time: 50mints, Total Time: 1 hr 5mints; Serving: 6
Ingredients
- 500g Minced Meat
- 1 Tbsp Dried Marjoram
- Salt, Pepper, and 2 Eggs
- 2 Buffalo Mozzarella
- 2 whole Leeks

Instructions
1. Heat up the stove to 180 degrees C
2. Clean the Leak, reduce approx 10cm from the white part and cut that into little pieces.
3. Rest of the leek separate right into solitary leaves
4. Heat chief pot with water until boiling.
5. When the water is bubbled, place leek leaves and leave for 3-4 minutes
6. In a bowl combine minced meat, pre-reduce white stop leeks, eggs, marjoram, salt, and pepper
7. Take a making ready dish preferably inside the state of a toast heating field; prepare the leek leaves on the bottom of the skillet with facets placing over
8. Add 2 mozzarellas and spread it with the rest of the beef combination
9. Heat it for 50 minutes then serve warm.

Nutrition Fact: Calories 183, Fat 18g, Carbs 3g, Sugar 1g, Protein 11g

DAY 13

Breakfast

HERB ROASTED BONE MARROW

Prep Time: 5mints, Cook Time: 15mints, Total Time: 20mints; Serving: 4

INGREDIENTS
- Marrow bones from grass-fed/pasture-raised beef, 1-2 per person
- Fresh rosemary
- Fresh thyme
- Unrefined salt and black pepper

Instructions
1. Preheat the stove to 400 degrees F. Put the bones in a preparing dish.
2. Finely chop equivalent pieces of fresh rosemary and thyme. Sprinkle the herbs over the marrow bones.
3. Broil for around 15 minutes, until pink inside isn't visible.
4. Season with salt and pepper and serve hot. Utilize a spoon to scoop out the marrow.

Nutrition Fact: Calories 332.2, Fat 8.3g, Carbs 10.4g, Sugar 1.4g, Protein 24g

Lunch

LOW CARB ONION RINGS

Prep Time: 15mints, Cooking Time: 15mints, Total Time 30 minutes; Servings: 2

Ingredients:
- 1 medium white onion
- 1/2 cup Coconut flour
- 2 large eggs
- 1 tbsp Heavy Whipping Cream
- 2 oz Pork Rinds
- 1/2 cup grated parmesan cheese

Instructions:
1. Cut onion into equal thick rings.
2. Utilize three unique dishes to make the coconut flour, egg wash, and whipping cream, and pork skin parmesan covering stations low carb onion rings stations
3. Beginning with coconut flour, covering onions with it and placing on tray.
4. When all onions are covered, backtrack and recoat them beginning with the egg wash.
5. Places twofold covered rings back on lubed heating rack and put in 425 degrees F stove for 15 minutes. Serve warm and enjoy!

Nutrition Facts: Calories 211, Fat 12.5g, Carbs 7.5g, Sugar 3g, Protein 16g

Dinner

KETO SALMON-FILLED AVOCADOS

Prep Time: 5mints, Total Time: 5mints; Serving: 2

Ingredients
- 2 avocados
- 6 oz. smoked salmon
- ¾ cup crème fraîche or sour cream
- Salt and pepper
- 2 tbsp lemon juice

Instructions
1. Cut avocados down the middle and remove the pit.
2. Put a bit of crème Fraiche or mayonnaise in the hollow of the avocado and add smoked salmon on top.
3. Season to taste with salt and lemon juice for additional flavor

Nutrition Fact: Calories 611, Fat 42g, Carbs 4.3g, Sugar 12.6g, Protein 23g

Dessert

KETO PIZZA CASSEROLE

Prep Time: 5mints, Cook Time: 30mints, Total Time: 35mints; Serving: 6

Ingredients
- 1.5-2 lb cooked chicken breast sliced
- 8 oz cream cheese
- 1 tsp dried minced garlic
- 1 cup marinara sauce
- 8 oz shredded mozzarella

Instructions
1. Preheat stove to 350 degrees F.
2. Put the chicken in the base of a 9x13 heating dish.
3. Join cream cheese and garlic. Drop little spoonfuls onto the chicken. Pour the sauce on top. Sprinkle with the shredded mozzarella.
4. Heat for 30 min or until the cheese is softened and bubbly

Nutrition Facts: Calories 153, Fat 7g, Carbs 4g, Sugars 3g, Protein 19g

DAY 14

Breakfast

GRILLED BEEF LIVER

Prep Time: 10mints, Cook Time: 7mints, Total Time: 17mints; Servings: 5
INGREDIENTS
- 1 lb beef liver
- ½ cup olive oil
- 1 clove garlic crushed
- 1 tbsp fresh mint
- ¼ tsp black pepper and 1 tsp salt

Instructions
1. Preheat a broil dish over medium-high heat.
2. Wash the liver altogether under cool running water. Try to clean out all the blood that follows. Pat dry with a kitchen paper, utilizing a sharp blade, evacuate every single extreme vein, assuming any. Cut across into slender cuts.
3. In a little bowl, add olive oil with squashed garlic, mint, salt, and pepper. Blend until very much mixed. Liberally brush the liver cuts with this blend and flame broil for 5-7 minutes on each side.
4. Serve and enjoy!

Nutrition Facts: Calories 315, Fat 25g, Carbs 4g, Sugar 1g, Protein 19g

Lunch

FARMHOUSE BEANS & SAUSAGE

Prep Time: 10mints, Cooking Time: 10mints, Total Time: 20mints; Serving: 4
Ingredients
- 2 cups gluten-free chicken broth
- 2 16 oz. frozen green beans
- 1 16 oz. chicken sausage
- 2 tsp Herbamare
- Salt, pepper, and 1/2 onion

Instructions
1. Put all ingredients in the Instant Pot. Put top on and close ensuring the steam vent is shut.
2. Utilize the manual setting and set it at 6 minutes.
3. At the point when cooking time is done utilizing the snappy discharge technique to release the pressure

Nutrition Fact: Calories 180; Fat 6g, Carbs 9g, Sugar 7g, Protein 24g

Dinner

KETO FRIED SALMON WITH GREEN BEANS

Prep Time: 5mints, Cooking Time: 10mints, Total Time: 15mints; Serving: 2
Ingredients
- 9 oz. fresh green beans
- 3 oz. butter
- 12 oz. salmon
- ½ lemon
- Salt and pepper

Instructions
1. Wash and trim the green beans.
2. Heat up the spread in a skillet tremendous enough to suit both the fish and greens
3. Fry the green beans collectively with the salmon over medium heat for around 3-4 minutes on every side. Season with salt and pepper
4. Crush the lemon squeezed over the fish and beans inside the skillet closer to the end. Mix the beans on occasion.

Nutrition Fact: Calories 705, Fat 58g, Carbs 6g, Sugar 25g, Protein 31g

Dessert

4-INGREDIENT PANCAKES

Prep Time: 10mints, Cooking Time: 5mints, Total Time: 15mints; Serving: 2
Ingredients
- 1 large banana
- 2 eggs
- 1/8 teaspoon baking powder
- 1/8 teaspoon ground cinnamon

Instructions
1. Heat a skillet on the stovetop to medium heat. While the container is warming, crush banana well and afterward blend in eggs, baking powder, and cinnamon.
2. When the dish is hot, spray container daintily with a non-stick spray. Pour 2 tablespoons of batter and cook until base seems set, flip with a spatula and cook an extra moment or less. Serve warm with butter and syrup.

Nutritional Fact: Calories: 22, Fat 1g, Carbs 2.6g, Sugar 0.2g, Protein 1.2g

SMOOTHIES & BREAKFASTS RECIPES

PERFECT KETO AVOCADO BREAKFAST BOWL

Prep Time: 5mints, Cook Time: 15mints, Total Time: 20mints; Serving: 1

INGREDIENTS
- 1 avocado
- 1 tbsp salted butter
- 3 large free-range eggs
- 3 rashers of bacon
- Pinch of salt and black pepper

INSTRUCTIONS
1. Start off by scooping out a large portion of the avocado substance, leaving about ½ inch around the avocado.
2. Put a huge pan on low heat and add the margarine. While the spread is dissolving, split the eggs into a container and beat them, including a put of salt and pepper.
3. Add the bacon to the other side of the container and let them fry for a few minutes all alone. At that point add the eggs to the opposite side of the container and mix routinely as they scramble. The eggs and bacon should both be completed 5 minutes after the eggs are added to the dish. In the event that you discover your eggs are done a little before the bacon, remove the fried eggs from the container and put them in a bowl.
4. Blend the bacon sorts and fried eggs out in a bowl, at that point spoon into the avocado dishes and get to eating'

Nutrition Fact: Calories: 500, Fat 40g, Carbs 11g, Sugar 1g, Protein 25g

SHEET PAN BRUSSELS SPROUTS WITH BACON

Prep Time: 10mints, Cook Time: 35mints, Total Time: 45mints; Serving: 6

INGREDIENTS
- 16 oz bacon
- 16 oz raw Brussels sprouts
- Salt
- Pepper

INSTRUCTIONS
1. Preheat stove to 400 degrees. Line heating sheet with parchment paper
2. Split Brussels grows.
3. Utilizing kitchen shears, cut bacon into little pieces the long way.
4. Add Brussels sprouts and bacon to arranged heating sheet and season with salt and pepper.
5. Heat for 35-40 minutes, until Brussels sprouts are somewhat caramelized, and bacon is firm.

Nutrition Fact: Calories: 113, Fat 6.9g, Carbs 6.8g, Sugar 4.3g, Protein: 7.9g

KALE AND CHIVES EGG MUFFINS

Prep Time: 10mints, Cook Time: 30mints, Total Time: 40mints; Serving: 4

INGREDIENTS
- 6 eggs
- 1/2 cup almond or coconut milk
- 1 cup kale
- 1/4 cup chives
- salt and pepper to taste

INSTRUCTIONS
1. Preheat the stove to 350
2. Whisk the eggs and add the hacked kale and chives. Additionally, add the almond/coconut milk, salt, and pepper. Blend well.
3. Oil 8 biscuit cups with coconut oil or line each cup with a prosciutto cut.
4. Gap the egg blend between the 8 biscuit cups. Fill just 2/3 of each cup as the blend rises when it's preparing.
5. Heat in the stove for 30 minutes
6. Let cool a couple of moments and afterward lift out cautiously with a fork. Note that the biscuits will sink a piece.

Nutrition Fact: Calories: 321, Fat 9g, Carbs 14g, Sugar 4.1g, Protein 24g

3-INGREDIENT BACON AND EGG BREAKFAST MUFFINS

Prep Time: 15mints, Cook Time: 25mints, Total Time: 40mints; Serving: 12 muffins

INGREDIENTS
- 8 bacon slices
- 8 large eggs
- 2/3 cup chopped green onion

INSTRUCTIONS
1. Preheat stove to 350 degrees. Coat biscuit tin cavities with nonstick cooking shower
2. In a huge container over medium heat, cook bacon until fresh.
3. Transfer cooked bacon to a paper towel-lined dish.
4. Enable bacon to cool marginally before cleaving bacon into little pieces.
5. In a blending bowl, whisk eggs together.
6. Add bacon and cleaved green onions and blend again until all ingredients are well-mixed.
7. Empty or scoop egg blend into pits of arranged biscuit tin until every depression is mostly full.
8. Move biscuit tin to stove and prepare until edges of biscuits are brilliant darker, around 20-25 minutes.

Nutrition Fact: Calories: 69, Fat 4.9g, Carbs 0.5g, Sugar 1.4g, Protein 5.6g

KETO MUSHROOM OMELET

Prep Time: 5mints, Cooking Time: 10mints, Total Time: 15mints; Serving: 1

INGREDIENTS

- 3 eggs
- 1 oz. butter
- 1 oz. shredded cheese
- ¼ yellow onion, salt, and pepper
- 4 large mushrooms

INSTRUCTIONS
1. Break the eggs into a blending bowl and add a touch of salt and pepper. Whisk the eggs with a fork until smooth and foamy.
2. Dissolve the margarine in a griddle, over medium heat. Add the mushrooms and onion to the dish, mixing until delicate, and afterward pour in the egg blend into the veggie mix.
3. When the omelet starts to cook but still has a little raw egg on top, sprinkle cheese over the egg.
4. Utilizing a spatula, cautiously ease around the edges of the omelet, and afterward overlap it over into equal parts. Once golden brown on both sides, remove skillet from the heat and slide the omelet on to a plate.

Nutrition Fact: Calories 517, Fat 44g, Carbs 5g, Sugar 3g, Protein 20g

COCONUT MACADAMIA BARS – BREAKFAST IN FIVE

Prep Time: 5mints, Total Time: 5mints; Servings: 6
INGREDIENTS
- 60 grams macadamia nuts
- 1/2 cup almond butter
- 1/4 cup coconut oil
- 6 Tsp unsweetened shredded coconut
- 20 drops Sweet leaf Stevia drops

INSTRUCTIONS
1. Squash the macadamia nuts a nourishment processor or by hand.
2. Join the almond margarine, coconut oil and destroyed coconut in a blending bowl. Add the macadamia nuts and Stevie drops.
3. Blend completely and empty the player into a 9×9 parchment paper lined preparing dish.
4. Refrigerate medium-term, cut and serve and enjoy.

Nutrition Fact: Calories 327, Fat 33g, Carbs 7g, Sugar 1g, Protein 5g

10-MINUTE KETO TOAST RECIPE

Prep Time: 5mints, Cook Time: 5mints; Serving: 2
INGREDIENTS
- 1/3 cup (35 g) almond flour
- 1/2 tsp (1 g) baking powder
- 1/8 tsp (1 g) salt
- 1 egg, whisked
- Tsp (37 ml) ghee

INSTRUCTIONS
1. Preheat stove to 400 F (200 C).
2. Put all the bread ingredients into a mug and blend well.
3. Put the mug into the microwave and microwave on high for 90 seconds.
4. Give the bread a chance to cool for a couple of moments and afterward fly out of the mug and cut into 4 cuts.
5. Put the cuts onto a heating plate and toast in the stove for 4 minutes.
6. Serve and enjoy with some extra ghee.

Nutrition Fact: Calories: 270, Fat 27g, Carbs 3g, Sugar 1g, Protein 6g

KETO SMOOTHIE - BLUEBERRY

Prep Time: 5mints, Total Time: 6mins; Servings: 1
INGREDIENTS
- 1 cup Coconut Milk or almond milk
- 1/4 cup Blueberries
- 1 tsp Vanilla Extract
- 1 tsp MCT Oil or coconut oil
- 30g Protein Powder optional

INSTRUCTIONS
1. Put all components right into a blender and mix until smooth.

Nutrition Facts: Calories 215, Fat 10g, Carbs 7g, Sugar 3g, Protein 23g

PERFECT KETO PEACHES AND CREAM FAT BOMBS

Prep Time: 10mints, Total Time: 10mints; Serving: 24
INGREDIENTS
- 4 tbsp unsalted Kerry gold butter
- 6 oz. organic cream cheese
- 1 cup frozen peaches, slightly warmed
- 3/4 scoop Perfect Keto Peach Base
- 3 1/2 tbsp. monk fruit sweetener

INSTRUCTIONS
2. In a medium-sized bowl with a hand blender, blend the margarine, cream cheddar, peaches, Peach Ketone Base, and 3 tbsp priest natural product sugar until well-joined.
3. Scoop blend into a silicone shape. Top each fat bomb with residual priest natural product sugar.
4. Put form in the cooler and stop for 4 hours.
5. When solidified, remove fat bombs from silicone form and serve and enjoy.

Nutrition Fact: Calories: 43, Fat 4.2g, Carbs 1g, Sugar 0.3g, Protein 0.5g

CREAMY TRIPLE CHOCOLATE KETO SHAKE

Prep Time: 2mints, Total Time: 2mints; Serving: 12 ounces
INGREDIENTS
- 1 cup dairy-loose milk
- 1 tsp almond butter
- 1/2 of tsp cacao powder
- scoop Perfect Keto Chocolate Collagen
- scoop Keto Chocolate Oil Powder

INSTRUCTIONS
1. Add all ingredients to a rapid blender.
2. Blend on high until simply mixed.

3. Add ice and mix until cover or present ice.
4. Top with chocolate chips or cacao nibs whenever wanted.
Nutrition Fact: Calories: 282, Fat 22g, Carbs 4g, Sugar 3g, Protein 8g

FROZEN KETO BERRY SHAKE

Prep Time: 5mints, Total Time: 5mints; Serving: 1
INGREDIENTS
- 1/3 cup creamed coconut milk
- 1/2 cup water
- 1/2 cup mixed frozen berries
- 1 tbsp Virgin coconut oil
- Few ice cubes

INSTRUCTIONS
1. To "cream" the coconut milk, essentially place the can in the refrigerator medium-term. The following day, open, spoon out the set coconut milk and dispose of the fluids. Try not to shake before opening the can. One 400 gram can yield around 200 grams of coconut cream. Solidified Keto Berry Shake
2. Put the creamed coconut milk, berries, water or almond milk and ice into a blender. Solidified Keto Berry Shake
3. Add MCT oil and Stevie. Solidified Keto Berry Shake
4. Heartbeat until smooth and serve right away, alternatively, top with whipped cream or coconut milk.
Nutrition Fact: Calories 400, Fat 41g, carbs 6.7g, Sugar 3.2g, Protein 4g

MINTY GREEN PROTEIN SMOOTHIE SHAKE

Prep Time: 5mints, Total Time: 5mints; Serving: 1
INGREDIENTS
- 1 scoop perfect keto unflavored whey protein powder
- ¼ Cup of coconut milk
- 1 scoop keto matcha MCT oil powder
- 1 large handful spinach
- 1 small avocado

INSTRUCTIONS
1. Add all ingredients to a fast blender and mix on high.
2. Garnish with mint leaves and a few berries if needed.
Nutrition Fact: Calories: 334, Fat 24g, Carbs 13g, Sugar 8g, Protein 19g

KETO BEETROOT SHAKE FOR ATHLETES

Prep Time: 5mints, Total Time: 5mints; Servings: 1
INGREDIENTS
- 1 tsp Temple Beetroot Powder
- 1 Tbsp Temple Nutrition MCT Oil
- 1 tsp Vanilla Extract
- 1/4 tsp Cinnamon Ground
- 1 Cup Coconut Milk

INSTRUCTIONS
1. Put all ingredients into a rapid blender.
2. Mix for 30 seconds.
3. Fill a glass, or drink directly from the holder. Top with additional beetroot powder if needs be.
Nutrition Facts: Calories 300, Fat 19g, Carbs 6g, Sugar 1g, Protein 25g

HEALTHY CHOCOLATE PEANUT BUTTER LOW CARB SMOOTHIE

Prep Time: 5mints, Total Time: 5mints; Serving: 3
INGREDIENTS
- 1/4 cup Peanut butter
- 3 tbsp Cocoa powder
- 1 cup Heavy cream
- 1 1/2 cup unsweetened almond milk
- 6 tbsp Powdered erythritol

INSTRUCTIONS
1. Join all ingredients in a blender.
2. Puree until smooth. Alter sugar to taste whenever wanted
Nutrition Facts: Calories 435, Fat 41g, Carbs 10g, Sugar 3g, Protein 9g

MCKEE STRAWBERRY KETO MILKSHAKE

Prep Time: 3mints, Total Time: 5mints; Serving: 2
INGREDIENTS
- 3/4 cup Coconut Milk
- 1/4 cup Heavy Cream
- 7 Ice Cubes
- 2 tbsp. Sugar-free Strawberry Torani®
- 1/4 tsp. Xanthan Gum

INSTRUCTIONS
1. Add all ingredients on your blender.
2. Mix everything collectively for 1-2mins or till the consistency is beneficial for you.
3. Spill out and admire it!
Nutrition Fact: Calories 368, Fat 38.85g, Carbs 3.7g, Sugar 1.28g, Protein 1.69g

COCONUT MILK STRAWBERRY SMOOTHIE

Prep Time: 2mints, Total Time: 2mints; Servings: 2
INGREDIENTS
- 1 cup of strawberries frozen
- 1 cup unsweetened coconut milk
- 2 Tsp smooth almond butter
- 2 packets Stevie

INSTRUCTIONS
1. Add all ingredients to a blender.
2. Mix until smooth.
3. Fill a glass and serve and enjoy!
Nutrition Fact: Calories: 397, Fat 37g, Carbs 15g, Sugar 8g, Protein 6g

BLUEBERRY COCONUT YOGURT SMOOTHIE RECIPE

Prep Time: 5mints, Total Time: 5mints; Serving: 2
INGREDIENTS
- 1 pot of coconut yogurt
- 10 blueberries
- 1 cup coconut milk

- 1/2 tsp vanilla extract
- Stevie to taste

INSTRUCTIONS
1. Put every one of the ingredients into the blender and mix truly well.
2. Serve and enjoy for a speedy and nutritious breakfast or tidbit.

Nutrition Fact: Calories: 70, Fat 5g, Carbs 2g, Sugar 2g, Protein 2g

KETO CHOCOLATE SMOOTHIE

Prep Time: 3mints, Total Time: 8mints; Serving: 2
INGREDIENTS
- 1 Can full-fat coconut milk
- ¼ cup egg white protein powder
- ½ tsp vanilla Stevie
- ⅓ Cup chopped 85% dark chocolate
- 2-3 cups ice

INSTRUCTIONS
1. In a Vitamin, join coconut milk, protein powder, and Stevie
2. Mix in chocolate until smooth
3. Mix in ice 3D squares until blend is all around joined
4. Serve

Nutrition Facts: Calories 215, Fat 10g, Carbs 7g, Sugar 3g, Protein 23g

STRAWBERRY AVOCADO KETO SMOOTHIE WITH ALMOND MILK

Prep Time: 2mints, Total Time: 2mints; Serving: 5
INGREDIENTS
- 1 lb. Frozen strawberries
- 1 1/2 cup unsweetened almond milk
- 1 large Avocado
- 1/4 cup Erythritol

INSTRUCTIONS
1. Pure all ingredients in a blender, mix till it smooth.
2. Adjust sugar to taste as needed.

Nutrition Facts: Calories 106, Fat 7g, Carbs 12g, Sugar 4g, Protein 1g

LOW CARB BLUEBERRY PROTEIN POWER SMOOTHIE

Prep Time: 2mints, Total Time: 2mints; Servings: 1
INGREDIENTS
- ¼ cup fresh blueberries
- 1 tbs flaxseed meal
- 8 oz unsweetened almond milk
- 1 scoop vanilla whey protein
- low carb simple syrup optional

INSTRUCTIONS
1. Blend all ingredients in a container blender or inundation blender and mix until smooth.
2. Test for sweetness and add syrup as wanted.

Nutrition Facts: Calories 110, Fat 7g, Carbs 9g, Sugar 3g, Protein 3g

STRAWBERRY PROTEIN SMOOTHIE

Prep Time: 3mints, Total Time: 8mints; Serving: 1
INGREDIENTS
- Almond butter 1 tbsp
- Protein powder, vanilla 1/2 scoop
- Almond milk 1/2 cup
- Water 1/3 cup
- Frozen strawberries 1/3 cup

INSTRUCTION
1. Put all ingredients right into a blender and blend.
2. Add water whenever required to make the smoothie much less thick.

Nutrition Fact: Calories: 334, Fat 24g, Carbs 13g, Sugar 8g, Protein 19g

LOW-CARB BLUEBERRY VANILLA SMOOTHIE

Prep Time: 5mints, Total Time: 5mints; Serving: 2
INGREDIENTS
- 14 oz. canned, coconut milk
- 3 oz. frozen blueberries or fresh blueberries
- 1 tbsp lemon juice
- ½ tsp vanilla extract

INSTRUCTIONS
1. Put all ingredients in a blender and blend until smooth.
2. Taste, and add more lemon juice whenever wanted.

Nutrition Fact: Calories 417, Fat 43g, Carbs 23g, Sugar 6g, Protein 4g

DAIRY-FREE PEANUT BUTTER AND JELLY SMOOTHIE

Prep Time: 5mints, Total Time: 5mints; Serving: 2
INGREDIENTS
- 1 cup of frozen mixed berries
- 2 Tsp peanut butter powder
- 1 scoop dairy-free vanilla protein powder
- 1 ½ cups Dairy Free Organic Almond milk

INSTRUCTIONS
1. Blend all ingredients in a blender and beat until soft and creamy.

Nutrition Fact: Calories 140, Fat 4g, Carbs 11g, Sugar 5g, Protein 18g

KETO ORGANIC PEANUT SMOOTHIE

Prep Time: 5mints, Total Time: 5mints; Servings: 2
INGREDIENTS
- 1 1/2 cups coconut milk
- 2/3 Cup Ice
- 1 Tbsp natural organic peanut butter
- 2 Tsp of raw cacao powder
- 1 Tsp of organic Stevie extract

INSTRUCTIONS
1. In a blender, blend all ingredients and mix until smooth.
2. Serve and serve and enjoy it.

Nutrition Facts: Calories 110, Fat 7g, Carbs 9g, Sugar 3g, Protein 3g

ENERGIZING KETO SMOOTHIE

Prep Time: 2mints, Total Time: 2mints; Serving: 1
INGREDIENTS
- 1 cup unsweetened cashew milk
- 1 tsp Perfect Keto MCT Oil
- 1 tsp Perfect Keto Nut Butter
- 2 Tsp maca powder
- 1 handful of ice

INSTRUCTIONS
1. Join all ingredients in a fast blender and mix until smooth.

Nutrition Fact: Calories: 250, Fat 26g, Carbs 4g, Sugar 3g, Protein 7g

KETO BLUEBERRY GINGER SMOOTHIE

Prep Time: 5mints, Total Time: 5mints; Serving: 2
INGREDIENTS
- 15 blueberries
- 1/2 cup of coconut yogurt
- 3 slices of ginger
- 2 slices of apple
- 1/2 Tsp collagen powder

INSTRUCTIONS
1. Blend all the ingredients well together.

Nutrition Fact: Calories 168, Fat 15g, Carbs 5g, Sugar 2g, Protein 4g

REFRESHING CUCUMBER CELERY LIME SMOOTHIE

Prep Time: 5mints, Total Time: 5mints; Serving: 2
INGREDIENTS
- 4 stalks of celery heart
- 1 small cucumber
- Juice from 1/2 lime
- 1/2 cup water
- 1/2 cup ice

INSTRUCTIONS
1. Put everything into a decent blender and mix well.
2. In the event that you need it to be a juice, at that point simply strain the smoothie.

Nutrition Fact: Calories: 107, Fat 9g, Carbs 4g, Sugar 2g, Protein 1g

SLEEP IN" SMOOTHIE

Prep Time: 5mints, Total Time: 5mints; Serving: 1
INGREDIENTS
- 1 raw egg
- 1/4 cup of kombucha
- 1 cup of fruit
- 2 cups of fresh spinach
- 1/4 avocado

INSTRUCTIONS
1. Toss everything into a blender together and star until very much mixed and smooth.

Nutrition Fact: Calories 165, Fat 14g, Carbs 11g, Sugar 2g, Protein 2g

KETO CHOCOLATE PEPPERMINT SMOOTHIE RECIPE

Prep Time: 10mints, Total Time: 10mints, Serving: 2
INGREDIENTS
- 2 cups of dairy-free milk
- 1 small avocado
- 1 cup ice
- 2 scoops of CoBionic Indulgence
- 1/2 tsp of vanilla extract

INSTRUCTIONS
1. Add all ingredients to your mix and mix until totally smooth.
2. Fill glasses and trimming with crisp peppermint leaves.

Nutrition Fact: Calories: 185, Fat 14g, Carbs 7g, Sugar 0.4g, Protein 10g

KETO RASPBERRY AVOCADO SMOOTHIE

Prep Time: 5mints, Total Time: 5mints; Serving: 2
INGREDIENTS
- 1/4 cup of fresh raspberries
- 1/4 avocado
- 2 scoops of CoBionic Foundation
- 1 cup coconut milk
- 1 cup of cold water

INSTRUCTIONS
1. Essentially mix every one of the ingredients in a blender and gap the smoothie between two glasses. On the off chance that the smoothie is excessively thick, add extra cool water until it is dainty just as you would prefer.

Nutrition Fact: Calories 135, Fat 6g, Carbs 20g, Sugar 3g, Protein 1g

EASY KETO AVOCADO TOAST RECIPE

Prep Time: 5mints, Cook Time: 2mints, Total Time: 7mins; Serving: 2
INGREDIENTS
- 2 slices Easy Keto Sandwich Bread
- 4 oz prosciutto
- 1 avocado and 1 tsp chives
- 1/2 cup arugula
- 1/4 cup sweet piquillo peppers

INSTRUCTIONS
1. Toast cuts of bread.
2. At the point when the bread is toasted, spread a portion of the avocado on one bit of bread
3. Top with arugula, peppers, prosciutto, and chives.
4. Serve and enjoy!

Nutrition Fact: Calories 330, Fat 15g, Carbs 15g, Sugar 1g. Protein 17g

CHOCOLATE PROTEIN WAFFLES

Prep Time: 2mints, Cook Time: 3mints, Total Time: 5mints; Serving: 1

INGREDIENTS
- 1 scoop Low carb chocolate protein powder
- 1 Teaspoon Coconut Flour
- 1 Teaspoon Baking Powder
- 1 egg and 2-3 Tsp Water
- 1 Teaspoon Coconut Oil

INSTRUCTIONS
1. Preheat waffle iron.
2. Add protein powder, coconut flour, baking powder, and egg.
3. Utilize a hand blender to mix until the dry ingredients become wet.
4. Add water, each tablespoon in turn until the blend turns into the consistency of a thick flapjack batter.
5. Lubricate waffle iron with oil to get ready for the batter.
6. Spoon batter onto hot iron
7. Cook waffles until fresh per producer's guidelines and serves quickly with a dab of butter or low carb syrup of your choice.

Nutrition Fact: Calories: 230, Fat 8g, Carbs 8g, Sugar 3g, Protein 29g

KETO LEMON GINGER GREEN JUICE SHOTS RECIPE

Prep Time: 10mints, Total Time: 10mints; Serving: 2
INGREDIENTS
- 1 oz of kale
- 5 stalks of trimmed celery
- 2 tsps. of lemon juice
- Generous handful of mint leaves
- 1 tsp of fresh ginger
- 1 tsp of erythritol

INSTRUCTIONS
1. Put everything, apart from the sugar, into a juicer and switch the juicer on.
2. When done, dispose of the mash.
3. Mix the sugar into the juice and blend well. Add ice for an extra refreshing sensation.

Nutrition Fact: Calories: 51, Fat 0.4g, Carbs 11g, Sugar 2g, Protein 3g

KETO RED VELVET SMOOTHIE RECIPE

Prep Time: 10mints, Total Time: 10mints; Serving:
INGREDIENTS
- 6 raspberries
- 2 Tsp of cacao powder
- 1/2 cup of coconut milk
- 1/2 cup of water
- 1/2 cup crushed ice

INSTRUCTIONS
1. Put every one of the ingredients into a blender and mix well.

Nutrition Fact: Calories: 148, Fat 12g, Carbs 9g, Sugar 2g, Protein 2g

KETO SPINACH AVOCADO GREEN SMOOTHIE

Prep Time: 5mints, Total Time: 5mints; Serving: 2
INGREDIENTS
- 2 cups spinach
- 1 cup coconut milk
- 1 ripe avocado
- 2 Tsp vanilla extract
- Sweetener

INSTRUCTIONS
1. Blend well and enjoy.

Nutrition Fact: Calories 190, Fat 17g, Carbs 10g, Sugar 1g, Protein 3g

STRAWBERRY AVOCADO COCONUT SMOOTHIE

Prep Time: 2mints, Total Time: 2mints; Servings: 2
INGREDIENTS
- 75 grams of frozen strawberries
- 1 medium avocado
- 1 1/2 cups coconut milk
- 1 tsp lime juice
- 2 stevia packets
- 1/2 cup ice more or less

INSTRUCTIONS
1. Add all ingredients into a blender and mix until smooth.

Nutrition Fact: Calories 165, Fat 14g, Carbs 11g, Sugar 2g, Protein 2g

CINNAMON CHOCOLATE BREAKFAST SMOOTHIE RECIPE

Prep Time: 5mints, Total Time: 5mints; Serving: 1
INGREDIENTS
- 3/4 cup coconut milk
- 1/2 ripe avocado
- 2 Tsp unsweetened cacao powder
- 1 tsp cinnamon powder
- 1/4 tsp vanilla extract
- Stevie to taste

INSTRUCTIONS
1. Mix every one of the ingredients together well.

Nutrition Fact: Calories 300, Fat 30g Carbs 14g, Sugar 2g, Protein 3g

STRAWBERRY & MINT SMOOTHIE

Prep Time: 2mints, Total Time: 2mints; Serving: 2
INGREDIENTS
- 100 grams of Strawberries
- 15 grams of Cream Cheese
- Few fresh mint leaves
- 100 ml Fresh Cream
- 150 ml Unsweetened Coconut Milk
- Stevie to taste

INSTRUCTIONS
1. Mix the strawberries with the cream cheddar and mint leaves
2. Add the cream, coconut milk, and Stevie
3. Mix together
4. Topping with mint and serve chilled.

Nutrition Facts: Calories 268, Fat 17.2g, Carbs 8.3g, sugar 4.5g, Protein 22g

KETO CHOCOLATE RASPBERRY SPINACH GREEN SMOOTHIE

Prep Time: 2mints, Total Time: 2mints; Servings: 1
INGREDIENTS
- 1/4 cup raspberries
- 1/2 cup spinach
- 1 tbsp cocoa powder
- 1/2 cup heavy cream
- 1/2 cup water
- ice cubes

INSTRUCTIONS
1. Mix the entirety of the ingredients until they add and become smooth and rich.
2. Mix spinach, cream, water, cocoa powder
3. Move to a tall glass and serve and enjoy it while cold.

Nutrition Facts: Calories 442, Fat 45g, Carbs 11g, Sugar 2g, Protein 4g

KETO GINGER CILANTRO SMOOTHIE

Prep Time: 5mints, Total Time: 5mints; Servings: 2
INGREDIENTS
- 1 cup of cold water
- 1 cup baby spinach
- 1/2 cup cilantro
- 1-inch ginger peeled
- 3/4 English cucumber peeled
- 1/2-1 lemon peeled
- 1 cup frozen avocado

INSTRUCTIONS
1. Combine all ingredients to a blender and blend till smooth.
2. Store in an airproof slot, for as long as three days

Nutrition Facts: Calories 148, Fat 11g, Carbs 13g, Sugar 2g, Protein 2g

KETO SMOOTHIE RECIPE {WITH CHOCOLATE & CHIA SEEDS}

Prep Time: 10mints, Total Time: 10mints; Servings:1
INGREDIENTS
- 2 tbsp chia seeds
- 3/4 cup water
- 6 cubes ice
- 1/4 cup whole milk
- 1/3 cup full-fat Greek yogurt
- 2 tbsp cocoa dark chocolate

INSTRUCTIONS
1. Douse chia seeds in 1/3 cup water for 5 minutes.
2. Add remaining ingredients to a blender. Mix until smooth.
3. In the event that excessively thick, add more water or milk, 1 tbsp at once.

Nutrition Facts: Calories 268, Fat 17.2g, Carbs 8.3g, sugar 4.5g, Protein 22g

LOW-CARB 5 MINUTE MOCHA SMOOTHIE

Prep Time: 5mints, Total Time: 5mints; Servings: 3
INGREDIENTS
- 1/2 cup coconut milk
- 1 1/2 cup unsweetened almond milk
- 1 tsp vanilla extract
- 3 tsp granulated Stevie
- 3 tsp unsweetened cocoa powder
- 1 avocado

INSTRUCTIONS
1. Put coconut milk, almond milk, vanilla concentrate, sugar, and cocoa powder into a blender. Mix until smooth.
2. Scoop the avocado into the blend. Mix until smooth. Fill glasses and serve.

Nutrition Fact:Calories 176, Fat 16g, Carbs 10g, Sugar 6g, Protein 3g

SALTED CARAMEL KETO SMOOTHIE

Prep Time: 2mints, Total Time: 2mints; Servings: 1
INGREDIENTS
- 1 bag Bigelow Salted Caramel Tea
- 1 cup unsweetened almond milk
- 2 tbsp whipping cream
- 1 tbsp MCT oil
- 1/2 tsp stevia
- 8 ice cubes

INSTRUCTIONS
1. Soak 1 pack of Bigelow Salted Caramel Tea in 6 oz. water
2. Evacuate and dispose of the tea sack when done.
3. Join remaining ingredients in a blender and mix until smooth.
4. Fill a glass and serve.

Nutrition Facts: Calories 275, Fat 28g, Carbs 3g, Sugar 0.4g, Protein 1g

BUTTERY COCONUT FLOUR WAFFLES

Prep Time: 10mints, Cook Time: 20mints, Total Time: 30mints; Servings: 5
INGREDIENTS
- 4 tbsp coconut flour
- 5 eggs separate whites from yolks
- 4 tbsp granulated Stevie
- 1 tsp baking powder
- 2 tsp vanilla extract
- 3 tbsp milk full fat
- 1/2 cup butter melted

INSTRUCTIONS
1. In a bowl, blend the egg yolks, coconut flour, Stevie, and preparing powder.
2. Add the liquefied margarine gradually to the flour blend; blend well to guarantee smooth consistency
3. Add the milk and vanilla to the flour and spread blend makes certain to blend well.
4. In another container, flit the egg whites till smooth.

5. Tenderly crease spoons of the whisked egg whites into the flour blend.
6. Empty blend into waffle creator and cook until dark in color.

Nutrition Facts: Calories 278, Fat 26g, Carbs 7g, Sugars 4g, Protein 8g

VEGAN KETO PORRIDGE

Prep Time: 15mints, Cooking Time: 20mints, Total Time: 35mints; Serving: 4

INGREDIENTS
- 2 tablespoons coconut flour
- 3 tablespoons golden flaxseed meal
- 2 tablespoons vegan vanilla protein powder
- 1 ½ cups unsweetened almond milk
- Powdered erythritol

INSTRUCTIONS
1. In a bowl combine the coconut flour, golden flaxseed meal and protein powder.
2. Add to a pot, alongside the almond milk, and cook over medium heat.
3. At the point when it thickens you can mix in your favored measure of sugar. I like to use about ½ a tablespoon.
4. Present with your preferred garnishes.

Nutrition Fact: Calories 423, Fat 24g, Carbs 8g, Sugar 6g, Protein 24g

CINNAMON FAUX-ST CRUNCH CEREAL

Prep Time: 15mints, Cooking Time: 15mints, Total Time: 30mints; Serving: 4

INGREDIENTS
- 1/2 cup milled flax seed
- 1/2 cup hulled hemp seeds
- 2 Tbsp ground cinnamon
- 1/2 cup apple juice
- 1 Tbsp coconut oil

INSTRUCTIONS
1. Add the dry ingredients in a Magic Bullet, blender or nourishment processor. Add the squeezed apple and coconut oil and mix
2. Spread the participant out on a fabric coated parchment sheet until first rate and flimsy – round 1/16 of an inch thick.
3. Heat in a preheated 300-degrees F stove for 15mins, lower the heat to 250 and prepare for an additional 10 minutes.
4. Remove from the stove and utilizing a pizza shaper or blade, cut into squares about the scale of the keys on your PC keyboard.
5. Switch off the stove and set the oats back in for about 60mins or till it is done
6. Present with unsweetened almond or coconut milk

Nutrition Fact: Calories 129, Fat 9g, Carbs 1.3g, Sugar 1.1g, Protein 16g

COCONUT FLOUR CREPES

Prep Time: 15mints, Cook Time: 10mints, Total Time: 25mints; Serving: 6 crepes

INGREDIENTS
- 4 eggs
- 1 tsp extra virgin coconut oil melted
- 1/4 cup almond milk or water
- 1/4 cup coconut cream melted
- 2 Tsp coconut flour
- 1 tsp almond meal also known

INSTRUCTIONS
1. In an enormous blending bowl, add every one of the ingredients in a specific order: eggs, softened coconut oil, almond milk, coconut cream, vanilla concentrate, coconut flour, and almond dinner, utilizing a whisk or electric blender, beat until a smooth player structure without any knots
2. Heat gentle oil smaller than expected egg skillet over medium/high heat
3. Pour 1/4 cup of the crepe hitter onto the dish, at that pointed tip and turn the skillet delicately to spread player as daintily as could reasonably be expected. Darker on one side first, cook 2-3 minutes until the sides are firm and un-stick effectively from the dish. The inside ought to be set and dry before you flip over to maintain a strategic distance from the crepe to break.
4. Dark colored on different sides around 1-2 minutes and serve hot with your preferred fillings - see formula note for motivation.

Nutrition Facts: Calories 108, Fat 8.9g, Carbs 2.5g, Sugar 0.3g, Protein 4.6g

KETO FOUR-INGREDIENT PANCAKE WITH ALMOND FLOUR RECIPE

Prep Time: 10mints, Cook Time: 30mints, Total Time: 40mints; Serving: 4

INGREDIENTS
- 1 1/4 cups of almond flour
- 2 Tsp erythritol, or to taste
- ½ cup unsweetened almond or coconut milk
- 2 eggs, whisked
- ¼ cup ghee

INSTRUCTIONS
1. Combine the almond flour, erythritol, almond or coconut milk, and eggs together.
2. Dissolve a portion of the ghee in a non-stick container and cautiously pour 1/4 cup of the player into the griddle.
3. Cook on medium heat until the flapjack starts rising on top. At that point utilize a spatula to poke the base of the hotcake to ensure it's cooked.
4. Cautiously flip and cook the opposite side for a couple of moments.

Nutrition Fact: Calories 321, Fat 31g, Carbs 7g, Sugar 1g, Protein 9g

KETO BACON ASPARAGUS MINI FRITTATA RECIPE

Prep Time: 10mints, Cook Time: 30mints, Total Time: 40mints; Serving: 12 muffins
INGREDIENTS
- 1 cup chopped asparagus
- 4 slices bacon
- 2 Tsp chopped onions
- 8 eggs
- 1/2 cup coconut milk
- Salt and pepper to taste

INSTRUCTIONS
1. Preheat stove to 350 F (175 C).
2. Cook the diced bacon in a skillet.
3. Blend all the slashed vegetables, cooked bacon, whisked eggs, and coconut milk together in a huge blending bowl.
4. Empty the player into biscuit cups.
5. Heat for 25-30 minutes until the center of the biscuits isn't liquid any longer.

Nutrition Fact: Calories: 460, Fat 41g, Carbs 4g, Sugar 2g, Protein 19g

PALEO EGG FRITTATA MUFFINS RECIPE [KETO, DAIRY-FREE]

Prep Time: 10mints, Cook Time: 30mints, Total Time: 40mints; Serving: 12
INGREDIENTS
- 1 cup chopped broccoli
- 2 Tsp chopped onions
- 1/4 cup chopped red bell pepper
- 8 eggs
- 1/2 cup coconut milk
- Salt and pepper to taste

INSTRUCTIONS
1. Preheat stove to 350 F (175 C).
2. Blend every one of the vegetables and whisked eggs and coconut milk together in a huge blending bowl.
3. Empty the hitter into biscuit cups.
4. Prepare for 25-30 minutes until the center of the biscuits isn't fluid any longer.

Nutrition Fact: Calories: 312, Fat 11g, Carbs 17g, Sugar 8g, Protein 34g

KETO OATMEAL: 5-MINUTE LOW-CARB OATMEAL

Prep Time: 5mints, Cook Time: 15mints, Total Time: 20mints; Serving: 1
INGREDIENTS
- 1 cup unsweetened almond milk
- 1/2 cup hemp hearts
- 1 tsp flax meal
- 1 tsp chia seeds
- 1 tsp coconut flakes
- 1 tsp cinnamon

INSTRUCTIONS
1. Join the entirety of the ingredients in a little saucepot, mix to add.
2. Bring to a stew until thickened just as you would prefer, mix infrequently.

3. Serve and enhancement with solidified berries

Nutrition Fact: Calories: 584, Fat 44g, Carbs 17g, Sugar: 6g, Protein 31g

MEAT-LOVER PIZZA CUPS

Prep Time: 15mints, Cook Time: 11mints, Total Time: 26mints ; Serving: 12
INGREDIENTS
- 12 deli ham slices
- 1 lb. bulk Italian sausage
- 12 Tbsp sugar-free pizza sauce
- 3 cups grated mozzarella cheese
- 24 pepperoni slices
- 1 cup cooked and crumbled bacon

INSTRUCTIONS
1. Preheat stove to 375 F. Dark-colored Italian frankfurters in a skillet, depleting abundance oil.
2. Line 12-cup biscuit tin with ham cuts. Partition wiener, pizza sauce, mozzarella cheddar, pepperoni cuts, and bacon disintegrate between each cup, in a specific order.
3. Heat at 375 for 10 minutes, cook for 1 moment until cheddar air pockets and tans and the edges of the meat ingredients look firm.
4. Remove pizza cups from biscuit tin and set on a paper towels to keep the bottoms from getting wet. Serve and enjoy promptly or refrigerate and warm in toaster stove or microwave.

Nutrition Fact: Calories 165, Fat 14g, Carbs 11g, Sugar 2g, Protein 2g

COLD BREW PROTEIN SHAKE SMOOTHIE

Prep Time: 10mints, Total Time: 10mints; Serving: 1
INGREDIENTS
- 8 oz cold brew coffee
- 1/3 cup almond milk
- 1 scoop Rootz Paleo Chocolate Banana
- A handful of ice cubes

INSTRUCTIONS
1. Join all ingredients in milk frothier or a shaker bottle. Blend until ingredients are integrated.

Nutrition Fact: Calories: 188; Fat 5g, Carbs 10g, Sugar 6g, Protein 24g

COCO-NUTTY GRAIN-FREE GRANOLA

Prep Time: 5mints, Cook Time: 20mints, Total Time: 25mints; Serving: 15
INGREDIENTS
- 3 cups unsweetened coconut flakes
- 2 cups raw nuts
- 2 tablespoons chia seeds
- 1 teaspoon ground cinnamon
- 5 tablespoons coconut oil

INSTRUCTIONS
1. Preheat stove to 250°F and line an oven tray with parchment paper.
2. Join all ingredients in a bowl, blend completely, and spread equally on the sheet.

3. Heat 30-40 minutes until done, turning part of the way through cooking time
4. Remove from stove and permit to cool.
5. Serve and eat will still fresh.
Nutritional Fact: Calories 388, Fat 14g, Carbs 2g, Sugar 1g, Protein 60g

KETO SAUSAGE AND EGG BREAKFAST SANDWICH

Prep Time: 5mints, Cook Time: 10mints, Total Time: 15mints; Serving: 1
INGREDIENTS
- 1 tbsp butter and 2 large eggs
- 1 tbsp mayonnaise
- 2 sausage patties
- 2 slices sharp cheddar cheese
- Avocado

INSTRUCTIONS
1. Heat the margarine in a huge skillet over medium heat
2. Put softly oiled artisan box jewelry or silicone egg molds into the skillet.
3. Split the eggs into the earrings and use a fork to break the yolks and delicately whisk.
4. Cover and cook dinner for 3-4mins or until eggs are cooked via.
5. Put one of the eggs on a plate and pinnacle it with 1/2 of the mayonnaise.
6. Top the frankfurter patty with a cut of cheddar and avocado.
7. Put the second frankfurter patty over the avocado and pinnacle it with the rest of the cheddar.
8. Spread the rest of the mayonnaise on the second one cooked egg and put it over the cheddar. Serve and admire
Nutrition Fact: Calories: 880, Fat 82g, Carbs 8g, Sugar 2g, Protein 32g

EASY LOW CARB KETO BREAKFAST CASSEROLE

Prep Time: 10mints, Cook Time: 45mints, Total Time: 55mints; Serving: 12
INGREDIENTS
- 1-pound breakfast sausage
- 1 tsp Garlic and 12 Eggs
- 1/2 cup Yellow onion
- 3 cups Spinach
- 1/8tsp salt, pepper, 2 cups peppers
- 1/2 cup Cheddar cheese

INSTRUCTIONS
1. Preheat stove to 350 degrees F and set up a heating dish with non-stick cooking shower and put aside.
2. Ground and cook wiener in a skillet until completely cooked. Add garlic, peppers, and onions to the skillet and sauté with frankfurter for 2 minutes. Put this in your readied heating dish.
3. In a different bowl whisk eggs with salt and pepper, pour egg wash over vegetables in a heating dish and tenderly blend to ensure eggs are covering the whole dish.
4. Top with cheddar and heat for 45 minutes or until a fork can confess all and eggs are cooked completely through.
Nutrition Facts: Calories 210, Fat 16g, Carbs 3g, Sugar 2g, Protein 13g

LOW CARB ORANGE DREAMLIKE SMOOTHIE

Prep Time: 5mints, Total Time: 5mints; Serving: 1
INGREDIENTS
- 16 ounces unsweetened almond milk
- 1 packet artificial sweetener
- 4 ounces heavy cream
- 1 scoop Jay Robb Tropical Dreamlike Whey powder
- 1/2 cup crushed ice

INSTRUCTION
1. Put all ingredients in blender and mix until smooth. This formula duplicates well.
Nutrition Fact: Calories 290, Fat 25g, Carbs 4g, Sugar 2g, Protein 15g

HOLLEY'S HAM AND SWISS BREAKFAST MUFFINS

Prep Time: 10mints, Cooking Time: 25mints, total Time: 35mints; Serving: 4
INGREDIENTS
- Eggs
- 1/2 cup grated Swiss cheese
- oz. Canadian Bacon
- 1/4 Cup Salsa, Salt, and Pepper
- 3 Baby Bella Mushrooms

INSTRUCTIONS
1. Preheat stove to 350° and shower a biscuit skillet with a non-stick cooking spray or gently oil.
2. In an enormous blending bowl, pound up the 3 cheddar wedges with a fork. Split every one of the 6 eggs into the bowl and blend well in with the cheddar.
3. Add Canadian bacon, mushrooms, salsa, and a touch of salt and pepper to the bowl and combine all ingredients.
4. Spoon blend into biscuit dish – This clump will fill 8 of the 12 puts in the biscuit skillet.
5. Heat for 25 minutes. Serve and Enjoy
Nutrition Fact: Calories: 250, Fat 26g, Carbs 4g, Sugar 3g, Protein 7g

CHEESY EGG WHITE VEGGIE BREAKFAST MUFFINS

Prep Time: 10mints, Cook Time: 20mints; Serves: 12
INGREDIENTS
- 3 eggs
- 2 1/2 cups egg whites
- 3/4 cup shredded cheese
- 2 tsp of skim milk
- Salt and pepper

INSTRUCTIONS
1. Preheat stove to 350 ranges F. Shower 12-cup biscuit tin with a nonstick cooking spray, you can likewise restore with biscuit tins, in reality, make sure you bathe within the biscuit tins.
2. Fill each biscuit tin 1/four-1/3 complete with vegetables and herbs of decision.
3. In a medium bowl together egg whites, eggs, and milk/yogurt
4. Fill every biscuit to the top with egg combo, pouring over the vegetables as of now in each tin. Heat for 20-half-hour or until risen and marginally awesome on the pinnacle
5. Let cool for a couple of moments, at that factor remove from the tin.
Nutrition Fact: Calories: 63, Fat 2.8g, Carbs 0.9g, Sugar 0.6g, Protein 9.3g

CINNAMON "RICE" BREAKFAST PUDDING

Prep Time: 15mints, Cooking Time: 15mints, Total Time: 30mints; Serving: 2
INGREDIENTS
- 2 cups caulis-rice
- 1 2/3 cup coconut milk
- 5 Tbsp Swerve sweetener
- 1/2 tsp cinnamon
- 1/2 tsp vanilla extract
- 3 Tbsp chia seeds

INSTRUCTIONS
1. In a medium pot over medium warm temperature, add the caulis-rice, coconut milk, and sugar.
2. Cook for 8-10 minutes or until the caulis-rice is delicate
3. Off the warm temperature, which add the cinnamon and vanilla and mix to fuse
4. Next, encompass the chia seeds and mix to add. Let sit down for five minutes
5. Mix one very last time and serve heat.
Nutrition Fact: Calories: 51, Fat 0.4g, Carbs 11g, Sugar 2g, Protein 3g

HIGH PROTEIN LOW CARB BREAKFAST CASSEROLE

Prep Time: 15mints, Cook Time: 50mints, Total Time: 1hr 5mints; Serving: 6
INGREDIENTS
- 24 eggs
- 1/2 lb. turkey bacon
- 6 sausage patties frozen

INSTRUCTIONS
1. Preheat stove to 375 and oil the base and sides of a 9x13 meal dish.
2. Cut 1/2 pound of turkey bacon into scaled-down pieces and fill the base of the lubed meal dish.
3. Break 24 eggs in a different bowl and beat with a whisk. Pour over your turkey pieces.
4. Add 6 frankfurter patties top of your eggs. They will drift on top. He spaces them out so the meal can without much of a stretch be cut into 6 servings.
5. Prepare for roughly 45-50 minutes.
6. He cuts his into 6 servings and just re-warms them in the microwave every morning. He cherishes adding hot sauce to his.
Nutrition Fact: Calories: 113, Fat 6.9g, Carbs 6.8g, Sugar 4.3g, Protein: 7.9g

EVERYTHING BUT THE BAGEL

Prep Time: 5mints, Total Time: 5mints; Serving: 1
INGREDIENTS
- 4 tsp poppy seeds
- 1/4 cup toasted sesame seeds
- 4 tsp minced onions
- 2 tsp coarse sea salt
- 4 tsp dried garlic flakes

INSTRUCTIONS
1. Combine the entirety of the ingredients and store in a hermetically sealed holder or flavor container. Shake before utilizing it.
Nutrition Fact: Calories: 61, Fat 1.5g, Carbs 3.5g, Sugar 0.9g. Protein 0.8g

POULTRY RECIPES

BAKED PESTO CHICKEN

Prep Time: 5mints, Cook Time: 35mints, Total Time: 40mins; Serving: 4

Ingredients
- 4 chicken breasts about 1.5 lb
- 3 tbsp basil pesto
- 8 oz mozzarella
- 1/2 tsp salt
- 1/4 tsp black pepper

Instructions
1. Preheat stove to 350 degrees.
2. Place the chicken in dish at even layers and sprinkle with salt and pepper.
3. Spread the pesto on the chicken. Put the mozzarella on top.
4. Heat for 35-45 minutes until the meat is a hundred and sixty deg. and the cheese is bubbly.
5. Serve and enjoy!

Nutrition Facts: Calories 471, Fat 22g, Carbs 2g, Sugar 4g, Protein 61g

SIMPLE BONE BROTH

Prep Time: 10mints, Cooking Time: 10hrs, Total Time: 10hrs 10mints; Serving: 4

Ingredients
- 3–4 lbs. of bones
- 1-gallon water
- 2 Tsp apple cider vinegar

Instructions
1. Add everything to the slow cooker.
2. Cook on a low setting in the slow cooker for 10 hours.
3. Cool the juices, strain and empty stock into the holder.
4. Store in the fridge
5. Scoop out the coagulated fat over the stock.
6. Heat juices when required.

Nutrition Fact: Calories: 368, Fat 14g, Carbs 4g, Sugar 6g, Protein 25g

SPRING SOUP WITH POACHED EGG

Prep Time: 5mints, Cook Time: 15mints, Total Time: 20mints; Serving: 2

Ingredients
- 2 eggs
- 32 oz chicken broth
- 1 head of romaine lettuce
- Salt to taste

Instructions
1. Heat the chicken soup to the point of boiling.
2. Turn down the heat and poach the 2 eggs in the soup for 5 minutes.
3. Remove the eggs and put each into a bowl.
4. Add the slashed romaine lettuce into the juices and cook for a couple of moments until marginally withered.
5. Scoop the stock with the lettuce into the dishes and serve.

Nutrition Fact: Calories 150, Fat 5g, Carbs 11g, Sugar 5g, Protein 16g

BOILED EGGS WITH BUTTER AND THYME

Prep Time: 10mints, Cook Time: 6mints, Total Time: 16mints; Servings: 1

Ingredients
- 3 large eggs
- 1 tbsp good quality unsalted butter
- Freshly ground black pepper
- Salt
- 1/4 tsp thyme leaves

Instructions
1. Fill a medium pan most of the way with water and heat until boiling.
2. When water is bubbling, tenderly put eggs in water and flip using a large spoon.
3. While your eggs are cooking, place one tsp of margarine in a microwave-safe bowl and microwave until dissolved, for around 20 seconds.
4. In the meantime, take the pan and cautiously spill out the excessive temp water carefully.
5. Cautiously strip every egg, wash to remove any shell parts, and add in the softened margarine.
6. Add the thyme leaves as well as the salt and pepper to flavor.

Nutrition Fact: Calories: 159, Fat 18g, Carbs 9g, Sugar 4g, Protein 8g

KETO DIJON SMOTHERED CHICKEN DRUMSTICKS

Prep Time: 15mints, Cook Time: 30mints, Total Time: 45mints; Serving: 2

Ingredients
- 1/4 cup of ghee
- 4 chicken drumsticks
- 1/4 cup of chicken broth
- 1/4 cup of coconut cream
- 2 Tsp of Dijon mustard

Instructions
1. Liberally season the chicken drumsticks with salt and pepper.
2. In a huge nonstick skillet, liquefy the ghee over medium-high heat.
3. Put the drumsticks in the skillet and dark-colored on all sides, around 5 to 7 minutes. Remove from skillet and put aside
4. Lessen the heat to medium-low and add the chicken juices, coconut cream, and mustard to the skillet. Return the drumsticks to the skillet. Season with salt and pepper, to taste
5. Spread and cook for 20 to 25 minutes, turning the drumsticks following 10 minutes until cooked through. Check with a meat thermometer that the inside temperature is 165 F.

Nutrition Fact: Calories: 537, Fat 46g, Carbs 1g, Sugar 1g, Protein 28g

KETO CRISPY ROSEMARY CHICKEN DRUMSTICKS

Prep Time: 10mints, Cook Time: 40mints, Total Time: 50mints; Serving: 4

Ingredients
- 12 chicken drumsticks
- 4 Tsp of olive oil
- 4 Tsp rosemary leaves
- 2 Tsp salt

Instructions
1. Preheat stove to 450 F.
2. Focus on salt on every chicken drumstick the blend and put on a lubed heating plate.
3. Ensure the drumsticks are not contacting each other on the plate. Shower the olive oil or avocado oil over the chicken drumsticks.
4. Prepare for 40 minutes until the skin is firm.

Nutrition Fact: Calories: 473, Fat 32g, Carbs 6g, Sugar 4g, Protein 42g

CHICKEN BREAST WITH OLIVE TAPENADE

Prep Time: 5mints, Cook Time: 10mints, Total Time: 15mints; Serving: 1

Ingredients
- 1 chicken breast
- 3 cloves garlic
- 1/2 cup olive tapenade
- 2 Tsp coconut oil for cooking

Instructions
1. Cut the hen bosom into 3 flimsy cutlets at the off risk that you have not simply accomplished as such.
2. Strip 3 cloves of garlic and squash softly with the level facet of a blade.
3. Soften 2 Tsp of coconut oil in a skillet on medium heat and add the 3 cloves of garlic.
4. Cook the garlic for 2mins, at that factor, consisting of the bird cutlets.
5. Cook each aspect of the chicken cutlets for 3-4mins.
6. Top with a half a cup of olive tapenade.

Nutrition Fact: Calories: 391, Fat 23.3g, Carbs 7.4g, Sugar 8.3g, Protein 35.5g

PAN-SEARED BEEF TONGUE

Prep Time: 35mints, Cooking Time: 1hr 5mints, Total Time: 1hr 40mints; Serving: 4

Ingredients
- Whole Beef Tongue
- 3 cups of water
- 1 tbsp olive oil
- Desired seasoning

Instruction:
1. Wash tongue in the sink.
2. Put tongue in a weight cooker alongside 3 cups of water.
3. Weight cook on the "stew" setting for 35 minutes
4. Enable strain to discharge normally for 30 minutes.
5. Remove from the weight cooker and skin tongue.
6. Cut tongue into emblems.
7. Season tongue with salt pepper
8. Skillet burn with olive oil for 2-3 minutes for each side

Nutrition Fact: Calories 463, Fat 6g, Carbs 5g, Sugar 4g, Protein 34g

BEEF TONGUE INTO DELICIOUS CRISPY BEEF

Prep Time: 15mints, Total Time: 15mints

Ingredients
- 1 beef tongue
- 3 cups of water
- 2-3 Tsp lard
- 2-3 Tsp sea salt
- Freshly ground black pepper

Instructions
1. Put the entire tongue and water into Instant Pot. Seal top and close valve. Select Stew setting. Enable strain to discharge normally for 30 minutes, at that point put a drying towel over the valve and discharge pressure.
2. Cut tongue beginning at the tip, in 1/2" cuts, at a slight point to get bigger pieces at the tip. Meat tongue into firm hamburger cutting before fricasseeing
3. Heat huge cast-iron skillet or another dish over medium-high heat, add 1 Tsp fat to the skillet, spreading it around. Put meat cuts firmly together. Sprinkle with 1 tsp. ocean salt, crisply ground pepper, to taste, and discretionary flavors. Cook for 5 minutes, at that point, diminishes heat to the vehicle for an extra 3 minutes. Check the surface that is searing. At the point when it's firm flip each piece, hamburger tongue into fresh meat browning
4. Remove meat to a cutting board and cut into flimsy strips, as wanted. Serve in Mexican nourishment settings, for example, tacos, enormous servings of mixed greens, over eggs with green chilies, inside delicate tortillas, and so forth with backups: new cilantro, sweet onions, salsa, and avocado, harsh cream, cheddar, crisp radishes, and so forth.

Nutrition Fact: Calories 432, Fat 4g, Carbs 6g, Sugar 9g, Protein 43g

KETO CROCKPOT SHREDDED CHICKEN

Prep Time: 5mints, Cook Time: 6hrs, Total Time: 6hrs 5mints; Serving: 8

Ingredients
- 4 chicken breasts
- 1 cup chicken broth
- 4 cloves garlic

- 1/2 onion, Salt, and pepper
- 1 Tsp Italian seasoning

Instructions
1. Add everything to the slow cooker.
2. Cook on low for 6 hours.
3. Shred the meat with your forks.
4. Serve and enjoy quickly in different dishes or stop in individual packs for some time later.
5. Serve and enjoy with Keto guacamole or over a plate of mixed greens with Keto Caesar dressing.

Nutrition Fact: Calories: 201, Fat 10g, Carbs 1g, Sugar 0.3g, Protein 24g

KETO BUFFALO CAULIFLOWER WINGS

Prep Time: 5mints, Cook Time: 24mints, Total Time: 29mints; Serving: 4

Ingredients
- 3-4 tbsp hot sauce
- 1 tbsp almond flour
- 1 tbsp avocado oil
- Salt to taste
- 1 medium head of cauliflower

Instructions
1. Preheat air fryer to 400F/200C
2. Combine hot sauce, almond flour, avocado oil and salt in an enormous bowl.
3. Add the cauliflower and blend until covered.
4. Add a large portion of the cauliflower into the air fryer and fry for 12-15 min.
5. Try to open the air fryer and shake the searing bin midway through to turn the cauliflower. Expel and put aside.
6. Add the subsequent group, however, cook it for 2-3mins less.
7. Serve warm with some extra hot sauce for plunging.

Nutrition Fact: Calories: 48, Fat 4g, Carbs 1g, Sugar 5g, Protein 10g

SMOKED PAPRIKA CHICKEN

Prep Time: 2mints, Cook Time: 14mints, Total Time: 16mints; Serving: 6

Ingredients
- 2 lbs. boneless, skinless chicken thighs
- 2 tbsp smoked paprika
- 1 tbsp + 1 tsp garlic salt
- 3 tbsp extra virgin olive oil

Instructions
1. Preheat the grill on high. On the off chance that you put the rack directly under the fire, the chicken will consume outwardly before it's cooked through.
2. Line an oven tray with foil and spread the chicken thighs out level. Sprinkle each side liberally with the garlic salt and smoked paprika; if the sums above don't appear enough, utilize more. Try not to hold back on the garlic salt, regardless whether your salt-phobic - it's essential and still will have far less sodium than any chicken dish you will ever eat in a café.
3. Sear the chicken around 7 minutes on each side, until the thighs are cooked through and have built up a decent hull. Grills will in general shift as far as quality; if your chicken is by all accounts consuming or cooking excessively quick, move the rack down an indent or two.
4. When the chicken has cooked through, serve right away.

Nutrition Facts: Calories 248, Fat 13g, Carbs 1g, Sugar 2g, Protein 29g

SLOW COOKER PALEO CHICKEN BROTH

Prep Time: 35mints, Cooking Time: 5hrs, Total Time: 5hrs 35mints; Serving: 4

Ingredients
- 1 whole chicken
- 2 Tsp of salt
- 1/2 Tsp of black pepper
- 1/4 cup of goji berries

Instructions
1. Put every one of the ingredients into the moderate cooker.
2. Add enough water to cover the chicken.
3. Cook on low heat for 5 hours.
4. Separate the stock from the chicken and goji berries. Let cool and store the soup and the chicken meat independently.

Nutrition Fact: Calories 447, Fat 31.6g, Carbs 1.2g, Sugar 1.1g, Protein 38g

LEMON PARSLEY CHICKEN

Prep Time: 20mints, cooking Time: 25mints, Total Time: 45mints; Serving: 4

Ingredients
- ¼ cup fresh curly-leaf parsley
- Zest and juice of one lemon each
- ¼ cup duck fat
- 8-12 chicken drumsticks
- Salt and pepper to taste

Instructions
1. Preheat stove to 375 degrees F. Liquefies duck fat in a pan over low heat.
2. Mastermind chicken in a preparing dish. Salt and pepper the drumsticks to taste.
3. Add lemon juice to the fat and pour this blend over the chicken.
4. Coat the drumsticks with the blend. Sprinkle lemon get-up-and-go over drumsticks.
5. Sprinkle parsley over drumsticks.
6. Go chicken to cover. Prepare at 375 degrees F for 15 minutes.
7. Turn the drumsticks over, cautiously.
8. Keep cooking until interior temp arrives at 165 degrees

Nutrition Fact: Calories: 575, Fat 40g, Carbs 5g, Sugar 3g, Protein 57g

BBQ CHICKEN LIVERS AND HEART

Prep Time: 25mints, Cooking Time: 20mints, Total Time: 45mints; Serving: 4
Ingredients
- 1 lb. chicken hearts
- 1 lb chicken livers
- sea salt
- black pepper
- bamboo skewers

Instructions
1. The liver and hearts may come solidified in little parcels. Defrost and bring to room temperature.
2. The heart's extreme top parts can be evacuated with a sharp blade.
3. Meanwhile set up the BBQ – ideally utilize just charcoals; however, you can utilize gas, and bring to high heat.
4. Presently string the hearts on the sticks, 5 to 7 minutes each, depending on their size.
5. Cleaning the livers, focusing not to break or smash them, lay level on an adaptable barbecuing bushel
6. Season both liver and hearts with ocean salt and naturally ground dark pepper.
7. The livers will stick on the barbecue generally and effectively break separated currently set on the flame broil and cook until the ideal doneness is come to.
8. Some tahini sauce is an incredible garnish for the two kinds of meat!

Nutrition Fact: Calories: 361, Fat 28g, Carbs 15g, Sugar 8g, Protein 23g

KETO CROCKPOT GARLIC CHICKEN

Prep Time: 10mints, Cook Time: 3hrs, Total Time: 3hrs 10mints; Serving: 4
Ingredients
- 1 Tsp of olive oil
- 4 chicken thighs
- 1 head of garlic and chives
- 1 1/2 cups of chicken broth, warm
- Salt and freshly ground black pepper

Instructions
1. Heat the oil in a container and dark colored the chicken skin-side down until brilliant and fresh.
2. Meanwhile, strip every one of the cloves from one head of garlic. Split everyone and add them to a simmering pot at that point pour in the warm chicken soup. When the chicken pieces have caramelized on the skin side, use tongs to remove them from the dish to the stewing pot, skin-side up. Cook for 3 hours on high.
3. Evacuate the chicken and season with salt and naturally ground dark pepper.
4. The mollified cloves can be served close by whenever wanted.

Nutrition Fact: Calories: 241, Fat 18g, Carbs 2g, Sugar 0.4g, Protein 16g

SLOW COOKER CHICKEN ADOBO KETO

Prep Time: 5mints, Cook Time: 8hrs, Total Time: 8hrs 5mints; Serving: 4
Ingredients
- 10–12 chicken drumsticks
- 1 onion and green onion
- 10 cloves garlic
- 1 cup gluten-free tamari soy sauce
- 1/4 cup apple cider vinegar

Instructions
1. Put chicken drumsticks, onion, garlic, tamari sauce, and vinegar into your moderate cooker for 6-8 hours until the chicken is delicate.
2. Serve over cauliflower rice. Sprinkle cleaved green onions on top for decorate.

Nutrition Fact: Calories: 432, Fat 8g, Carbs 2g, Sugar 4g, Protein 32g

SLOW COOK CHICKEN CURRY

Prep Time: 10mints, cooking Time: 5hrs, Total Time: 5hrs 10mints; Serving: 5
Ingredients
- 2-3 lbs. boneless chicken thighs
- 1 can coconut milk
- 3 Tsp green curry paste

Instructions
1. Add chicken, coconut milk and curry glue to the moderate cooker.
2. Utilize a fork to blend in the curry glue.
3. Cook on low for 4-5 hours.
4. Utilize 2 forks to pull separated the chicken. Utilize an opened spoon to remove the chicken from the fluid. Serve and serve and enjoy!

Nutrition Fact: Calories: 123, Fat 12g, Carbs 4g, Sugar 5g, Protein 24g

SPLIT CHICKEN BREAST WITH ONIONS AND MUSHROOMS

Prep Time: 5mints, Cooking Time: 8hrs, Total Time: 8hrs 5mints; Serving: 2
Ingredients
- 1 Sliced Onions
- 1 cup Sliced Mushrooms
- 2 Large Chicken Breasts
- 1 cup Chicken Broth
- Thyme, Salt, and Pepper

Instructions
1. Line base of slight cooker with onions
2. Put hen bosoms over the onions
3. Top Chicken Breasts with mushrooms
4. Pour the Chicken Broth around the threshold of the moderate cooker
5. Add Thyme, Salt, and Pepper
6. Cook on low for 6-eight hours

Nutrition Fact: Calories: 231, Fat 8g, Carbs 4g, Sugar 7g, Protein 32g

CROCK POT CHICKEN STOCK

Prep Time: 5mints, Cook Time: 12hrs, Total Time: 12hrs 5mins; Serving: 4

Ingredients
- 1 organic chicken carcass
- 1 medium onion quartered
- 3 carrots quartered
- 3 celery stalks quartered
- 1 tsp apple cider vinegar and water

Instructions
1. Add all ingredients to a moderate cooker.
2. Set to low and cook for 12 - 18 hours.
3. Strain stock and refrigerate or solidify.

Nutrition Fact: Calories: 233, Fat 6g, Carbs 7g, Sugar 3g, Protein 32g

CROCKPOT CHICKEN STOCK

Prep Time: 5mints, Cook Time: 8hrs, Total Time: 8hrs 5mints; Servings: 4

Ingredients
- 1 chicken carcass
- 1 onion
- 3-4 bay leaves
- 2-3 TBSP salt
- Water

Instructions
1. Put the body into your moderate cooker.
2. Add the onion, inlet leaves, and salt and pepper, whenever wanted.
3. Add enough water to come up to around 1" under the lip of the pot.
4. Spread and cook for 8-10 hours.
5. When done, utilize an opened spoon or strainer to evacuate the bones and veggies.
6. I, for the most part, add some meat toward the finish of the chicken, however, you can simply leave it as juices in the event that you like!
7. I solidify in glass containers - simply ensure you leave enough room at the top for extension, or the glass will break!

Nutrition Fact: Calories: 321, Fat 17g, Carbs 12g, Sugar 9g, Protein 34g

BBQ CHICKEN LIVERS AND HEARTS

Prep Time: 25mints, Cooking Time: 15mints, Total Time: 40mints; Serving: 5

Ingredients
- 1 lb. chicken hearts
- 1 lb. chicken livers
- Sea salt and black pepper
- Bamboo skewers

Instructions
1. The liver and hearts may come solidified in little parcels. Defrost and bring to room temperature.
2. The heart's intense top parts can be evacuated with a sharp blade.
3. Meanwhile set up the BBQ - we utilize just charcoals; however, you can utilize gas, and bring to drug/high heat.
4. Presently string the hearts on the sticks, 5 to 7 each, contingent upon their size.
5. In the wake of cleaning the livers, focusing not to break or smush them, lay level on an adaptable flame broiling bin
6. Season both liver and hearts with ocean salt and crisply ground dark pepper.
7. The livers will stick on the flame broil generally and effectively break separated currently set on the barbecue and cook until the ideal doneness is come to.
8. We like our hearts very much done and the livers still delicate.

Nutrition Fact: Calories 264, Fat 9g, Carbs 8g, Sugar 5g, Protein 27g

HEALTHY BUFFALO CHICKEN DIP

Prep Time: 35mints, Cooking Time: 4hrs 30mints, Total Time: 5hrs 5mints; Serving: 4

Ingredients
- 10 oz Neufchatel cream cheese
- 1 cup 0% Greek yogurt
- 2/3 cup frank's red hot
- 2 cups cooked shredded chicken
- 1 cup mozzarella cheese

Instructions
1. Put all the ingredients into your crockpot
2. Set crockpot on low for 3-4 hours, stirring up every hour.
3. If you don't have a crockpot, you can set your oven to 350 and prepare this in a glass dish covered with foil, bake for 25-30 min.

Nutrition Fact: Calories: 324, Fat 17g, Carbs 6g, Sugar 3g, Protein 43g

2 INGREDIENT PALEO CROCKPOT CHICKEN

Prep Time: 5mints, Cook Time: 5hrs, Total Time: 5hrs 5mints; Serves: 4

Ingredients
- 2-3 lbs. of chicken breasts
- 1 16 oz of salsa Verde
- Optional: onions and peppers

Instructions
1. Add chicken and salsa Verde to crockpot.
2. Cook on low for 5-6 hours.
3. Shred with a fork.

Nutrition Fact: Calories: 143, Fat 2.1g, Carbs 5g, Sugar 1.4g, Protein 28g

LEMON PEPPER CHICKEN

Prep Time: 20mints, Cooking Time: 45mints, Total Time: 1hr 5mints; Serving: 2

Ingredients
- 1 whole chicken
- 2 medium lemons
- salt
- 2 tsp freshly ground black pepper

Instructions
1. Preheat stove to 375 F.

2. Design the chicken pieces in a 9" x 13" heating dish and pour the lemon squeeze over the chicken. Sprinkle generously with salt, at that point the lemon pizzazz, lastly the pepper, covering the pieces well. Fold the held lemon skins under and around the chicken pieces.
3. Prepared, revealed, for 30 to 45 minutes, treating a few times with the amassed fluid, or until the chicken is brilliant dark colored and the juices run clear when pierced with a fork.
4. Dispose of the lemon skins before serving.
Nutrition Fact: Calories 336, Fat 24.1g, Carbs 4.4g, Sugar 1g, Protein 26.4g

JUICY RANCH CHICKEN

Prep Time: 10mints, Cook Time: 1hr 45mints, Total Time: 1hr 55mints ; Serving: 4
Ingredients
- 4-5 lb. chicken
- 1-1/2 tbsp. Dry Ranch Seasoning
- 4 tbsp. salted butter
- 1/2 lemon
- Salt/pepper

Instructions
1. Preheat stove to 425 degrees F.
2. Mix dry farm flavoring with relaxed margarine until all-around mixed and put aside.
3. Force the skin away from the bosom and utilizing a spoon, place Ranch Butter between the skin and meat. Attempt to spread the margarine over the whole bosom to appropriate the seasonings uniformly.
4. Spread any outstanding Ranch Butter over the outside of the whole chicken.
5. Put half of the lemon inside the chicken depression.
6. Put chicken on simmering skillet and heat for 1 hour 15 minutes or until inward temperature arrives at 165 degrees F.
7. Cautiously remove broiling skillet from stove and permit to rest for 10 minutes before cutting.
Nutrition Fact: Calories: 376, Fat 26g, Carbs 6g, Sugar 1g, Protein 27g

WORLD'S MOISTEST CHICKEN

Prep Time: 35mints, Cooking Time: 55mints, Total Time: 1hr 30mints; Serves: 9
Ingredients
- 3 large split chicken breasts
- salt and pepper
- 1 cup mayonnaise
- 1/4 cup Sriracha hot sauce

Instructions
1. Preheat stove to 350 F. In a little bowl, mix together the mayonnaise and Sriracha.
2. Pat the chicken bosoms dry with a paper towel and sprinkle softly with salt and pepper. Spread the mayonnaise blend equitably over each bosom. Prepare for 45 to 50 minutes, or until the chicken is brilliant and the juices run clear when pierced with a fork.
3. Enable the chicken to rest for 5 minutes; cut each bosom into thirds and serve.
Nutrition Fact: Calories 447, Fat 31.6g, Carbs 1.2g, Sugar 1.1g, Protein 38g

AVOCADO CHICKEN SALAD

Prep Time: 15mints, Cooking Time: 20mints, Total Time: 35mints; Serving: 3
Ingredients
- 3 avocados
- 1 lb. chicken
- 1 medium tomato and onions
- 4 limes
- Sea salt and fresh ground black pepper

Instructions
1. In an enormous bowl pound, the avocados until smooth.
2. Add the chicken, onions, tomatoes, lime squeeze, salt, and pepper.
3. Blend well.
Nutrition Fact: Calories: 665, Fat 38g, Carbs 17g, Sugar 4g, Protein 55g

CHICKEN LIVER WITH RAW GARLIC AND THYME

Prep Time: 10mints, Cook Time: 7mints, Total Time: 17mints; Serves: 4
Ingredients
- 1-pound chicken liver, sliced thinly
- 3 Tsp extra-virgin olive oil
- 1 lemon
- 4 cloves garlic
- Sea salt and Thyme for garnish

Instructions
1. Set up the livers by washing and drying them altogether. You need them to be as dry as conceivable before cooking them to ensure they get decent and fresh.
2. At the point when you are prepared, heat a skillet on medium-without a friend in the world fry the livers for 3-4 minutes before flipping. Cook another 2-3 minutes on the opposite side, until never again pink inside.
3. Remove from the container and coat with olive oil, crude garlic, ocean salt, and thyme.
Nutrition Fact: Calories 534, Fat 15g, Carbs 10g, Sugar 6g, Protein 34g

BACON-WRAPPED TAHINI AND SUN-DRIED TOMATO STUFFED CHICKEN BREASTS

Prep Time: 5mints, Cook Time: 35mints, Total Time: 40mints; Servings: 2
Ingredients
- 2 boneless skinless chicken breasts
- 4 slices nitrate-free bacon
- Sun-dried tomatoes

- Tahini
- Salt and pepper to taste

Instructions
1. Preheat your stove to 375 Degrees F
2. Rinse your chicken bosoms under chilly water and pat dry with paper towels
3. Cautiously butterfly open your chicken bosoms guaranteeing not to cut completely
4. Season within the bosoms with salt and pepper, with as much tahini as you like, spread it everywhere throughout within the filleted bosoms
5. Next, take the same number of sun-dried tomatoes as you like and sprinkle them everywhere throughout within
6. Overlap the chicken bosoms shut back onto itself and fold two cuts of bacon over every chicken bosom
7. Put the chicken in a Pyrex heating dish and prepare for 30 minutes or until your chicken is nearly done
8. Evacuate your chicken, set your stove to cook on high and afterward place your chicken on the best in a class of your stove for 5-10 minutes to get your bacon pleasant and dark-colored

Nutrition Fact: Calories: 376, Fat 26g, Carbs 6g, Sugar 1g, Protein 27g

PALEO CRISPY GARLIC CURRY CHICKEN DRUMSTICKS RECIPE

Prep Time: 5mints, Cook Time: 40mints, Total Time: 45mints; Serving: 2

Ingredients
- 10 chicken drumsticks
- 1–2 Tsp salt
- 3 Tsp curry powder
- 3 Tsp garlic powder
- 1/2 Tsp of coconut oil

Instructions
1. Preheat stove to 450F (230C).
2. Oil a huge heating plate with coconut oil.
3. Blend the salt, curry powder, and garlic powder together in a bowl.
4. Ensure the drumsticks are not very wet.
5. Coat every drumstick with the blend and put it on the preparing plate. Ensure the drumsticks are not contacting each other on the plate.
6. Heat for 40 minutes

Nutrition Fact: Calories: 414, Fat 33g, Carbs 3g, Sugar 0.3g, Protein 26g

POMEGRANATE CHICKEN SALAD RECIPE

Prep Time: 10mints, Total Time: 10mints; Serving: 2

Ingredients
- 1/4 cup pomegranate seeds
- 1 cup of chicken meat
- 1 avocado
- 1/2 lb. spinach
- Sea salt and virgin olive oil

Instructions
1. Blend the juice from the 2 orange portions together with 2-3 Tsp of additional virgin olive oil.
2. Mix the dressing together with the chicken meat, spinach, and ocean salt.
3. Sprinkle on the pomegranate seeds
4. At that point add the avocado cuts top.

Nutrition Fact: Calories: 470, Fat 37g, Carbs 16g, Sugar 3g, Protein 24g

CHICKEN PEPPER POPPERS FOR BBQS AND POTLUCKS

Prep Time: 20mints, Total Time: 45mints; Servings: 4

Ingredients
- 2 pounds boneless chicken thighs
- 4-6 Anaheim chilies
- 1/2-pound bacon finds sugar-free bacon
- 1 tsp smoked paprika
- 1/2 tsp sea salt and black pepper

Instructions
1. In the event that flame broiling, absorb wooden sticks water for 20 minutes or more.
2. In the event that heating, this progression isn't fundamental.
3. Stop the chicken for 20 minutes so it is simpler to cut.
4. Sprinkle chicken pieces equitably with smoked paprika, ocean salt, and dark pepper.
5. Preheat stove to 425 C or the flame broil to medium-high.
6. Push the move upright to the end and afterward proceed with the chicken/pepper/bacon wraps, dispersing them around 1/8 – ¼ inch separated on the stick, 4-6 to a stick.
7. Heat for 35mins or until chicken is cooked through and bacon is firm, check at regular intervals and pivot, moving sticks as expected to more sultry pieces of the barbecue to cook uniformly. Cook for roughly 30 minutes altogether.

Nutrition Facts: Calories 533, Fat 28g, Carbs 1g, Sugar 1g, Protein 64g

PALEO GARLIC CHICKEN NUGGETS

Prep Time: 10mints, Cook Time: 15mints, Total Time: 25mints; Serving: 2

Ingredients
- 2 chicken breasts
- 1/2 cup coconut flour
- 1 egg and 1 Tsp garlic
- 2 Tsp garlic powder
- 1/4–1/2 cup ghee for shallow frying

Instructions
1. 3D squares the chicken bosoms in the event that you haven't done so as of now.
2. In a bowl, combine the coconut flour, garlic powder, and salt. Taste the blend to check whether you'd like progressively salt.
3. In a different bowl, whisk 1 egg to make the egg wash.
4. Put the ghee in a pan on medium heat.

5. Plunge the cubed chicken in the egg wash and afterward drop into the coconut flour blend to cover it with the "breading."
6. Cautiously place a portion of the "breaded" chicken 3D squares into the ghee and fry until brilliant. Ensure there's just a solitary layer of chicken in the dish so they would all be able to cook in the oil. Turn the chicken pieces to ensure they get cooked consistently.
7. Put the cooked chicken pieces onto paper towels to absorb any excessive oil.
Nutrition Fact: Calories: 665, Fat 38g, Carbs 17g, Sugar 4g, Protein 55g

KETO LEMON PEPPER ROAST CHICKEN

Prep Time: 10mints, Cook Time: 1hr 45mints, Total Time: 1hr 55mints; Serving: 6

Ingredients
- 1 whole chicken, remove giblets
- 2 lemons
- 1/2 cup ghee
- 2 sprigs of thyme
- Salt and pepper

Instructions
1. Preheat stove to 350 F (175 C).
2. Wash and pat dry the chicken and put into an enormous cooking skillet.
3. Get-up-and-go 1 of the lemons, and rub the get-up-and-go over the outside of the chicken
4. Season the chicken with a lot of salt and pepper. Don't under season!
5. Stuff within the chicken with 1/2 lemon, the 2 sprigs of thyme, and 1/4 cup of ghee.
6. Rub the remainder of the ghee outwardly of the chicken.
7. Cut the remainder of the lemons and put around the chicken in the cooking skillet.
8. Cook in the stove for 85-120 minutes. For a 4 lb. (2 kg) chicken, cook for 105 minutes
9. Supplement a thermometer into the thickest piece of the thigh and check the temperature is 165 F (74 C).
Nutrition Fact: Calories: 575, Fat 40g, Carbs 5g, Sugar 3g, Protein 57g

CHICKEN CAESAR

Prep Time: 48hrs 5mints, Cook Time: 1hr 25mints, Total Time: 49hrs 30mints; Serving: 6

Ingredients
- 1 Whole Pastured Chicken
- 1 cup Caesar salad dressing
- 1/4 cup olive oil
- 5–6 Romaine Hearts
- 12 Parmesan Crisps and Sea Salt

Instructions
1. First, spatchcock your chicken. This will make it simpler to marinate and it will cook quicker and all the more equitably.
2. Next salt the chicken generously with ocean salt, get each niche and corner.
3. Put your chicken in a cozy holder of the heating dish, presently slather it with dressing. Spread, marinate as long as 48 hours.
4. At the point when prepared to cook, pre-heat stove to 375F. Lay chicken bosom side up on a sheet skillet or preparing dish.
5. Sprinkle with a little olive oil. Broil for 1 hour to 1 hour + 15 minutes.
6. Remove from the stove; let rest for a couple of moments before cutting separated.
7. Meanwhile, slash romaine, sprinkle with olive oil and disintegrate parmesan crisps
8. To segment off your chicken cut the leg quarters off, these will break apart effortlessly. Serve
Nutrition Fact:: Calories: 391, Fat 23.3g, Carbs 7.4g, Sugar 8.3g, Protein 35.5g

CHICKEN, BACON, AND APPLE MINI MEATLOAVES RECIPE

Prep Time: 15mints, Cook Time: 25mints, Total Time: 40mints; Serving: 12

Ingredients
- 1 1/2 apples
- 2 chicken breasts
- 8–10 slices of bacon
- 3 Tsp olive oil
- 1 tsp salt

Instructions
1. Preheat stove to 400F.
2. Nourishment process the chicken bosom if it's not as of now minced.
3. Cook the bacon.
4. Bones the apple.
5. Combine every one of the ingredients in an enormous bowl.
6. Oil a biscuit container and load up with the meat blend or utilize this non-stick silicone biscuit skillet
7. Heat for 20-25 minutes – check with a meat thermometer that the inside temperature arrives at 170F.
Nutrition Fact: Calories: 385, Fat 31g, Carbs 7g, Sugar 5g, Protein 20g

GARLIC LEMON CHICKEN BREAST

Prep Time: 25mints, Total Time: 1hr; Serving: 4

Ingredients
- 3 boneless, skinless chicken breasts
- 3 cloves garlic
- 2 small lemons
- 1-2 Tsp cooking oil
- Salt and pepper

Instruction
1. Warm cooking oil in a dish over medium/medium-low heat, pulverize and slash garlic. Add the garlic to the oil and cook for about a moment.
2. Garlic Lemon Chicken Breast Recipe from domesticsoul.com

3. Cut the lemons and add a portion of the cuts to the base of the container. Salt and pepper the two sides of the chicken bosoms and lay them over the garlic/lemon cuts in the base of the container. Top the chicken bosoms with the remainder of the cuts.
4. Garlic Lemon Chicken Breast Recipe from domesticsoul.com
5. Spread the container with a top and go down to medium-low. Cook until the chicken bosoms are cooked through, turning once. The measure of time this will take will rely upon how thick the chicken bosoms are.
6. Garlic Lemon Chicken Breast Recipe from domesticsoul.com
7. When they're set, either serve and serve and enjoy or cut them up and store in the cooler to serve and serve and enjoy later

Nutrition Fact: Calories 447, Fat 31.6g, Carbs 1.2g, Sugar 1.1g, Protein 38g

EASY 5 INGREDIENT PALEO ROAST CHICKEN

Prep Time: 40mints, Cooking Time: 1hr, Total Time: 1hr 40mints; Serving: 4

Ingredients
- 1 organic pastured chicken
- 2 Tbsp organic paprika
- 1-2 Tbsp high-quality sea salt
- 1-2 Tbsp organic black pepper
- 2 Tbsp organic garlic powder

Instruction
1. Preheat the stove to 350.
2. Wash off a defrosted chicken.
3. Haul out the sack of giblets and put something aside for some other time.
4. Combine every one of the flavors in a little bowl.
5. Rub the entire chicken with the flavor rub.
6. Put the chicken in a stove safe dish.
7. Cook for an hour on 350.
8. You will realize it is done when the juices run clear.

Nutrition Fact: Calories 447, Fat 31.6g, Carbs 1.2g, Sugar 1.1g, Protein 38g

SIMPLE MARINATED CHICKEN HEARTS

Prep Time: 1hr 15mints, Cook Time: 5mints, Total Time: 1hr 20mints; Serving: 3-4

Ingredients
- 2 lbs. chicken hearts
- 2 Tbsp. extra virgin olive oil
- 1 clove garlic
- 2 Tbsp. coconut amino
- 1 Tbsp. sherry vinegar and 1 tsp. ground ginger

Instructions
1. Set up the hearts by removing the greasy tops and external films.
2. At that point rinse to remove any blood. Put the cleaned hearts in a bowl.
3. Place the olive oil, alongside the remainder of the ingredients, in a little bowl
4. Mix with a fork and pour over the hearts.
5. When prepared to cook, heat the remaining tbsp of olive oil in a huge skillet over medium-high heat.
6. Utilize an opened spoon to move the hearts from the bowl to the skillet.
7. Sauté 5 minutes, mixing occasionally, to be certain they cook equally

Nutrition Fact: Calories: 575, Fat 40g, Carbs 5g, Sugar 3g, Protein 57g

KETO ALMOND BUTTER CHICKEN SAUTE

Prep Time: 1hr, Cook Time: 15mints, Total Time: 1hr 15mints; Serving: 4

Ingredients
- 2 chicken breasts
- 1/4 cup almond butter and olive oil
- 2 Tsp lime juice
- 1 Tsp dried oregano
- Salt and pepper

Instructions
1. Combine the marinade ingredients (almond spread, olive oil, lime juice, oregano, salt, and pepper).
2. Marinate the diced chicken for 60 minutes.
3. Empty the chicken and marinade into a skillet on medium heat and cook until the chicken is cooked through.
4. Present with a plate of mixed greens.

Nutrition Fact: Calories: 414, Fat 33g, Carbs 3g, Sugar 0.3g, Protein 26g

HOMEMADE THAI CHICKEN BROTH

Prep Time: 5mints, Cook Time: 8hrs, Total Time: 8hrs 5mints; Serving: 10

Ingredients
- 1 whole chicken
- 1 stalk of lemongrass
- 20 fresh basil leaves
- 5 thick slices of fresh ginger and lime
- 1 Tsp salt

Instructions
1. Put the chicken, lemongrass, 10 basil leaves, ginger, and salt into the moderate cooker.
2. Top off the moderate cooker with water.
3. Cook on low for 8-10 hours.
4. Scoop the stock into a bowl; add salt to taste, crush in new lime juice to taste, and trimming with slashed basil leaves.

Nutrition Fact: Calories 447, Fat 31.6g, Carbs 1.2g, Sugar 1.1g, Protein 38g

GARLIC GHEE BAKED CHICKEN BREAST

Prep Time: 5mints, Cook Time: 30mints, Total Time: 35mints; Serving: 1

Ingredients
- 1 chicken breast
- 1 tsp garlic powder
- 1 Tsp ghee
- 2 cloves garlic
- 1 tsp of sea salt

Instructions
1. Preheat stove to 350F (180C).
2. Put the chicken bosom on a bit of aluminum foil and put the garlic powder, ghee, hacked crisp garlic, and ocean salt over it. Rub everything over the chicken bosom.
3. Crease up the foil with the goal that it covers the chicken bosom. Put it on a preparing plate and heat for 30 minutes. The chicken bosom ought to be cooked through.
4. Cut the chicken bosom down the middle or into cuts and sprinkle diced chives on top.
5. Present with more ghee and salt to taste.

Nutrition Fact:: Calories: 391, Fat 23.3g, Carbs 7.4g, Sugar 8.3g, Protein 35.5g

GRILLED CHICKEN DRUMSTICKS WITH GARLIC MARINADE

Prep Time: 2hrs 20mints, Cook Time: 1hr, Total Time: 3hrs 20mints; Serving: 4

Ingredients
- 10 chicken drumsticks
- 1 ½ cups of olive oil
- 1 head of garlic
- Juice from 1 lemon
- 1 tsp of sea salt and ½ tsp of pepper

Instructions
1. Put the olive oil, garlic, lemon juice, ocean salt, and pepper into a blender or nourishment processor and puree. This is the marinade.
2. Focus on the chicken drumsticks the marinade. At that point place the chicken with the marinade into Ziploc sacks and put in the icebox. Marinade for in any event 2 hours.
3. Flame broils the chicken drumsticks.

Nutrition Fact: Calories: 660, Fat 56g, Carbs 4g, Sugar 3g, Protein 36g

BAKED CHICKEN MEATBALLS - HABANERO & GREEN CHILI

Prep Time: 10mints, Cook Time: 25mints, Total Time: 35mints; Servings: 15 meatballs

Ingredients
- 1-pound ground chicken
- 1 poblano pepper, habanero pepper, jalapeno pepper, and salt
- 1/2 cup cilantro
- 1 tbsp vinegar
- 1 tbsp olive oil

Instructions
1. Preheat stove to 400 degrees Fahrenheit.
2. In an enormous blending bowl, join chicken, minced peppers, cilantro, salt and vinegar with your hands. Structure 1-inch meatballs with the blend
3. Coat every meatball with olive oil, at that point place on a rimmed heating sheet or meal dish.
4. Heat for 25 minutes

Nutrition Fact: Calories: 54, Fat 3g, Carbs 5g, Sugar 1.3g, Protein 5g

GRILLED CHICKEN WITH CHIMICHURRI SAUCE

Prep Time: 2mints, Cook Time: 13mints, Total Time: 45mints; Serving: 8

Ingredients
- 8 bone-in chicken thighs
- 1 recipe chimichurri sauce

Instructions
1. Coat the bird in 1/3 cup of chimichurri sauce and marinate for in any occasion half-hour.
2. Remove bird and take away the marinade.
3. Preheat flame broil and fish fry hen, skin facet down for 6- 8mins.
4. Turn hen over and flame broil 4 - five minutes, until internal temperature arrives at 165 tiers.
5. Present with greater chimichurri sauce.

Nutrition Fact: Calories: 361, Fat 28g, Carbs 15g, Sugar 8g, Protein 23g

BALSAMIC, GARLIC, AND BASIL MARINATED CHICKEN BREASTS

Prep Time: 5mints, Cook Time: 15mints, Total Time: 20mints; Servings: 4

Ingredients
- 1/4 cup of olive oil
- 1/4 cup of balsamic vinegar
- 2 cloves of garlic
- 1 tbsp fresh basil
- Sea salt and freshly cracked pepper
- 4 skinless boneless chicken breasts

Instructions
1. Join the olive oil, balsamic vinegar, garlic, basil, ocean salt, and newly break up pepper, to flavor, together in a full-size zip lock percent.
2. Blend till all-around joined at that point upload the fowl bosoms to it, seal and notice into the fridge for 2-24 hours.
3. Remove the chook from the fridge 20 minutes preceding flame broiling.
4. Coat the fish fry rack with cooking bathes at that point heat on excessive.
5. Put the fowl on the flame broil rack and prepare dinner 4-6mins for every facet or until cooked thru and the juices run clear.
6. Let the hen rest for 5-7mins earlier than cutting and presenting with rather extra slashed basil sprinkled on the pinnacle. Serve and enjoy.

Nutrition Fact: Calories: 391, Fat 23.3g, Carbs 7.4g, Sugar 8.3g, Protein 35.5g

KETO GOLDEN CHICKEN BACON FRITTER BALLS RECIPE

Prep Time: 10mints, Cook Time: 30mints, Total Time: 40mints; Serving: 6
Ingredients
- 1 chicken breast
- 4 slices of bacon
- 1 egg
- 2 green onions
- 2 cloves of garlic
- 1/4 cup olive oil

Instructions
1. Preheat stove to 350 F (175 C).
2. Line a preparing plate with parchment paper.
3. Nourishment processes the chicken, bacon, egg, green onions, and garlic together.
4. Structure 12 chicken bacon balls.
5. Plunge the balls into the olive oil.
6. Put on the lined heating plate and prepare for 30 minutes until brilliant outwardly.

Nutrition Fact: Calories: 287, Fat 26g, Carbs 2g, Sugar 0.3g, Protein 13g

EASY PALEO CHICKEN PEPPER STIR-FRY

Prep Time: 5mints, Cook Time: 10mints, Total Time: 15mints; Serving: 2
Ingredients
- 2 bell peppers
- 2 cooked and shredded chicken breasts
- 1 tsp gluten-free tamari soy sauce
- 1/4 tsp chili powder
- Salt and pepper to taste
- 1 Tsp coconut oil

Instructions
1. Add 1 tsp coconut oil into a skillet on medium heat.
2. Put the cut chime peppers into the skillet.
3. After the chime peppers mollify, add the cooked chicken meat.
4. Add the soy sauce, stew powder, salt, and pepper.
5. Blend well and pan-fried food for a couple of more minutes.

Nutrition Fact: Calories: 159, Fat 18g, Carbs 9g, Sugar 4g, Protein 8g

KETO MACADAMIA CRUSTED CHICKEN BREAST

Prep Time: 10mints, Cook Time: 20mints, Total Time: 30mints; Serving: 4
Ingredients
- 1/2 cup of macadamia nuts
- 1/4 cup of shredded coconut
- 2 Tsp of garlic powder
- Salt and pepper
- 1 egg
- 2 chicken breasts

Instructions
1. Preheat stove to 400 F (200 C).
2. In a huge bowl, blend the squashed macadamia nuts, destroyed coconut, and garlic powder. Season the blend with salt and pepper, to taste.
3. Put the whisked egg in a different bowl.
4. Dunk every chicken piece into the whisked egg. At that point dunk, the chicken cuts into the nut blend. Put the chicken pieces on a lubed rimmed heating plate.
5. Heat for 20 minutes until the chicken is completely cooked. Check with a meat thermometer that the inward temperature of the chicken is 165 F (75 C).

Nutrition Fact: Calories: 376, Fat 26g, Carbs 6g, Sugar 1g, Protein 27g

KETO CROCKPOT GARLIC CHICKEN

Prep Time: 10mints, Cook Time: 3hrs, Total Time: 3hrs 10mints; Serving: 4
Ingredients
- 1 Tsp of olive oil
- 4 chicken thighs
- 1 head of garlic
- 1 1/2 cups of chicken broth
- Salt and ground black pepper
- Chives, to garnish

Instructions
1. Heat the oil in a skillet and dark-colored the chicken skin-side down until brilliant and fresh
2. Meanwhile, strip every one of the cloves from one head of garlic. Divide everyone and add them to a stewing pot at that point pour in the warm chicken juices. When the chicken pieces have caramelized on the skin side, use tongs to remove them from the container to the slow cooker, skin-side up. Cook for 3 hours on high.
3. Remove the chicken and season with salt and naturally ground dark pepper. Trimming with chives. The relaxed cloves can be served close by whenever wanted.

Nutrition Fact: Calories: 241, Fat 18g, Carbs 2g, Sugar 0.3g, Protein 16g

BACON AVOCADO RANCH CHICKEN BURGER AND TABASCO SAUCE

Prep Time: 15mints, Cooking Time: 10mints, Total Time: 25mints; Serving: 5
Ingredients
- 1 lb. ground chicken
- 1 tsp dry ranch mix
- 3 strips bacon
- 1 tsp fresh parsley
- 8 dashes TABASCO Sauce
- 1 Avocado from Mexico

Instructions
1. In a blending, bowl adds the ground chicken, dry farm blend, diced bacon, minced parsley, and

TABASCO Sauce and mix until very much joined. Structure 5 3"wide patties and set onto a plate.

2. Put a skillet over medium-high heat. Add the burgers when the skillet is hot and cook for 8 to 10 minutes for every side, at that point flip and repeat.

3. Serve on your preferred bun or lettuce wrapped with Avocado on top

Nutrition Fact: Calories: 257, Fat 4g, Carbs 5g, Sugar 2g, Protein 18g

STUFFED CHICKEN WITH ASPARAGUS & BACON

Prep Time: 5mints, Cook Time: 40mints, Total Time: 45mints; Serving: 4

Ingredients
- 8 chicken tenders
- 1/2 tsp salt
- 1/4 tsp pepper
- 12 asparagus spears
- 8 pieces of bacon

Instructions
1. Preheat stove to 400.
2. Lay two bits of bacon out on an oven tray. Put 2 chicken fingers on top. Season with somewhat salt and pepper. Add 3 lances of asparagus. Fold the bacon over the chicken and asparagus to hold everything together. Repeat.
3. Prepare for 40 minutes until the chicken is cooked through, the asparagus is delicate, and the bacon is fresh.

Nutrition Facts: Calories 377, Fat 25g, Carbs 3g, Sugars 1g, Protein 32g

EASY MOZZARELLA & PESTO CHICKEN CASSEROLE

Prep Time: 5mints, Cook Time: 25mints, Total Time: 30mints; Serving: 8

Ingredients
- 1/4 cup pesto
- 8 oz cream cheese
- 1/4-1/2 cup heavy cream
- 8 oz mozzarella
- 2 lb. cooked cubed chicken breasts
- 8 oz mozzarella shredded

Instructions
1. Preheat stove to 400. Shower a huge meal dish with a cooking spray.
2. Join the initial three ingredients and blend until smooth in an enormous bowl. Add the chicken and cubed mozzarella. Move to the meal dish. Sprinkle the destroyed mozzarella on top.
3. Heat for 25-30 minutes. Present with zoodles, spinach, or pounded cauliflower.

Nutrition Facts: Calories 451, Fat 30g, Carbs 3g, Sugars 1g, Protein 38g

BACON-WRAPPED CHICKEN TENDERS WITH RANCH DIP

Prep Time: 5mints, Cook Time: 35mints, Total Time: 40mins; Servings: 12 pieces

Ingredients
- 12 chicken tenderloins
- 12 slices of bacon
- 1/3 cup sour cream
- 1/3 cup mayo
- 1 tsp garlic powder onion powder
- 1/2 tsp salt

Instructions
1. Preheat the stove to 400.
2. Wrap every chicken delicate firmly in a bit of bacon. I extended the bacon as I folded it over the chicken.
3. Put on an oven tray. Heat for 35-45 minutes until the bacon is fresh and the chicken is completely cooked.
4. In the interim, mix together the elements for the plunge. Present with the cooked chicken.

Nutrition Facts: Calories 204, Fat 15g, Carbs 0.1g, Sugars 2g, Protein 13g

CHILI ROASTED CHICKEN THIGHS

Prep Time: 5mints, Cook Time: 15mints, Total Time: 20mints; Serving: 8

Ingredients
- 2 pounds boneless chicken thighs
- 1 tsp organic extra virgin olive oil
- 1 tsp chili powder
- Sea salt, Ground pepper, and fresh cilantro
- Lime wedges

Instructions
1. Preheat stove to 375 degrees.
2. Put chicken on a sheet skillet or an enormous preparing dish. Shower with olive oil and go to cover. Rub with stew powder, salt, and pepper.
3. Broil the chicken thighs in the stove until cooked through, around 15 minutes.
4. Sprinkle with cilantro and present with lime wedges.

Nutrition Fact: Calories: 266, Fat 20g, Carbs 0.2g, Sugar 0.3g, Protein 18g

SUPER EASY SPICY BAKED CHICKEN

Prep Time: 5mints, Cook Time: 33mints, Total Time: 38mints; Servings: 3

Ingredients
- 4 ounces cream cheese cut into large chunks
- 1/2 cup salsa
- 1/2 teaspoon sea salt
- 1/4 teaspoon black pepper freshly ground
- 1-pound boneless, skinless chicken breasts

Instructions
1. Preheat stove to 350º Fahrenheit.
2. Put cream cheddar and salsa in a little, overwhelming weight pot. Put over low heat and cook, mixing much of the time, until cream cheddar

melts and adds with the salsa. Mix in ocean salt and pepper. Remove from heat.
3. Organize chicken bosoms in a preparing dish. Pour arranged cream cheddar sauce over top, covering the bosoms.
4. Heat in the preheated stove for 40-45 minutes, or until the focal point of chicken bosoms arrives at 180º Fahrenheit. Remove from the stove and sprinkle with parsley, whenever wanted, before serving.
Nutrition Fact: Calories: 291, Fat 17g, Carbs 4g, Sugar 1g, Protein 34g

CHICKEN AL FORNO WITH VODKA SAUCE & TWO KINDS OF CHEESE

Prep Time: 5mints, Cook Time: 25mints, Total Time: 30mints; Serving: 6
Ingredients
- 2 pounds of chicken breast
- 1 1/2 cups vodka sauce jarred
- 1/2 cup parmesan cheese
- 16 oz fresh mozzarella
- Fresh spinach

Instructions
1. Preheat the stove to 400. Spray a goulash dish with a cooking shower. Add the cooked chicken.
2. Top with the vodka sauce, parmesan cheddar, and pieces of new mozzarella.
3. Prepare until hot and bubbly. Around 25-30 minutes.
4. You can serve this over child spinach. The heat from the sauce shrivels the spinach.
Nutrition Facts: Calories 446, Fat 23g, Carbs 3g, Sugars 3g, Protein 52g

EASY MEXICAN CHICKEN CASSEROLE WITH CHIPOTLE

Prep Time: 5mints, Cook Time: 20mints, Total Time: 25mints; Serving: 8
Ingredients
- 3 cups of chicken shredded
- 8 oz cream cheese softened
- 16 oz salsa
- 8 oz shredded cheddar cheese
- 3/4 tsp ground chipotle pepper

Instructions
1. Preheat stove to 4 hundred. Oil a nine x 13 heating dish.
2. Join the hen, cream cheddar, salsa, a large portion of the destroyed cheddar, and half tsp ground chipotle pepper.
3. Blend nicely. Put in the readied goulash dish.
4. Prepare for 20 min or until warm and bubbly.
Nutrition Facts: Calories 319, Fat 25g, Carbs 5g, Sugars 3g, Protein 17g

RANCH CHICKEN

Prep Time: 5mints, Total Time: 5mints; Serving: 6
Ingredients
- 1/3- cup plain yogurt
- tbsp dill
- tbsp parsley
- tbsp onion powder and 1 tsp salt
- tbsp garlic powder

Instructions
1. Blend all ingredients in a bowl or gallon size Ziploc sack. Add 2.5 lbs. of chicken strips.
2. Marinade in the icebox for in any event 4 hours before flame broiling.
Nutrition Facts: Calories 170, Fat 9g, Carbs 2g, Sugar 4g, Protein 5g

CHICKEN BACON RANCH CASSEROLE

Prep Time: 30mints, Cook Time: 45mints, Total Time: 1hr 15mins; Serving: 6
Ingredients
- 1 pound shredded chicken
- 1 medium onion
- 1 head cauliflower
- 10 oz package bacon
- 1 tsp salt and 1 cup ranch dressing

Instructions
1. Preheat the stove to four hundred°. Spread the bacon out level on a heating sheet. Put within the four hundred° stove for 15 minutes or until firm.
2. Sprinkle with the salt and mix to enroll in. Remove the bacon from the range and placed apart to chill.
3. Put the bird on the heating sheet and put together within the stove for a half-hour or till by no means once more purple.
4. At the point whilst chook is completed, decrease up or shred in your stand blender with the oar connection at a low pace.
5. Add the chicken to the dish with the cauliflower, onion, and bacon.
6. Heat at 350° secured for half-hour, at that factor reveal and prepares 10 minutes more. Throughout the preceding five minutes, flip the stove at the prepare dinner and clean up the top, observing near ignite positive it does not!
7. Serve proper away. Top with additional bacon, additional farm, or crisp herbs for additional focuses!
Nutrition Fact: Calories: 412, Fat 7g, Carbs 7g, Sugar 2g, Protein 28g

5 INGREDIENT BACON WRAPPED CHICKEN BREAST

Prep Time: 5mints, Cook Time: 40mints, Total Time: 45mints; Serving: 6
Ingredients
- 5-6 chicken breasts
- 2 tbsp seasoning rub
- 1/2 lb. bacon cut strips in half
- 4 oz shredded cheddar

- Sugar-free barbecue sauce

Instructions
1. Preheat stove to 400. Spray a huge rimmed oven tray with a cooking shower.
2. Rub the two sides of chicken bosoms with flavoring rub. Top each with a bit of bacon. Prepare for 30 min on the top rack until the chicken is 160 degrees and the bacon look firm.
3. Remove plate from the stove and sprinkle the cheddar over the bacon. Set back in the stove for around 10 min until the cheddar is bubbly and brilliant. Present with grill sauce.

Nutrition Facts: Calories 345, Fat 23g, Carbs 1g, Sugars 0.3g, Protein 29g

PARMESAN CHICKEN TENDERS

Prep Time: 20mints, Cooking Time: 30mints, Total Time: 50mints; Serving: 2

Ingredients
- 1 2.5 lb. bag chicken tenderloins
- ¾ cup butter
- 1⅛ cup parmesan cheese
- ¾ tsp. garlic powder
- Salt

Instructions
1. Liquefy the margarine in a skillet and add the parmesan cheddar and garlic powder. Dunk the chicken in the blend and put on a treat sheet. Prepare at 325 degrees F for 20-30 minutes. Don't overbake!
2. We have likewise utilized these for Sunday lunch. My mother set them up for the congregation, at that point heated them on our stove's "warm" setting for about 3½ hours while we were no more. Worked extraordinarily!

Nutrition Fact: Calories 188; Fat 5g, Carbs 10g, Sugar 6g, Protein 24g

BROILED CHICKEN THIGHS WITH ARTICHOKES AND GARLIC

Prep Time: 10mints, Cook Time: 20mints, Total Time: 30mints; Serving: 4

Ingredients
- pounds chicken thighs
- 1-2 jars artichoke hearts
- 2 tablespoons dried oregano
- 2 tablespoons minced garlic
- Salt and pepper to taste

Instructions
1. Blend chicken thighs and artichoke hearts in an enormous bowl. Permit marinating for 20-30 minutes.
2. Channel the fluid.
3. Add oregano, minced garlic, salt and pepper.
4. Blend.
5. Sear on high for 18-25 minutes or until chicken is cooked through

Nutrition Fact: Calories: 300, Fat 28g, Carbs 7g, Sugar 1g, Protein 11g

ROSEMARY GARLIC CHICKEN KABOBS

Prep Time: 15mints, Cook Time: 15mints, Total Time: 30mints; Servings: 8 kabobs

Ingredients
- 8 bamboo skewers
- 3 chicken breasts
- 1/4 cup olive oil
- 2 tablespoons rosemary
- 3 cloves garlic
- 1 tsp kosher salt and black pepper

Instructions
1. Spray bamboo sticks in water for in any event 15 minutes to shield them from consuming on the barbecue.
2. Add remaining ingredients – chicken through pepper – in a huge bowl. Mix to cover all sides of chicken pieces.
3. Amass kabobs by isolating chicken pieces and stringing them on to 8 sticks. Spread sticks and refrigerate until you're prepared to flame broil.
4. Preheat the flame broil to 375°F. Barbecue chicken for 3 minutes for each side for a sum of 12 to 15 minutes, or until cooked through and still damp. Serve.

Nutrition Fact: Calories: 280, Fat 31g, Carbs 2.8g, Sugar 2.2g, Protein 1g

KETO HONEY MUSTARD CHICKEN

Prep Time: 5mints, Cook Time: 30mints, Total Time: 35mints; Serving: 4

Ingredients
- 4 boneless skinless chicken breasts
- 1 cup Keto Honey Mustard Dressing
- 2 tablespoons olive oil

Instructions
1. Add the bird and 1/2 cup of the nectar mustard dressing in a bowl and remove the chook, protecting it in the dressing.
2. Let marinate inside the cooler for 60mins, or as long as 24 hours.
3. Preheat the stove to 350°F.
4. Heat the olive oil in an enormous stove affirmation skillet over medium-excessive heat
5. When the skillet is warm, consist of the hen, and container singe caramelizing on the 2 aspects. Around 3 to 4 minutes on every aspect.
6. Pour the staying nectar mustard dressing over the bird.

Nutrition Fact: Calories: 242, Fat 9.5g, Carbs 1g, Sugar 0.2g, Protein 34g

CROCKPOT GREEN CHILE CHICKEN

Prep Time: 5mints, Cook Time: 3hrs 30mints, Total Time: 3hrs 35mints; Serving: 6

Ingredients
- 3 pounds Boneless Chicken Thighs fresh
- 4 ounces Green Chiles
- 2 teaspoons Garlic Salt
- ½ cup White Onions

Instructions
1. Cook chicken in the slow cooker on HIGH for 3 hours or LOW for 6 hours
2. Following 3 hours on HIGH or 6 hours on LOW, channel juices from slow cooker
3. Combine green chilies and garlic salt.
4. Pour blend over chicken, and cook on HIGH for 30 additional minutes
5. Remove chicken from stewing pot, and shred with a fork.
6. Present with everything on the side for tacos or enveloped with burritos. YUM!

Nutrition Facts: Calories 449, Fat 31g, Carbs 3g, Sugar 1g, Protein 38g

BLACKENED DIJON CHICKEN

Prep Time: 10mints, Cook Time: 30mints, Total Time: 40mints; Serving: 4

Ingredients
- 1 ½ lbs. chicken breasts
- ¼ cup Dijon mustard
- 3 tbsp Blackened Seasoning
- 2 tbsp olive oil

Instructions
1. Preheat stove to 400°
2. Generously cover every chicken bosom with darkened flavoring.
3. Brush each piece with Dijon mustard on the two sides.
4. Heat olive oil in an enormous skillet over medium-high heat
5. Burn the chicken for 3 minutes on each side.
6. Remove the chicken from the skillet and put on a heating sheet. Prepare for 20 minutes.

Nutrition Fact: Calories: 220, Fat 3g, Carbs 1g, Sugar 2g, Protein 38g

BLACKENED RANCH PAN-FRIED CHICKEN THIGHS

Prep Time: 5mints, Cook Time: 25mints, Total Time: 30mints; Serving: 4

Ingredients
- 1 tablespoon vegetable oil
- 4 chicken thighs
- 2 tablespoons dry ranch dressing mix
- Salt to taste
- 1 pinch fresh cracked black pepper

Instructions
1. Heat oil in a cast-iron skillet over medium heat, rub 1 tablespoon dry farm dressing, salt, and new cut up pepper onto 1 aspect of chook thighs.
2. Flip and repeat on the other facet.
3. Put chicken thighs, skin face down, into the hot oil. Cook over medium heat without transferring to darken skin, around 12 minutes.
4. Turn bird thighs and cook until he is in no way again pink in the inner and the juices run clear around 12 extra minutes.
5. A moment examine thermometer embedded into the center must peruse in any event a 165 degrees F.

Nutrition Facts: Calories 194, Fat 13.1g, Carb 1.9g, Sugar 5.3g, Protein 15.9g

KETO SLOW COOKER GREEK CHICKEN

Prep Time: 5mints, Cook Time: 6hrs, Total Time: 6hrs 5mints; Serving: 3

Ingredients
- 3-4 boneless chicken breasts
- 3 Tbsp. Greek Rub
- 1½ Tbsp. garlic
- 3 Tbsp. lemon juice and 1½ cups hot water
- 2 chicken bouillon cubes

Instructions
1. Line moderate cooker with liner or cooking shower
2. Rub every fowl bosom with Greek Rub to cover liberally on every facet.
3. Next, rub about ½ Tablespoon of garlic on every bird bosom.
4. Put hen bosom inside the mild cooker and shower lemon squeeze over the pinnacle.
5. Disintegrate and mix 2 hen bouillon stable shapes in 1½ cups of boiling water.

Nutrition Facts: Calories 401, Fat 24g, Carbs 2g, Sugar 1g, Protein 42g

INSTANT POT KETO CRACK CHICKEN

Prep Time: 15mints, Cooking Time: 20mints, Total Time: 35mints; Serving: 4

Ingredients
- 2 lbs. chicken breasts
- 12 oz cream cheese
- 2 1 oz Dry Ranch Seasoning
- 8 oz bacon crumbles and 1/2 cup Cheddar Cheese
- 1 cup bone broth

Instructions
1. Put 1 cup of fluid in the base of the weight cooker
2. Prep the cream cheddar by cutting the squares into huge blocks.
3. Add the chicken to the weight cooker.
4. Add the cream cheddar and seasonings over the chicken.
5. Set the weight cooker to high for 10 minutes for chicken strips or 12 minutes for full chicken breasts.
6. Cautiously evacuate the chicken and shred it utilizing two forks, place the destroyed chicken back in the fluid squeezes that are held in the weight cooker.
7. Add the cheddar and bacon disintegrates into the destroyed chicken and combine the ingredients.
8. Put the top back on the weight cooker for around 5 minutes. Giving the ingredients a chance to

sit for a few moments will enable the sauce to thicken.
Nutrition Fact: Calories: 440, Fat 41.1g, Carbs 3.5g, Sugar 2.2g, Protein 41.1g

CREAMY MEXICAN SLOW COOKER KETO CHICKEN

Prep Time: 5mints, Cook Time: 6hrs, Total Time: 6hrs 5mints\; Serving: 6
Ingredients
- 1 cup sour cream
- 1/2 cup chicken stock
- 14 oz tomatoes and green chilies
- 1 batch homemade taco seasoning
- 2 lbs. chicken breast

Instructions
1. Heat moderate cooker on low setting
2. To the moderate cooker, add the sharp cream, chicken stock, diced tomatoes with green chilies and taco flavoring. Blend until all ingredients are all around mixed.
3. Add the chicken's bosoms to the moderate cooker. Cover and cook on low for 6 hours

Nutrition Fact: Calories: 262, Fat 13g, Carbs 8.3g, Sugar 2.5g, Protein 32g

BASIL STUFFED CHICKEN BREASTS

Prep Time: 5mints, Cook Time: 45mints, Total Time: 50mints; Serving: 2
Ingredients
- 2 bone-in, skin-on chicken breasts
- 2 tbs cream cheese
- 2 tbs shredded cheese
- ¼ tsp garlic paste
- 3-4 fresh basil leaves and black pepper

Instructions
1. Preheat the stove to 375F.
2. Make the stuffing by consolidating the cream cheddar, cheddar, garlic glue, basil, and dark pepper.
3. Delicately strip back the skin on one side of the chicken bosom and put the half stuffing inside. Smooth it down and supplant the skin. Repeat for the other bit of chicken.
4. Broil on a preparing plate for 45 minutes or until an inward temperature of 165F has been come to.

Nutrition Fact: Calories: 405, Fat 9g, Carbs 1g, Sugar 3g, Protein 41g

LOW CARB CHICKEN NUGGETS KETO

Prep Time: 5mints, Cook Time: 13mints, Total Time: 20mints; Serving: 6
Ingredients
- 2 cups cooked chicken
- 8 oz cream cheese
- 1 egg
- 1/4 cup almond flour
- 1 tsp garlic salt

Instructions
1. Shred chicken with an electric blender. This works best with a blend of dim and white meat that is still warm. On the off chance that you are utilizing extra chicken warm it up somewhat first. When the chicken is destroyed add the remainder of the ingredients and blends until altogether joined.
2. Drop scoops onto a lubed heating sheet and smooth it into a chunk shape.
3. Heat at 350 for 12-14 min until marginally brilliant and firm

Nutrition Facts: Calories 243, Fat 17g, Carbs 2g, Sugars 1g, Protein 18g

KETO HONEY MUSTARD CHICKEN

Prep Time: 5mints, Cook Time: 30mints, Total Time: 35mints; Serving: 4
Ingredients
- 4 boneless skinless chicken breasts
- 1 cup Keto Honey Mustard Dressing
- 2 tablespoons olive oil

Instructions
1. Join the hen and half of cup of the nectar mustard dressing in a bowl and remove the hen, covering it in the dressing.
2. Let marinate within the fridge for 60mints, or so long as 24 hours.
3. Preheat the range to 350°F.
4. Heat the olive oil in a massive range verification skillet over medium-high warm temperature
5. When the skillet is warm, add the chicken, and box burn, sautéing on the 2 aspects. Around 3 to four minutes on every side.
6. Pour the staying nectar mustard dressing over the chook. Move the skillet to the stove and heat for 20mins or till the hen is cooked completely via.

Nutrition Fact: Calories: 242, Fat 9.5g, Carbs 1g, Sugar 0.5g, Protein 34g

PORK, BEEF & LAMB RECIPES

VEGGED UP PALEO BEEF BURGERS

Prep Time: 15mints, Cook Time: 30mints, Total Time: 45mints; Serving: 15 burgers

Ingredients
- 3 lbs. of ground beef
- 2 leeks
- 3 Tsp of parsley
- 3 eggs
- Salt and pepper

Instructions
1. Combine every one of the ingredients well.
2. Structure into meat patties
3. Barbecue or sauté

Nutrition Fact: Calories: 69, Fat 4.9g, Carbs 0.5g, Sugar 1.4g, Protein 5.6g

SLOW COOKER PORK

Prep Time: 5mints, Cook Time: 8hrs, Total Time: 8hrs 5mints; Serving: 4

Ingredients
- 2 lb. pork shoulder
- 1 tsp salt
- 1 tsp ginger powder
- 1 tsp Szechuan peppercorns
- 4 prunes

Instructions
1. Put the pork into the moderate cooker.
2. Sprinkle the flavors onto the meat.
3. Add the prunes.
4. Set moderate cooker for 8 hours on low heat setting.
5. Turn meat over following 6 hours however don't pull separated meat.

Nutrition Fact: Calories: 422, Fat 28g, Carbs 15g, Sugar 10g, Protein 40g

PALEO SLOW COOKER PORK RECIPE

Prep Time: 5mints, Cook Time: 10hrs, Total Time: 10hrs 5mints; Serving: 6-8

Ingredients
- 4 lb. pork shoulder or butt
- 1/2–3/4 cup Cajun seasoning
- 1/2 cup water
- Salt to taste

Instructions
1. Ensure all the pork fits into the moderate cooker.
2. Spread the meat with the Cajun flavoring and put into the moderate cooker.
3. Add the 1/2 cup of water into the base of the moderate cooker.
4. Cook for 10 hours on low.
5. Add salt to taste when you shred the pork.

Nutrition Fact: Calories 176, Fat 16g, Carbs 10g, Sugar 6g, Protein 3g

WORLD'S EASIEST CROCKPOT PORK ROAST

Prep Time: 5mints, Cook Time: 4hrs, Total Time: 4hrs 5mints; Servings: 4

Ingredients
- 3-4 lb. pork butt roast
- 1/4 cup coconut amino
- Favorite spice blend

Instructions
1. Put broil into the moderate cooker.
2. Pour coconut amino over it.
3. Sprinkle liberally on all sides with the flavor blend.
4. Spread and let cook on low for 4-6 hours.
5. Shred and fill in as wanted

Nutrition Facts:Calories 215, Fat 10g, Carbs 7g, Sugar 3g, Protein 23g

KETO ROASTED BONE MARROW RECIPE

Prep Time: 5mints, Cook Time: 20mints, Total Time: 25mints; Serving: 2

INGREDIENTS
- 4 bone marrow halves
- Sea salt flakes and freshly ground black pepper

Instructions
1. Preheat the stove to 350 F.
2. Put the bones marrow side-up onto a profound preparing plate.
3. Put in the stove for 20-25 minutes until brilliant and firm and the vast majority of the excessive fat has rendered off.
4. Season the marrow with ocean salt chips and naturally ground dark pepper.
5. Serve without anyone else as a starter or scoop out the marrow and spread on flame-broiled steak.

Nutrition Fact: Calories: 440, Fat 48g, Carbs 0.2g Sugar 0.4g, Protein 4g

EASY SLOW COOKER KETO POT ROAST

Prep Time: 10mints, Cook Time: 8hrs, Total Time: 8hrs 10mints; Serving: 8

Ingredients
- 3 lb. beef roast
- 3 stalks of celery
- 1 carrot and 1 onion
- 4 cloves of garlic
- 2 Tsp Italian seasoning

Instructions
1. Put everything into the moderate cooker and cook for 8 hours until the hamburger is delicate.

Nutrition Fact: Calories: 468, Fat 36g, Carbs 3g, Sugar 1g, Protein 29g

ROSEMARY LIVER BURGERS

Prep Time: 15mints, Cook Time: 15mints, Total Time: 30mints; Serving: 15
INGREDIENTS
- 2 lbs. ground grass-fed beef
- 1 lb. ground liver
- 1/4–1/2 cup rosemary
- 1 tsp chili pepper flakes and black pepper
- 2 Tsp oregano

Instructions
1. Combine every one of the ingredients well.
2. Structure slim burger patties with your hands.
3. Flame broils the burgers until completely cooked through.

Nutrition Fact: Calories 324, Fat 21g, Carbs 16g, Sugar 3g, Protein 6g

KETO OVEN-BAKED STEAK WITH GARLIC THYME PORTABELLA MUSHROOMS

Prep Time: 10mints, Cook Time: 15mints, Total Time: 25mints; Serving: 2
Ingredients
- 2 Tsp of olive oil
- 4 portabella mushrooms
- 4–6 sprigs of thyme
- 2 beef filet mignons
- 1 Tsp of garlic powder
- Salt and pepper

Instructions
1. Preheat stove to 320°F (160°C).
2. Put the portabella mushrooms on a lubed broiling plate and shower a tsp of olive oil over it. Sprinkle the garlic powder equally over every one of the four and disperse over the picked thyme leaves. Season with salt and newly ground dark pepper and put in the stove for 15 minutes
3. Season the steaks with salt.
4. Add one tsp olive oil to a huge skillet and singe the two sides of the steaks with the goal that a brilliant hull frames on all sides. Put the steaks on a rimmed heating plate and put into the preheated stove for 8-10 minutes until the focal point of the steak arrives at 130 F for medium-uncommon or 140 F for medium. Rest for 10 minutes before serving

Nutrition Fact: Calories: 733, Fat 56g, Carbs 10g, Sugar 1g, Protein 42g

LOW-CARB STUFFED POBLANO PEPPERS

Prep Time: 15mints, Cook Time: 30mints, Total Time: 45mints; Serving: 1
Ingredients
- 1 poblano pepper
- 1/3 cup finely chopped cauliflower
- 1/3 lb. ground beef
- 1 tsp onion
- 3 tsp tomato sauce

Instructions
1. Cut the poblano pepper down the middle and take out the seeds.
2. Dark colored the ground hamburger and onion in a little skillet.
3. Blend the ground hamburger blend with the cauliflower and tomato sauce.
4. Spoon into the pepper parts

Nutrition Facts: Calories 344, Fat 25g, Carbs 12g, Sugar 4g, Protein 28g

MINI ZUCCHINI AVOCADO BURGERS

Prep Time: 10mints, Cook Time: 15mints, Total Time: 25mints; Serving: 2
Ingredients
- 1 large zucchini
- 1/2 lb ground beef
- 1/4 avocado
- 2 Tbsp olive or avocado oil for greasing a baking tray
- 2 Tsp salt

Instructions
1. Preheat stove to 400°F (200°C).
2. Oil a heating plate with olive or avocado oil and sprinkle 1 tsp of salt.
3. Put the zucchini cuts on the heating plate.
4. Structure little balls starting from the earliest stage and press into patties – around 7 or 8 patties – and place on the preparing plate.
5. Put the heating plate into the stove and prepare for 15 minutes. On the other hand, rather than heating them, you can flame bake the zucchini and hamburger patties or sauté them in some olive or avocado oil.
6. Then, cut the avocado into little dainty cuts.
7. Set up the scaled-down burgers together utilizing the zucchini cuts as buns – add a cut of avocado to every burger and top with toppings like Paleo mayo and mustard.

Nutrition Fact: Calories: 370, Fat 30g, Carbs 9g, Sugar 4g, Protein 23g

KETO INSTANT POT ROASTED BONE BROTH RECIPE

Prep Time: 10mints, Cook Time: 2hrs, Total Time: 2hrs 10mints; Serving: 8
Ingredients
- 4 lb grass-fed beef bones
- 2 carrots
- 4 stalks of celery
- 1 onion and 2 Tsp sea salt
- 2 Tsp apple cider vinegar

Instructions
1. Preheat stove to 450 F.
2. Put the bones on a rimmed heating plate and dish for 30-40 minutes until sautéed.
3. Put the bones with the remainder of the ingredients into the Instant Pot.
4. Top off with cold water.
5. Select the soup alternative and set the clock for 120 minutes.

6. At the point when it blares, you can utilize the stock as is or you can set it for an additional 120 minutes to make thicker juices
7. Allow the two pots to depressurize.
8. Strain the stock and spoon into artisan containers to refrigerate. Remove that top layer of cemented fat before utilizing it in case you're drinking it straight away.

Nutrition Fact: Calories: 30, Fat 1.2g, Carbs 3g, Sugar 0.2g, Protein 6g

PALEO CROCK POT OXTAIL WITH MUSTARD GRAVY

Prep Time: 5mints, Cook Time: 10hrs, Total Time: 10hrs 5mints; Serving: 4-6

Ingredients
- 4 lb. oxtail
- 4 cups of chicken broth
- 8 Tsp of Dijon mustard
- salt to taste

Instructions
1. Put the oxtail and the chicken juices in the slow cooker and cook on low for 10 hours. You would then be able to store the meat and juices in the cooler until you're prepared to eat it.
2. At the point when you're prepared to eat, heat the oxtail in a stockpot on low heat with what's left of the juices to lessen the soup into a sauce.
3. At the point when the stock comes down and turns thicker, mix in the mustard.
4. Add salt to taste and serve.

Nutrition Fact: Calories: 141, Fat 8g, Carbs 4g, Sugar 0.5g, Protein 21g

COWBOY BURGERS (KETO)

Prep Time: 20mints, Cooking Time: 15mints, Total Time: 35mints; Serving: 4

Ingredients
- 4 slices bacon
- 1 lb ground beef
- 1/2 cup shredded cheese
- 1 Tsp sea salt
- 1/2 tsp ground black pepper

Instructions
1. Put the bacon in your nourishment processor and procedure until crisp. Scoop this into a bowl with the remainder of the ingredients.
2. With your hands combine the ingredients until all-around mixed and structure into 4 huge patties, approximately 4" x ½" thick. Put a skillet over medium-high heat and place the burgers.
3. Cook until caramelized on one side, for about 5 minutes then flip. Serve on lettuce leaves with sauces of decision.

Nutrition Fact: Calories: 421, Fat 28g, Carbs 1g, Sugar 0.3g, Protein 38g

LAMB & LEEK BURGERS

Prep Time: 10mints, Cooking Time: 10mints, Total Time: 20mints; Serving: 4

Ingredients
- 1 lb ground lamb
- 1/2 cup leeks
- 1 tbl coconut oil
- 1/2 tbl garlic powder
- 1/2 tsp fine sea salt

Instructions
1. Place leeks and 1/2 of the coconut oil in a dish and prepare over medium heat until the leeks for around three-five minutes.
2. Move the leeks to a bowl.
3. In another large bowl, place the ground lamb, garlic powder and salt
4. When the leeks are cool, place in 2nd bowl and blend till the mixed evenly. Form into four patties.
5. Over low-medium heat, cook patties until caramelized, around 5 minutes on each side.
6. Ensure the lamb is cooked thoroughly.

Nutrition Fact: Calories 140, Fat 12g, Carbs 5g, Sugar 2.1g, Protein 8g

EASY BROILED TABLE SEASONED MINI BEEF PATTIES

Prep Time: 15mints, Cooking Time: 20mints, Total Time: 35mints; Serves 4

Ingredients:
- 1 tsp coconut oil
- 1 pound ground meat
- 3 large shallots
- 6 garlic cloves
- 1 tsp table seasoning and 2/3 tsp kosher salt

Instructions
1. Preheat your oven and ensure the top rack is around 5 crawls from the warming component.
2. Next, line a oven tray with uncompromising aluminum foil and oil well with coconut oil.
3. Put the ground meat in a medium-sized bowl. Rush the shallots in your nourishment processor.
4. Add the shallots, minced garlic, Table flavoring, and salt to the ground meat. Utilize your hands to blend everything admirably.
5. Structure meat into patties, ensuring they're not exactly an inch thick.
6. Put patties on a heating sheet and stick under the oven. Sear on one side for 4 minutes, at that point flip over and cook for an additional 2 minutes or cooked through.

Nutrition Fact: Calories: 100, Fat: 9.5g, Carbs 2g, Sugar 5g, Protein 1g

CORNED BEEF HASH

Prep Time: 10mints, Cooking Time: 15mints, Total Time: 25mints; Serving: 4

Ingredients

- 2 cups chopped cooked corned beef
- 1 small onion, Salt and pepper
- 1 lb. radishes
- 2 cloves garlic
- 1/2 cup beef broth

Instructions
1. Heat 1 Tbsp of oil over medium-high heat
2. Add the onions and sauté for 3-4 minutes.
3. Add the radishes and sauté for 5 minutes.
4. Add the garlic and sauté for an additional 1 moment.
5. Add the meat stock, spread freely, and cook for 5 minutes or until the radishes are delicate and the fluid has been consumed.
6. Add the corned meat and season and mix to join.
7. Season with salt and pepper to taste

Nutrition Fact: Calories: 432, Fat 20g, Carbs 10g, Sugar 5g, Protein 28g

SLOW-COOKED KETO CORNED BEEF BRISKET

Prep Time: 35mints, Cooking Time: 6hrs, Total Time: 6hrs 35mints; Serving: 3

Ingredients
- 2½ lb. corned beef brisket
- ½ medium Onion
- 1 carrot
- 1 celery stalk
- 1 cup chicken or beef stock

Instructions
1. Slash onion, carrot, and celery stalk coarsely and place in the base of a moderate cooker.
2. Pour chicken stock over onion, carrot, and celery and put corned hamburger brisket over veggies in the moderate cooker.
3. Put the highest point of the moderate cooker and cook on low for 6-8 hours. That is it!

Nutrition Fact: Calories: 324, Fat 16g, Carbs 12g, Sugar 8g, Protein 36g

KETO STEAK AU POIVRE

Prep Time: 5mints, Cook Time: 10mints, Total Time: 15mints; Serving: 1

INGREDIENTS
- 1 filet mignon
- 1 Tsp salt 2 Tsp peppercorns
- 1 sprig of thyme
- 2 cloves of garlic
- 2 Tsp ghee

Instructions
1. Remove steaks from the cooler, season with salt and let sit for 30 minutes.
2. Smash the peppercorns, utilizing a mortar and pestle or a level board or container.
3. Press the squashed peppercorns onto the two sides of the steak.
4. In a hot skillet, add the ghee, thyme, and garlic.
5. Cook the steak for 3-4 minutes for every side. This ought to get it to medium-uncommon.

Nutrition Fact: Calories: 696, Fat 58g, Carbs 2g, Sugar 0.3g, Protein 42g

HIDDEN LIVER MEATBALLS

Prep Time: 15mints, Cook Time: 15mints, Total Time: 30mints; Serving 4 to 6 servings

Ingredients
- 1-pound ground pork
- 1-pound US Wellness Meats Liverwurst
- Solid fat of choice for frying

Instruction
1. In a nourishment processor, join the ground pork and liverwurst until smooth.
2. Fold the blend into 1/2-inch wide meatballs and put aside.
3. Heat 1 to 2 Tsp of fat of decision in an enormous hardened steel skillet over medium heat, add meatballs to the skillet, being certain to not pack.
4. Fry on all sides until sautéed and cooked through around 13 to 15 minutes all out.
5. Remove from heat and let rest 5 minutes before presenting with your most loved plunging sauce.

Nutrition Fact: Calories 232, Fat 9g, Carbs 21g, Sugar 12g, Protein 43g

KETO SPICY BEEF AVOCADO CUPS

Prep Time: 5mints, Cook Time: 15mints, Total Time: 20mints; Serving: 2

Ingredients
- 1 beefsteak
- 2 chili peppers
- 1/2 medium onion
- 2 Tsp avocado oil and 1 large ripe avocado
- 2 Tsp gluten-free tamari sauce

Instructions
1. Add the avocado oil to a skillet on excessive heat and cook dinner the steak 3-d shapes until performed exactly as you would prefer.
2. At that point consist of the bean stew peppers and onions to the skillet and cook dinner until comfy.
3. Utilize an increasing number of avocado oil if essential. Return the steak 3-d shapes to the griddle and season with tamari sauce.
4. Spoon the hamburger combo over the avocado elements and serve.

Nutrition Fact: Calories: 570, Fat 50g, Carbs 13g, Sugar 2g, Protein 19g

SIMPLE BEEF TENDERLOIN FILET MIGNON

Prep Time: 15mints, Total Time: 35mints; Serving: 4

Ingredients
- 1 tsp of sea salt
- 1 tsp ground pepper
- 1 tsp smoked paprika
- 1-pound beef tenderloin filet mignon

- 2 tsp ghee or organic butter

Instructions
1. In a touch bowl, add salt, pepper, and paprika.
2. Rub this mixture over the beef, top, and base.
3. Preheat range to 400 ranges F.
4. Singe meat 1 moment for every facet stovetop.
5. Put meat in a heating dish. Rub with margarine and heat till the appropriate doneness.
6. A meat thermometer is your closest companion while cooking meat.
7. Let rest for 5mins.
8. Cut and serve.

Nutrition Fact: Calories: 242, Fat 18g, Carbs 12g, Sugar 8g, Protein 43g

KETO SKIRT STEAK

Prep Time: 5mints, Cooking Time: 15mints, Total Time: 20mints; Servings: 2

Ingredients
- 1 lb Skirt Steak
- 1 Tbsp Paleo Adobo Seasoning
- 1 Tbsp Coconut Vinegar
- 1 Tbsp Olive Oil

Instructions
1. Heat up the stove pan.
2. Flame broils the steaks for 3-4 minutes on each side. Let rest for 5 minutes, at that point cut the meat over the grain.

Nutritional Fact: Calories: 362, Fat 5g, Carbs 7g, Sugars: 2g, Protein 32g

THREE INGREDIENT KETO STEAK SAUTÉ

Prep Time: 10mints, Cook Time: 20mints, Total Time: 30mints; Serving: 1

Ingredients
- 1 beef ribeye steak
- 1/2 onion
- 2 cloves of garlic
- 2 Tsp avocado oil

Instructions
1. Add avocado oil to a griddle and sauté the steak, onion, and garlic.

Nutrition Fact: Calories: 798, Fat 70g, Carbs 7g, Sugar 3g, Protein 35g

EASY MARINATED GRILLED STEAK TACOS

Prep Time: 1hr 50mints, Cooking Time: 35mints, Total Time: 2hrs 25mints; Serving: 6

Ingredients:
- 9-ounce skirt steak or flank steak
- ½ tsp sea salt and black pepper
- 1 tbsp lime juice
- ½ tsp cumin
- 6 Romaine lettuce cups or these low carb tortillas

Instructions
2. Sprinkle every aspect of steak with salt and pepper.
3. In a bit, bowl adds lime juice and cumin.
4. Put steak in a large skillet or dish.
5. Pour a few lime marinades over the 2 sides of steak and rub into meat softly.
6. Preheat flame broil or stove-top barbecuing skillet to medium-high.
7. Flame broils steak for around 3 to 5 minutes on each side.
8. Remove from flame broil and let it rest for 10 minutes before cutting it.
9. Cut steak into little reduced down strips.
10. Burden into a lettuce cup or tortillas and top with discretionary: salsa, harsh cream, cilantro, avocado, tomato or cheeses.

Nutritional Fact: Calories: 168, Fat 6g, Carbs 1g, Sugars: 0.2g, Protein 24g

PALEO-ITALIAN CARPACCIO

Prep Time: 1hr 30mints, Cooking Time: 1hr, Total Time: 2hrs 30mints; Serving: 4

Ingredients
- 8 ounces of grass-fed, grass-finished filet mignon
- 1 bunch fresh organic Arugula
- 4 tsp truffle infused extra virgin olive oil
- 1 tsp unrefined sea salt
- Freshly ground black pepper to taste

Instructions
1. Put the meat in the cooler for around 2 hours. This will make it firm enough to cut with a sharp gourmet specialist's blade or with a meat slicer.
2. Cut meagerly and isolate the individual cuts laying them on 4 individual plates.
3. Organize the arugula over the meat, separating it similarly
4. Shower the oil on the plates, at that point sprinkle with salt and pepper
5. In the event that you are utilizing cheddar, mastermind the shaved parmesan on top
6. You can add extra naturally ground dark pepper to decorate the top.
7. Plates can be chilled in the icebox for 30 minutes before serving.

Nutrition Fact: Calories: 437, Fat 28g, Carbs 4g, Sugar 6g, Protein 31g

BUTTER COFFEE RUBBED TRI-TIP STEAK

Prep Time: 20mints, Cook Time: 10mints, Total Time: 30mints; Serving: 2

Ingredients
- 2 Tri-tip steaks
- 1 tsp coarse black pepper and sea salt
- 1 package of Coffee Blocks
- 1/2 tbsp garlic powder
- 2 tbsp olive oil

Instructions
1. Give the beef a danger to sit down at room temperature for around 20mins.

2. In a bowl, add all ingredients aside from steaks.
3. Rub combination throughout steaks along with top, base, and aspects.
4. Heat a skillet with olive oil to medium-high warm temperature
5. Add steaks to skillet and cook dinner on one side for around 5mins.
6. Flip and cook dinner on the alternative aspect for a further five minutes or until it's, in any event, one hundred forty degrees for medium-uncommon
7. Remove from the dish and permit sit down in its own juices for in any occasion a moment
8. Cut your steak into cuts contrary to what would be expected, and respect!
Nutrition Fact: Calories: 451, Fat 27g, Carbs 2g, Sugar 1g, Protein 48g

PALEO RIB EYE STEAK

Prep Time: 10mints, Cooking Time: 15mints, Total Time: 25mints; Serving: 2
Ingredients
- 1 lb., 1" thick Grass-fed Rib Eye Steak
- 1 Tbsp Extra Virgin Olive Oil
- Paleo Adobo Seasoning
- Sea Salt and Pepper

Instructions
1. To begin with, I'm certain you're pondering… 1 entire pound of meat??! Are these individuals insane? We like to prepare extra and have it for lunch the following day. See our Perfect Steak Cooking Guide for additional information on cooking time which depends on thickness.
2. At any rate, I like to place the steak in a bowl and shower a tad bit of the oil on the two sides. Next, dust the seasonings on the two sides and rub them into the meat.
3. I let the meat sit for brief time Angel warms up the flame broil. In the event that you need a little direction on the ideal method to cook your steak, go to our Perfect Steak Cooking Guide for a total rundown – both on the flame broil and in the stove!
Nutrition Fact: Calories: 258, Fat 18g, Carbs 15g, Sugar 14g, Protein 37g

KETO SPICY BEEF AVOCADO CUPS

Prep Time: 5mints, Cook Time: 15mints, Total Time: 20mints; Serving: 2
Ingredients
- 1 beefsteak, chopped into small cubes
- 2 chili peppers and 1/2 medium onion
- 2 Tsp avocado oil
- 2 Tsp gluten-free tamari sauce or coconut amino
- 1 large ripe avocado

Instructions
1. Add the avocado oil to a skillet on excessive heat and cook the steak three-D shapes till accomplished simply as you will prefer.
2. At that factor consist of the bean stew peppers and onions to the skillet and prepare dinner until mellowed.
3. Utilize regularly avocado oil if vital. Return the steak blocks to the skillet and season with tamari sauce.
4. Spoon the beef combination over the avocado components and serve.
Nutrition Fact: Calories: 570, Fat 50g, Carbs 13g, Sugar 2g, Protein 19g

KETO ROSEMARY ROAST BEEF AND WHITE RADISHES

Prep Time: 10mints, Cook Time: 60mints, Total Time: 1hr 10mints; Serving: 8
Ingredients
- 3 lb. boneless beef roast
- 2 white daikon radishes
- 3 Tsp rosemary
- 2 Tsp salt, to taste
- 2 Tsp olive oil

Instructions
1. Preheat grill to 400 F.
2. Spread olive oil, rosemary, and salt over the cheeseburger.
3. Detect the stripped and severed radishes at the base of a warming dish.
4. Detect the burger over the radishes and heat for an hour.
5. Wrap the burger by utilizing foil and permit unwinding for 20mins sooner than serving.
Nutrition Fact: Calories: 492, Fat 39g, Carbs 4g, Sugar 2g, Protein 29g

KETO BROCCOLI BEEF STIR-FRY

Prep Time: 10mints, Cook Time: 10mints, Total Time: 20mints; Serving: 2
Ingredients
- 1/2 lb. broccoli florets
- 1/2 lb. beef steak
- 2 Tsp Easy Stir-Fry Sauce
- 4 Tsp avocado oil
- Salt, pepper, and 1/4 onion

Instructions
1. Put 2 tsp of avocado oil into a skillet or pan on medium heat. Add the broccoli florets into the skillet and sauté until marginally delicate. Remove and put on a plate.
2. Add 2 more tsp of avocado oil into the skillet and turn the heat to high.
3. Add the onion and meat cuts and sauté until the hamburger is cooked. Add the broccoli and the pan-fried food sauce. Sautéed food for 2-3 additional minutes
4. Season with salt and pepper, to taste
Nutrition Fact: Calories: 573, Fat 51g, Carbs 9g, Sugar 3g, Protein 22g

CUBE STEAK

Prep Time: 2mins, Cook Time: 5mins, Total Time: 7mins; Serving: 1

Ingredients
- Cube Steak
- Seasoning of some kind
- Favorite kind of fat
- Salt + Pepper

Instructions
1. Gets a major oil skillet warming up with your preferred fat.
2. While that is warming, sprinkle your flavoring, salt + pepper on one side of the solid shape steak I attempt to do it while it's still in the bundle in the event that it'll fit since I loathe destroying an additional cutting board. Yet, in the event that you can't in the bundle, simply spread it out on a cutting board and you're good to go!
3. With a couple of tongs put the steaks prepared side down into the hot skillet w/liquefied fat.
4. While it begins to get all beautiful on that side, season the side confronting you.
5. Flip it over a few moments later, let it cook on the opposite side and blast. You're finished.

Nutrition Fact: Calories: 274, Fat 21g, Carbs 9g, Sugar 5g, Protein 29g

BEEF (HEART) STEAK

Prep Time: 20mints, Cooking Time: 15mints, Total Time: 35mints; Serving: 3

Ingredients
- 1 tsp ghee
- 4 slices of beef heart 1" thick
- 2 tsp rosemary-infused olive oil
- salt and pepper to taste

Instructions
1. Cheer up cuts from the marinade and pat dry.
2. Heat a cast-iron skillet with the ghee on a high fire for ⅔ minutes
3. Lay meat in the skillet. The temperature ought to be sufficiently high to sizzle.
4. Cook for 5 min on each side until pleasantly seared outwardly yet at the same time pink in the center.
5. Shower with the rosemary-injected olive oil.
6. Present with a plate of mixed greens of decision.

Nutrition Fact: Calories 241, Fat 13g, Carbs 5g, Sugar 7g, Protein 25g

KETO CORNED BEEF AND HASH RECIPE

Prep Time: 10mints, Cook Time: 15mints, Total Time: 25mints; Serving: 4

Ingredients
- 2 Tsp of olive oil
- 3 cloves of garlic and 4 green onions
- 3/4 lb. of cauliflower florets, processed into rice-like pieces
- 3/4 lb. of corned beef
- Salt and freshly ground black pepper

Instructions
1. Heat the olive oil in a significant nonstick box and fry the garlic till mollified.
2. Add the white portions of the reduce serving of mixed vegetable onions and cook for more than one moment earlier than together with the rice cauliflower.
3. Add the diced corned meat and tenderly crease through the combo, cooking until the corned hamburger has warmed through.
4. Taste the blend and change the flavoring with salt and newly ground darkish pepper.
5. Trimming the dish with the staying reduce inexperienced onions and serve.

Nutrition Fact: Calories: 307, Fat 25g, Carbs 5g, Sugar 2g, Protein 16g

KETO SOUS-VIDE FILLET STEAK RECIPE

Prep Time: 20mints, Cook Time: 50mints, Total Time: 1hr 10mints; Serving: 2

Ingredients
- 2 fillet steaks
- 3 Tsp of olive oil
- 2 sprigs of rosemary
- 2 sprigs of thyme
- Salt and freshly ground black pepper

Instructions
1. Fill a water shower with water and preheat it to 130°F.
2. Put each steak into singular sous-vide packs and add a tsp of olive oil, a twig of rosemary, and a spray of thyme into every sack.
3. Utilize a vacuum sealer to seal the two packs underneath complete weight.
4. Put the packs into the preheated water bathe, making sure they're absolutely submerged underneath the water. Leave within the water shower for 35mins.
5. Remove the sacks from the water bathe and allow resting for 10 minutes earlier than establishing.
6. To complete, heat a little olive oil in a skillet and once warm, singe the outside of the two steaks for 20-30 seconds on each side to get a few notable shading and caramelization
7. Season with salt and crisply floor dark pepper, serve quick with your selected aspect dish

Nutrition Fact: Calories: 512, Fat 47g, Carbs 0.6g, Sugar 0.2g, Protein 21g

KETO BEEF LIVER WITH ASIAN DIP

Prep Time: 10mints, Cook Time: 15mints, Total Time: 25mints; Serving: 10

Ingredients
- 1 lb. beef liver, whole
- 1/4 cup tamari sauce
- 2 cloves garlic
- 1 tsp fresh ginger

- 1 tsp sesame oil

Instructions
1. Put the meat liver into a pot secured with water and heat to the point of boiling. Bubble for 2-3 minutes and afterward pour the water with the filth out. Top off with new water and bubble for 10 minutes.
2. In the interim, make the plunge by combining all the plunge ingredients.
3. Let the hamburger liver cool, at that point cut it daintily and serve and enjoy with the plunge.

Nutrition Fact: Calories: 66, Fat 2g, Carbs 2g, Sugar 0.2g, Protein 9g

PAN SEARED DUCK BREAST

Prep Time: 15mints, Cooking Time: 20mints, Total Time: 35mints; Serving: 2

INGREDIENTS
- 1 medium duck breast
- Salt and pepper to taste

INSTRUCTIONS
1. Pat the duck breast dry. Cut the skin in a mismatched design with a sharp edge. This will help discharge the fat that is situated under the skin and will bring about a crispier skin.
2. Sprinkle the duck breast with salt and pepper, and place on a skillet, skin facing down. Turn the heat up to medium-heat and cook the duck breast until the skin turns golden and dark in color, which should take around 6-8 minutes, depending on the thickness of the skin.
3. Turn the breast over and cook for an extra 3 to 5 minutes (interior temperature should show 125°F – 130°F)
4. Remove the duck from the stove and let it lay on a cutting board, skin side up for around 5 minutes to rest.
5. Cut in slices and serve.

Nutrition Facts: Calories 460, Fat 36g, Carbs 0.2g, Sugars 0.4g, Protein 34g

KETO STEAK AU POIVRE

Prep Time: 5mints, Cook Time: 10mints, Total Time: 15mints; Serving: 1

Ingredients
- 1 filet mignon or similar steak
- 1 Tsp salt
- 2 Tsp peppercorns
- 1 sprig of thyme
- 2 cloves of garlic and 2 Tsp ghee

Instructions
1. Remove steaks from the cooler, season with salt and allow sit down for 30 minutes.
2. Pound the peppercorns, utilizing a mortar and pestle or a stage board or box.
3. Press the squashed peppercorns onto the 2 facets of the steak.
4. In a hot skillet, consist of the ghee, thyme, and garlic.
5. At the point whilst the ghee is hot, add the steak.
6. Cook the steak for 3-4mins for each side. This need to get it to medium-unusual

Nutrition Fact: Calories: 696, Fat 58g, Carbs 2g, Sugar 2g, Protein 42g

KETO OVEN-BAKED STEAK WITH GARLIC THYME PORTABELLA MUSHROOMS

Prep Time: 10mints, Cook Time: 15mints, Total Time: 25mints; Serving: 2

Ingredients
- 2 Tsp of olive oil
- 4 portabella mushrooms
- 4–6 sprigs of thyme
- 2 beef filet mignons
- 1 Tsp of garlic powder
- Salt and pepper

Instructions
1. Preheat stove to 320°F.
2. Put the portabella mushrooms on a lubed cooking plate and sprinkle a tsp of olive oil over it. Sprinkle the garlic powder equally over each of the four and dissipate over the picked thyme leaves. Season with salt and newly ground dark pepper and put in the stove for 15 minutes Season the steaks with salt.
3. Add one tsp olive oil to a huge griddle and singe the two sides of the steaks with the goal that a brilliant outside layer shapes on all sides. Put the steaks on a rimmed heating plate and put into the preheated stove for 8-10 minutes until the focal point of the steak arrives at 130 F for medium-uncommon or 140 F for medium.

Nutrition Fact: Calories: 733, Fat 56g, Carbs 10g, Sugar 1g, Protein 42g

KETO SOUS-VIDE FILLET STEAK RECIPE

Prep Time: 20mints, Cook Time: 50mints, Total Time: 1hr 10mints; Serving: 2

Ingredients
- 2 fillet steaks
- 2 Tsp of olive oil
- 2 sprigs of rosemary
- 2 sprigs of thyme
- 1 Tsp of olive oil
- Salt and freshly ground black pepper

Instructions
1. Fill a water shower with water and preheat it to 130°F.
2. Put every steak into singular sous-vide packs and add a tsp of olive oil, a sprig of rosemary.
3. Utilize a vacuum sealer to seal the two-packs under the complete weight.
4. Put the packs into the preheated water shower, guaranteeing they may be completely submerged below the water.
5. Leave in the water shower for 35mins.

6. Remove the packs from the water bathe and allow relaxation for 10mins before beginning.
7. To complete, warmness some olive oil in a dish and as soon as extremely hot, singe the exterior of the two steaks for 20-30 seconds on each facet to get some incredible shading and caramelization. Season with salt and obviously floor darkish pepper
Nutrition Fact: Calories: 512, Fat 47g, Carbs 0.5g, Sugar 01g, Protein 21g

TUSCAN-STYLE GRILLED RIB EYE STEAK

Prep Time: 5mints, Cook Time: 15mints, Total Time: 20mints; Servings: 4

Ingredients
- 2 Rib Eye Steaks
- 2 tbsp. Fresh Rosemary
- 2 Cloves Garlic
- 1/4 c. Extra Virgin Olive Oil
- 3 tbsp. Balsamic Vinegar
- 1 tsp. Kosher or Sea Salt and 1/2 tsp. Ground Black Pepper

Instructions
1. Add the rosemary, garlic, oil, vinegar, salt, and pepper to a little bowl and whisk together.
2. Add the steaks to a re-sealable plastic pack; at that point add the marinade blend. Seal the sack and coat the meat.
3. Refrigerate for in any event 2 hours or medium-term; at that point barbecue just as you would prefer.
Nutrition Fact: Calories: 321, Fat 12g, Carbs 15g, Sugar 8g, Protein 24g

CORNED BEEF AND CAULIFLOWER HASH

Prep Time: 20mints, Cooking Time: 15mints, Total Time: 35mints; Serving: 5

Ingredients
- 1 Tbsp olive oil
- 2 cups corned beef
- 2 cups raw cauli
- 1/2 cup chopped onion
- Salt & pepper

Instructions
1. Heat the olive oil in a medium sauté skillet, add the corned meat and cook for a couple of moments to render any fat out. Add the cauliflower and cook over medium heat for around 8 minutes, blending infrequently.
2. Add the onions and cook for an additional 5 minutes until relaxed and marginally caramelized.
3. Season with salt and pepper
Nutrition Fact: Calories: 135, Fat 8g, Carbs 6g, Sugar 4g, Protein 28g

EASY ZUCCHINI BEEF SAUTE, GARLIC, AND CILANTRO

Prep Time: 5mints, Cook Time: 10mints, Total Time: 15mints; Serving: 2

Ingredients
- 10 oz beef
- 1 zucchini
- 1/4 cup cilantro
- 3 cloves of garlic
- 2 Tsp gluten-free tamari sauce
- Avocado oil to cook with

Instructions
1. Put 2 Tsp of avocado oil into a griddle on high heat.
2. Add the pieces of meat into the griddle and sauté for a couple of moments on high heat.
3. At the point when the meat is caramelized, add the zucchini strips and keep sautéing.
4. At the point when the zucchini is delicate, add the tamari sauce, garlic, and cilantro.
5. Sauté for a few moments more and serve right away
Nutrition Fact: Calories: 500, Fat 40g, Carbs 5g, Sugar 2g, Protein 31g

EASY PALEO BROCCOLI BEEF RECIPE

Prep Time: 5mints, Cook Time: 15mints, Total Time: 20mints; Serving: 2

Ingredients
- 8oz or 2 cups of broccoli florets
- 1/2 lb. beef
- 3 cloves garlic
- 1 tsp freshly grated ginger
- 2 Tsp of coconut amino
- Coconut oil to cook in

Instructions
1. Put 2 Tsp of coconut oil into a skillet or pan on medium heat. Add the broccoli florets into the skillet.
2. At the point when the broccoli mollifies to the sum you need, add the meat.
3. Sauté for 2 minutes and afterward add the garlic, ginger, and coconut amino.
4. Serve right away.
Nutrition Fact: Calories: 132, Fat 6g, Carbs 13g, Sugar 4g, Protein 34g

LOW CARB PORK MEDALLIONS

Prep Time: 15mints, Cook Time: 20mints, Total Time: 35mints; Serving: 2

Ingredients
- 1 lb. pork tenderloin
- 3 medium shallots
- 1/4 cup oil

Instructions
1. Cut the red meat into half of inch thick cuts.
2. Cleave the shallots and notice them on a plate.
3. Warm the oil in a skillet
4. Press every bit of red meat into the shallots on the 2 aspects.
5. The shallots will adhere to the pork at the off chance which you press solidly.

6. Put the red meat cuts with shallots into the warm oil and cook till carried out.
7. You will find that a part of the shallots will eat at some point of cooking, but, they'll even now confer a heavenly taste to the red meat.
8. Panic don't as properly. Simply cook the beef until it's cooked through.
9. Present with vegetables.
Nutrition Facts: Calories 519, 36g, Fat 4g, Carbs 7g, Sugar 3g, Protein 46g

STUFFED PORK CHOPS – 5 INGREDIENTS

Prep Time: 5mints, Cook Time: 35mints, Total Time: 40mints; Servings: 6
Ingredients
- 12 thin-cut boneless pork chops
- 4 garlic cloves
- 1 1/2 tsp salt
- 2 cups baby spinach
- 12 slices provolone cheese

Instructions
1. Preheat the stove to 350.
2. Spread the garlic rub on one facet of the beef cleaves. Flip 6 hacks garlic side down onto a large rimmed making a ready sheet.
3. Gap the spinach between the ones 6 hacks. Overlap the cheddar cuts into identical components and placed them over the spinach.
4. Put a next pork hack over every with the garlic side up.
5. Heat for 20 minutes. Spread each pork cleaves with some other cut of cheddar.
6. Back for an extra 10-15 minutes or until the meat is 160 tiers whilst checked with a meat thermometer.
Nutrition Facts: Calories 436, Fat 25g, Carbs 2g, Sugar 7g, Protein 47g

CHIPOTLE STEAK BOWL

Prep Time: 15mints, Cook Time: 8mints, Total Time: 23mints; Servings: 6
Ingredients
- 16 oz. skirt steak
- 1 homemade guacamole
- 4 oz. pepper jack cheese and salt
- 1 cup sour cream
- 1 handful fresh cilantro
- 1 spray Chipotle Tabasco Sauce

Instructions
1. Season the steak with salt and pepper to flavor and warm up a cast-iron skillet on extremely high heat.
2. While it's heating, place the steak for 3-4 mins on every side.
3. Prepare the guacamole according to our Homemade Guacamole recipe.
4. Cut the steak contrary to what would be expected into small strips and partition into 4 divides.
5. Shred the pepper jack cheese utilizing a cheese grater and top every phase of the steak.
6. Add around 1/4 cup of guacamole to every section, followed by 1/4 cup of sour cream.
Nutrition Fact: Calories 180; Fat 6g, Carbs 9g, Sugar 7g, Protein 24g

BACON-WRAPPED PORK CHOPS

Prep Time: 10mints, Cook Time: 30mints, Total Time: 40mints ; Serving: 4
Ingredients
- 12 oz bacon package
- 6 to 8 boneless pork chops
- Salt and pepper

Instructions
1. Preheat your stove to 350 degrees and line a oven tray with parchment paper.
2. On a plate or cutting board fixed with paper towels, design your pork hacks and top them with new pepper.
3. Wrap every pork slash in uncooked bacon cuts.
4. Put every bacon-wrapped pork hack onto the oven tray.
5. Crush extra pepper over the highest point of the now bacon-wrapped pork cleaves.
6. Heat them for 30 minutes, flipping them at the 15-minute imprint. Serve promptly and serve and enjoy it!
Nutrition Fact: Calories: 35, Fat 2.8g, Carbs 0.4g, Sugar 1.4g, Protein 8g

SLOW COOKER KETO CORNED BEEF CABBAGE

Prep Time: 6mints, Cook Time: 6hrs, Total Time: 6hrs 6mints; Servings: 8
Ingredients
- 3 lb. corned beef brisket
- ½ large onion and 1 large carrot
- 3 ribs celery stalks
- ½ head of green cabbage
- 4 cups of water

Instructions
1. Add corned meat brisket and the flavors to a moderate cooker.
2. Pour 4 cups or enough water over brisket to simply cover the entire dish.
3. Add onions, carrots, and celery. Cover and moderate cook on low for 6 to 8 hours or on high for 4 to 5 hours
4. Add cabbage the last half hour of cooking time, Cover and keep on cooking the staying 30 minutes.
5. Evacuate vegetables and cabbage with an opened spoon from a slow cooker to deplete abundance fluid.
6. Evacuate corned hamburger and cut contrary to what would be expected. Serve.

Nutrition Fact: Calories: 158, Fat 6g, Carbs 4g, Sugar 1g, Protein 27g

SHREDDED TACO PORK

Prep Time: 10mints, Cook Time: 9hrs, Total Time: 9hrs 10mints; Serving: 10

Ingredients
- 2 cups chicken stock
- 4 pounds pork roast
- 1/4 cup grass-fed butter
- 1 batch homemade taco seasoning

Instructions
1. Heat moderate cooker on low setting
2. To the slight cooker, encompass chicken stock, beef meal, unfold and taco flavoring.
3. Cover and prepare dinner on low for 8-10 hours.
4. Utilize forks to shred the beef.

Nutrition Fact: Calories: 411.1, Fat 29g, Carbs 1.6g, Sugar 0.3g, Protein 33g

KALUA PORK

Prep Time: 5mints. Cook Time: 1hr 30mints. Total Time: 1hrs 35mints ; Serving: 4

Ingredients
- 4 pounds of pork shoulder
- 1 to 2 tablespoons oil
- 1/2 cup water
- 1 tablespoon hickory liquid smoke
- 2 teaspoons coarse kosher salt

Instructions
1. Select Sauté to preheat the pot. At the point when hot, including the oil and dark-colored every 50% of the meal independently. Darker every 50% of the pork broil on the two sides, around 3 minutes for each side. Evacuate to a platter when cooked.
2. Turn the weight cooker off, and add water and fluid smoke to the cooking pot. Mix to remove any caramelized bits from the base of the pot. Add the sautéed pork and any aggregated juices. Sprinkle the salt over the highest point of the pork cooks.
3. Lock the cover set up. Select High Pressure and an hour and a half cook time.
4. At the point when the clock sounds, utilize a characteristic weight discharge. At the point when the valve, drops cautiously evacuate the top.
5. Remove the meat from the weight cooker and shred with two forks.

Nutrition Fact: Calories: 117, Fat 10g, Carbs 4g, Sugar 1g, Protein 6g

COFFEE BARBECUE PORK BELLY

Prep Time: 15mints, Cook Time: 60mints, Total Time: 1hr 15mints; Serving: 4

Ingredients
- 1 1/2 cups beef stock
- 2 pounds of pork belly
- 4 tablespoons olive oil
- 1 batch Low Carb Barbecue Dry Rub
- 2 tablespoons Instant Espresso Powder

Instructions
1. Preheat the stove to 350°F.
2. Heat the hamburger stock in a little pan over medium heat until hot yet not bubbling
3. In a little bowl, combine the grill dry rub and coffee powder until very much joined.
4. Put the pork midsection, skin side up in a shallow dish and sprinkle 2 tablespoons of the olive oil over top, scouring it over the whole pork tummy.
5. Sprinkle the rub everywhere throughout the pork gut and focus on well to uniformly circulate.
6. Pour the hot stock around the pork midsection and spread the dish firmly with aluminum foil. Prepare for 45 minutes. Cut into 8 thick cuts.
7. Heat the staying olive oil in a skillet over medium-high heat and singe each cut for 3 minutes on each side or until the ideal degree of freshness is come to.

Nutrition Fact: Calories: 644, Fat 68g, Carbs 3.4g, Sugar 0.8g, Protein 24g

LOW CARB TORTILLA PORK RIND WRAPS

Prep Time: 10mints, Cook Time: 30mints, Total Time: 40mints; Serving: 8 wraps

Ingredients
- 4 large eggs
- 3 ounces pork rinds
- 1/2 teaspoon garlic powder
- 1/4 teaspoon ground cumin
- 1/4 to 1/2 cup water
- Avocado oil or coconut oil

Instructions
1. In a powerful blender or nourishment processor, add the eggs, pork skins, garlic powder, and cumin. Mix until smooth and very much joined. Add 1/4 cup of the water and mix once more. On the off chance that the blend is extremely thick, keep on including water until it is the consistency of hotcake hitter.
2. Heat a sparse 1/2 teaspoon of oil in an 8-inch nonstick skillet over medium-low heat, add around 3 tablespoons of the hitter and utilize an elastic spatula to spread it meagerly over the base of the dish, nearly to the edges.
3. Cook for about a moment, until the base is starting to dark-colored.
4. Repeat with the rest of the player, adding oil to the skillet just as essential
5. Add more water to the player as required; it will thicken as it sits.

Nutrition Fact: Calories: 94, Fat 5.6g, Carbs 0.4g, Sugar 0.2g, Protein 9.7g

KETO CHILI DOG POT PIE CASSEROLE

Prep Time: 15mints, Cooking Time: 35mints, Total Time: 50mints; Serving: 4

Ingredients
- One batch Kickin' Chili

- 2 tbsp butter
- 8 grass-fed beef hot dogs
- 1 1/2 cups cheddar cheese
- 1 1/2 cups mozzarella cheese

Instructions
1. Set up the bean stew early. You can definitely decrease the cooking time of this formula by changing over the bean stew to a stovetop formula.
2. Heat the margarine in a huge ovenproof skillet over medium heat. When the margarine is dissolved and the skillet is hot, add the cut wieners to the container and cook until they have a pleasant burn on them.
3. Pour the whole bunch of bean stew over the cooked franks.
4. Blend the cheddar and mozzarella cheeses and sprinkle them over top of the stew.
5. Set up the roll mixture as indicated by the headings
6. Preheat stove to 350°
7. Drop huge scoops of the bread mixture over the dish.
8. Prepare for 30 minutes or until the bread beating is brilliant darker.

Nutrition Fact: Calories: 500, Fat 40g, Carbs 11g, Sugar 1g, Protein 25g

KETO BARBECUE DRY RUB RIBS

Prep Time: 20mints, Cook Time: 2hrs 30mints, Total Time: 2hrs 50mints; Serving: 6

Ingredients
- 2 pounds pork baby back ribs
- 2 tablespoons olive oil
- 1 batch Barbecue Dry Rub

Instructions
1. Preheat the stove to 300°F. Line a rimmed making ready sheet with aluminum foil.
2. Remove the moderate layer from the lower back, or sunken side, of the ribs.
3. Start by means of slicing into the film with a pointy blade, at that factor pulls the pores and skin away from the ribs.
4. Pour the dry rub over the ribs and work it equally onto the two facets.
5. Prepare until the ribs are delicate and scrumptious within and respectable and sparkling outwardly around 2 half hours.
6. The keep remains within the cooler for so long as multi-week

Nutrition Fact: Calories: 400, Fat 43g, Carbs 3.8g, Sugar 1g, Protein 43g

EASY KETO INSTANT POT CHILE VERDE

Prep Time: 10mints, Cook Time: 40mints, Total Time: 55mints; Servings: 6

Ingredients
- 2 lbs. pork shoulder
- ½ tbsp avocado oil
- tsp sea salt and ½ tsp black pepper
- ½ cup salsa Verde
- cup chicken broth

Instructions
1. When the Instant pot is hot, singe red meat portions on all sides till cooked for around three to four minutes for each aspect.
2. In a huge bowl add salsa Verde and bird soup and mix.
3. Close and lock the cover. Turn the load discharge handle to Sealing.
4. When cooking time is finished, allow the load Naturally Release for 10mins and later on Quick Release the relaxation of the load.
5. When all weight is discharged, remove the cover.
6. Add the destroyed pork back to the sauce inside the Instant Pot, mix to sign up for and serve.

Nutrition Fact: Calories: 342, Fat 22g, Carbs 6g, Sugar 4g, Protein 32g

GARLIC BUTTER BAKED PORK CHOPS

Prep Time: 5mints, Cook Time: 18mints, Total Time: 23mints; Serving: 2

Ingredients
- 2 medium-sized pork chops
- kosher salt and freshly ground black pepper
- 4 tsp butter
- 1 tsp fresh thyme and 2 cloves garlic
- 1 tsp extra virgin olive oil

Instructions
1. Preheat stove to 375°F.
2. Season the pork with salt and pepper
3. In a cast-iron skillet, heat the olive oil over medium heat.
4. At the point when the skillet is extremely hot, add the pork cleaves.
5. Singe until brilliant, around 2 minutes for each side.
6. Pour the garlic spread blend over the pork slashes.
7. Put the skillet in the stove, and cook until the pork slashes arrive at an inner temperature of 145ºF, around 10-12 minutes.
8. Remove from the stove. Utilizing a spoon, pour a portion of the margarine sauce left in the skillet onto the pork slashes before serving.

Nutrition Fact: Calories: 371, Fat 35g, Carbs 1g, Sugar 1g, Protein 14g

STUFFED PORK CHOPS WITH BACON AND GOUDA

Prep Time: 10mints, Cook Time: 30mints, Total Time: 40mints; Servings: 4

Ingredients
- 4 2 inches thick boneless pork
- 4 slices thick-cut bacon
- 4 ounces Smoked gouda
- salt and pepper

Instructions

1. Preheat stove to 375F
2. Cut a wide opening into the side of every pork slash.
3. Cut the cut as wide and strip as you can without slicing through.
4. Season the exterior with salt and pepper.
5. Generally, blend the cooled bacon in with the Gouda and stuff into the pork hacks.
6. Put the pork cleaves stuffing side up on a stove-safe dish and puts a stove safe inside kitchen thermometer test into the thickest piece of the pork hacks.
7. Heat until the thermometer peruses 145F. Remove from the stove and let rest for 10 minutes. Serve.

Nutrition Fact: Calories: 280, Fat 31g, Carbs 2.8g, Sugar 2.2g, Protein 1g

ROSEMARY GARLIC BUTTER PORK CHOPS

Prep Time: 5mints, Cook Time: 25mints, Total Time: 30mints ; Serving: 3

Ingredients
- 3 Boneless Pork Chops
- 4 tbsp butter and 3 cloves Garlic
- 1 tsp Garlic Powder
- 1 tsp dried thyme
- 1 tsp Dried Rosemary
- Salt and pepper

Instructions
1. Start via flavoring the pork hacks on either side with salt and put them into a medium nonstick griddle and burn over medium to high heat.
2. Add the spread, thyme, rosemary; garlic powder and treat the pork on each side cooking till never again pink.
3. During the last moment of cooking add the minced garlic, sauté for one moment till fragrant.
4. When the pork slashes have completely cooked, place on a plate and enable them to sit for 5 minutes before serving. Serve and enjoy!

Nutrition Fact: Calories: 460, Fat 34g, Carbs 2g, Sugar 0.2g, Protein 37g

PECAN CRUSTED PORK CHOPS

Prep Time: 10mints, Cook Time: 30mints, Total Time: 40mints ; Serving: 6

Ingredients
- pounds boneless pork chops
- 1/4 cup Dijon mustard
- 2 cups pecans
- 2 large eggs
- 2-3 tablespoons olive oil

Instructions
1. Preheat stove to 350
2. Empty the walnuts into a nourishment processor and blend until you have got a decent piece consistency.
3. Dunk every red meat cleaver inside the egg, at that point the walnut combination.
4. Press the walnuts into the red meat cleaves gently to guarantee a first-rate robust hull.
5. Put your breaded red meat cleaves within the cooler for 10 minutes; I suppose this serves to really seal the overlaying so the walnuts stay on better.
6. Be that as it can, within the occasion which you are missing in time you may skirt this progression.
7. Preheat a skillet to medium warm temperature with the olive oil.
8. Cook two pork slashes one after some other within the skillet, 1-2 minutes on each side.
9. Put skillet singed pork hacks on a heating sheet and prepares dinner 15-20mins.

Nutrition Fact: Calories: 625, Fat 51.4g, Carbs 8g, Sugar 2g, Protein 38.5g

STUFFED PORK CHOPS – 5 INGREDIENTS

Prep Time: 5mints, Cook Time: 35mints, Total Time: 40mints; Servings: 6 stuffed pork chops

Ingredients
- 12- thin-cut boneless pork chops
- 4- garlic cloves
- 1 1/2- tsp salt
- 2- cups baby spinach
- 12- slices provolone cheese

Instructions
1. Preheat the stove to 350.
2. Press the garlic cloves thru a garlic press into a bit bowl. Add the salt and blend to join.
3. Spread the garlic rub on one facet of the red meat hacks. Flip 6 slashes garlic aspect down onto a large rimmed heating sheet.
4. Separation of the spinach among the ones 6 cleaves.
5. Overlap the cheddar cuts fifty-fifty and put them over the spinach. Put a subsequent beef cleave over each with the garlic aspect up.
6. Prepare for 20mins. Spread each red meat cut down with any other cut of cheddar.
7. Back for a further 10-15mins or until the beef is a hundred and sixty levels when checked with a meat thermometer.

Nutrition Facts: Calories 436, Fat 25g, Carbs 2g, Sugar 1.3g, Protein 47g

POT PORK CHOPS DINNER

Prep Time: 20mints, Cooking Time: 30mints, Total Time: 50mints; Serving: 6

Ingredients
- 2- lbs. sliced boneless pork chops
- Can of Diced Tomatoes
- Can of Tomato Sauce
- 16 oz bag of frozen green beans
- tsp Italian Seasoning
- tsp Garlic Salt

Instructions

1. Put pork cleaves in the Instant Pot. Pork slashes can be solidified in the event that you might want.
2. Put the green beans on top. Dump the tomatoes and tomato sauce on top.
3. Sprinkle in the seasonings. Add the top, lock, and set to ingredient.
4. Set the strain to 30 minutes. Do a brisk discharge. Mix and serve and enjoy it!
5. Salt and Pepper to taste.
Nutrition Facts: Calories 282, Fat 10g, Carbs 10g, Sugar 5g, Protein 35g

CRISPY PORK CHOPS KETO
Prep Time: 5mints, Cook Time: 12mints, Total Time: 17mints, Servings: 6
Ingredients
- 1 1/2 lbs. boneless pork chops
- 1/3 cup Almond Flour
- 1/4 cup grated Parmesan cheese
- 1 tsp garlic powder and 1 tsp Paprika
- 1 tsp Tony Chachere's Creole Seasoning

Instructions
1. Preheat your air fryer to 360 degrees F
2. In the meantime, place all ingredients, besides pork chops, into a large zip lock sack.
3. Put the pork chops into the sack and seal it, and later on shake to marinate the pork chops
4. Remove from the sack and place in fryer in a solitary layer. Cook for 8-12mins relying on the thickness of your red meat chops.
Nutrition Fact: Calories: 231, Fat 12g, Carbs 2g, Sugar 2g, Protein 27g

CARAMELIZED ONION AND BACON PORK CHOPS
Prep Time: 40mints, Cooking Time: 10mints, Total Time: 50mints, Serving: 4
Ingredients
- 4 oz. bacon
- 1 yellow onion
- ¼ tsp salt, ¼ tsp pepper, and 4 pork chops
- ½ cup chicken broth
- ¼ cup heavy whipping cream

Instructions
1. In a huge skillet, cook bacon over medium heat until fresh. Utilizing an opened spoon, remove to a bowl and save bacon oil.
2. Add onion to bacon oil and season with salt and pepper. Cook, blending every now and again, for 15 to 20 minutes, until onions are delicate and brilliant dark-colored, adds onions to bacon in the bowl.
3. Increment heat to medium-high and sprinkle pork cleaves with salt and pepper. Add slashes to containers and dark-colored on the primary side for 3 minutes. Flip slashes and decrease heat to medium, cooking on the second side until inside temperature arrives at 135° F, around 7 to 10 additional minutes.
4. Add soup to the skillet and scrape up any cooked bits. Add cream and stew until the blend is thickened, 2 or 3 minutes. Return onions and bacon to dish and mix to join. Top pork cleaves with onion and bacon blend and serve.
Nutrition Fact: Calories: 113, Fat 6.9g, Carbs 6.8g, Sugar 4.3g, Protein: 7.9g

KETO PORK BELLY
Prep Time: 10mints, Cooking Time: 2hrs, Total Time: 2hrs 10mints, Serving: 8
Ingredients
- 2lb. pork belly
- 2 teaspoons salt
- ½ tsp coarse ground mixed pepper
- 2 teaspoons olive oil

Instructions:
1. Preheat stove to 450F.
2. Cut the pork with a sharp blade. Season with salt and pepper.
3. Put the pork right onto a broiling plate for 30 minutes or until the skin is wrinkled.
4. Decrease temperature to 320F and leave to simmer for 1 hour 15 minutes.
5. Leave the pork meat to rest for 20mins, then serve.
Nutrition Fact: Calories 264, Fat 9g, Carbs 8g, Sugar 5g, Protein 27g

LEMON PEPPER PORK CHOPS
Prep Time: 10mints, Cooking Time: 15mints, Total Time: 25mints, Serving: 4
Ingredients
- 4 pork chops
- 1 tsp salt
- 2 tsp lemon pepper
- 2 tbsp oil

Instructions
1. With a paper towel, smudge the outside of the pork chops to remove dampness. Sprinkle the salt and lemon pepper on the pork and leave to sit on for 30 minutes.
2. Put oil in large skillet and heat over medium-high temp.
3. Put pork in the dish and allow to cook on each side for around 3-4 minutes, until it turns dark in color.
4. Remove skillet from the heat and allow the pork chops to sit and steam for 8-10 minutes before serving.
5. Presenting with crisp lemon cuts and herbs
Nutrition Fact: Calories: 132, Fat 6g, Carbs 3.3g, sugar 2.3g, Protein 28g

BONELESS PORK CHOPS RECIPE
Prep Time: 5mints, Cook Time: 5mints, Total Time: 10mints, Serving: 6
Ingredients

- 1 tablespoon coconut oil
- 4-6 boneless pork chops
- 1 stick of butter
- 1 package of ranch mix
- 1 cup of water

Instructions
1. Put the pork in the Instant pot with a tablespoon of coconut oil. Turn on the sauté setting until it turns dark in color on both sides.
2. Put the spread on top and sprinkle the ranch mix on top.
3. Pour water over the pork. Put the cover on and leave for ingredients to set in.
4. Fasten the lid and set it to 5 minutes.
5. Leave to discharge pressure for 5 minutes.
6. When cooked, serve.

Nutrition Facts: Calories 372, Fat 23g, Carbs 4g, Sugar 2g, Protein 38g

SLOW COOKER KETO MEATBALLS

Prep Time: 20mints, Cooking Time: 5hrs, Total Time: 5hrs 20mints, Serving: 4

Ingredients:
- 3lbs Ground Beef
- 1/4 cup spinach
- 1 tsp garlic salt, pepper, and 2 onions
- oil
- favorite pasta sauce

Instructions
1. In a bowl, place the ground meat, spinach, onion, garlic salt, salt, and pepper.
2. Combine all well with your hands.
3. Structure little meatballs and put on a plate.
4. In the interim, heat oil in a dish
5. Put Meatballs in the base of moderate heat
6. Spread with sauce of your choice
7. Cook on low for 4-5 hours.

Nutrition Fact: Calories: 324, Fat 14g, Carbs 12g, Sugar 8g, Protein 43g

EASY ZUCCHINI BEEF SAUTE, GARLIC, AND CILANTRO

Prep Time: 5mints, Cook Time: 10mints, Total Time: 15mints, Serving: 2

Ingredients
- 10 oz beef
- 1 zucchini
- 1/4 cup cilantro
- 3 cloves of garlic
- 2 Tsp gluten-free tamari sauce
- Avocado oil to cook with

Instructions
1. Put 2 Tsp of avocado oil into a griddle on high heat.
2. Add the pieces of meat into the griddle and sauté for a couple of moments on high heat.
3. At the point when the meat is caramelized, add the zucchini strips and keep sautéing.
4. At the point when the zucchini is delicate, add the tamari sauce, garlic, and cilantro.
5. Sauté for a few moments more and serve right away.

Nutrition Fact: Calories: 500, Fat 40g, Carbs 5g, Sugar 2g, Protein 31g

EASY KETO BROCCOLI BEEF RECIPE

Prep Time: 5mints, Cook Time: 15mints, Total Time: 20mints, Serving: 2

Ingredients
- 8oz or 2 cups of broccoli florets
- 1/2 lb beef
- 3 cloves garlic
- 1 tsp freshly grated ginger
- 2 Tsp of coconut amino
- Coconut oil to cook in

Instructions
1. Put 2 Tsp of coconut oil into a skillet or pan on medium heat. Add the broccoli florets into the skillet.
2. At the point when the broccoli mollifies to the sum you need, add the meat.
3. Sauté for 2 minutes and afterward add the garlic, ginger, and coconut amino.
4. Serve right away.

Nutrition Fact:: Calories: 132, Fat 6g, Carbs 13g, Sugar 4g, Protein 34g

THE BEST BUNLESS BURGER RECIPE BURGERS

Prep Time: 5mints, Cook Time: 10mints, Total Time: 15mints, Servings: 3

Ingredients
- 1 pound ground beef
- 1 tsp Worcestershire sauce
- 1 tsp Montreal Steak Seasoning
- Salt and pepper and 4 ounces the onion
- 2 tsps bacon drippings

Instructions
1. Blend tenderly together with your hands to bring the flavoring and shape into 3 balls. Tenderly press/pat into patties.
2. Oil the mesh. Season the burger patties with a light sprinkling of salt and pepper.
3. Present with your selected additional objects, however, do not forget to tally the carbs.
4. Heat 1 tablespoon of oil over medium-low flame, and when hot, add the onions and sauté until brown. Add half a teaspoon of erythritol and cook till it turns dark in color. This development can take as long as 10mins.

Nutrition Facts: Calories 479, Fat 40g, Carbs 2g, Sugar 1.3g, Protein 26g

KETO SLOW COOKER ONIONS

Prep Time: 40mints, Cooking Time: 6hrs, Total Time: 6hrs 40mints, Serving: 3

Ingredients

- 4 large onions
- 4 Tbsp butter
- 1/4 cup coconut amino
- Salt and pepper

Instructions
1. Cut the onions into 1/4" cuts and put into the bowl of a moderate cooker,
2. Top with the spread and coconut amino
3. Cook on low for 6-8 hours
4. Serve over flame-broiled pork hacks, chicken, pulled pork, or as a side dish

Nutrition Fact: Calories: 102, Fat 8g, Carbs 2g, Sugar 1g, Protein 4g

LAMB LOLLIPOPS WITH GARLIC AND ROSEMARY RECIPE

Prep Time: 10mints, Cook Time: 10mints, Total Time: 20mints; Serving: 2

Ingredients
- 8 lamb lollipops
- 2 garlic cloves
- 2–3 tablespoons olive oil
- 2–3 sprigs of fresh rosemary
- salt and pepper to taste

Instruction
1. Season every part of the lamb generously with salt and pepper.
2. Add a little rosemary onto each facet of the sheep lollipops.
3. Heat olive oil in a cast-iron skillet on a medium-high temperature. When hot, add garlic and a sprinkle of rosemary into the skillet and spread similarly.
4. Add the lamb and cook for 4-5 minutes on each side.
5. Serve right away.

Nutrition Fact: Calories: 117, Fat 10g, Carbs 4g, Sugar 1g, Protein 6g

GRILLED LAMB IN PALEO MINT CREAM SAUCE

Prep Time: 20mints, Cooking Time: 25mints, Total Time: 45mints; Serving: 4

Ingredients
- 1 rack of lamb
- 2 tbsp. fresh chopped dill
- 1/4 cup fresh mint
- 2 tbsp red pepper
- 1 tbsp lemon juice
- 1/8 cup coconut cream

Instructions
1. Add dill, mint, red pepper, lemon juice and coconut cream.
2. Blend well and refrigerate until prepared to serve
3. Give your lamb a chance to rest out before grilling; room temperature.
4. Fire up the grill, you need to cook the lamb quickly and at high heat to keep the juices in.
5. Put the rack on a hot barbecue and close the cover, cook approx. 4 min
6. Utilizing tongs to flip the meat
7. Plate and add a smidge of sauce on top

Nutrition Fact: Calories: 426, Fat 38g, Carbs 3g, Sugar 2g, Protein 17g

GRILLED LAMB CHOPS WITH DIJON-BASIL BUTTER

Prep Time: 10mints, Cooking Time: 10mints, Total Time: 20mints; Serving: 4

Ingredients
- 4 – 6 center-cut lamb chops
- 1 tbs olive oil
- 1/2 tsp garlic powder
- 1 tbs fresh basil and 1 clove garlic
- 1 tsp Dijon-style mustard
- 2 tbs soft butter

Instructions
1. Sprinkle chops with garlic powder, shower with oil and permit to sit until prepared to cook.
2. Cook on grill barbecue over medium-high heat for 2 – 5 minutes on every side.
3. Return them on grill if you feel they need more time to cook
4. Once cooked, add basil butter on top of each lamb chop and serve.

Dijon-Basil Butter:
Put garlic and basil into a little bowl, add mustard, butter and blend well. It very well may be made ahead, molded into a log, chilled and cut before putting on chops.

Nutrition Fact: Calories: 280, Fat 31g, Carbs 2.8g, Sugar 2.2g, Protein 1g

GARLIC & ROSEMARY LAMB CHOPS

Prep Time: 10mints, Cooking Time: 10mints, Total Time: 20mints; Servings: 6

Ingredients
- 8 Grass-fed Australian Lamb Chops
- 2 Tbsp Olive Oil
- 3 Garlic cloves
- Tbsp fresh Rosemary
- Tbsp Coarse Sea Salt

Instructions
1. Remove the leaves from the rosemary and generally chop it. I like to add mine with the coarse sea salt in a container and afterward jumble them, so the ocean salt takes on the oils for the rosemary that way it soaks the flavors into the meat.
2. Strip and mince the garlic.
3. Rub the lamb chops down with the ocean salt, rosemary, and garlic and afterward let sit, at room temperature for about 30 minutes.
4. Heat a dish enormous enough for the entire meat on the stove over medium heat, while the container is warming, just before cooking, rub the

lamb chops down with olive oil. When hot, add the meat to the stove.

5. Cook on each side for 3-4 minutes and make ensure that your dish is hot before you add the meat.
Nutrition Fact: Calories: 113, Fat 6.9g, Carbs 6.8g, Sugar 4.3g, Protein: 7.9g

GREEK LAMB CHOP MARINADE

Prep Time: 4hrs, Cooking Time: 2hrs, Total Time: 6hrs; Serving: 4
Ingredients
- 2- tsp Olive Oil
- 2- tsp Red Wine Vinegar
- 1/2- tsp Majoram
- 1/2- tsp Rosemary
- 1/2- tsp dried parsley
- 1/2- tsp Sea Salt, 1/4- tsp Pepper

Instructions
1. Add all marinade ingredients together.
2. Marinade 4 Lamb Chops for 4-12 hours.
3. Remove excessive marinade and flame grill lamb chops over high heat until cooked as wanted.
Nutrition Fact: Calories: 321, Fat 9g, Carbs 14g, Sugar 4.1g, Protein 24g

LAMB, RED ONION AND HERB KOFTAS

Prep Time: 35mints, Cooking Time: 45mints, Total Time: 1hr 20mints; Serving: 4
Ingredients
- 515g pack lamb minced
- red onion and 2 cloves garlic
- 5- fresh mint leaves
- 6-7 fresh parsley leaves
- Pinch of salt
- medium-sized wooden skewers

Instructions
1. Put the minced lamb into a bowl and mash in the red onion and garlic. Add the crushed herbs and the salt and delicately blend in with your hands.
2. Heat a frying pan or skillet to medium heat. Get a skewer with one hand and with the other hand get a little bunch of the lamb blend. Shape the meat around the skewer, pressing it so it's a uniform thickness all throughout, Put tenderly into the warmed skillet. Repeat with the remainder of the blend.
3. Turn the koftas normally, so they darken in color on all sides and keep on cooking for 10-12 minutes until no pinkness is gone.
4. Don't have skewers? Simply structure them into burgers and fry for 5-6 minutes on each side.
Nutrition Fact: Calories 264, Fat 9g, Carbs 8g, Sugar 5g, Protein 27g

SAUSAGE KALE SOUP WITH MUSHROOM

Prep Time: 10mints, Cook Time: 1hr, Total Time: 1hr 10mints; Servings: 6
Ingredients
- 29 ounces of chicken bone broth
- ounces fresh kale
- 1 pound sausage
- ounces sliced mushrooms
- 2 cloves garlic
- Salt & Pepper to taste

Instructions
1. Put the two jars of chicken stock in an enormous pot alongside two jars worth of water. Heat to the point of boiling over medium heat
2. Add the kale, sausage, mushrooms, and garlic. Season for taste with salt and pepper
3. Stew over low heat for about 60 minutes.
Nutrition Fact: Calories: 259, Fat 20g, Carbs 4g, Sugar 4g, Protein 14g

LAMB & LEEK BURGERS WITH LEMON CREAM

Prep Time: 15mints, Cooking Time: 20mints, Total Time: 35mints; Serving: 4
Ingredients
- 454g ground lamb
- 45g leeks
- 5g garlic powder and 1/2 tsp sea salt
- 120 ml coconut cream and 1 tbl coconut oil
- 5g lemon zest

Instructions
1. Add the crushed leeks and 1/2 of the coconut oil to a dish and cook over medium heat till the leeks are mollified, around 3 – 5 minutes.
2. Move the leeks to a bowl to cool. In a 2nd large bowl, cover the ground lamb with garlic powder and salt.
3. When the leeks are cool, add to the meat bowl and mix delicately until the combination is mixed. Partition into 4 patties
4. Add the rest of the coconut oil to a skillet. Over low-medium warmness, add the patties and cook evenly till completely seared, around 5mins for every area. Ensure the lamb is cooked thoroughly.
5. Utilize a smaller than regular nourishment processor to add the blended coconut cream and lemon zest.
Nutrition Fact: Calories: 696, Fat 58g, Carbs 2g, Sugar 0.3g, Protein 42g

GUILT-FREE SLOW COOKED SHOULDER OF LAMB

Prep Time: 5mints, Cook Time: 5hrs, Total Time: 5hrs 5mints; Serving: 4
Ingredients
- 500 g Lamb Shoulder
- 1 Tbsp Olive Oil
- Handful Fresh Rosemary
- Salt & Pepper

Instructions
1. Put the olive oil at the base of the tray and utilizing your hand to move it around with the goal that the entire of base is covered in it.
2. Cover the lamb shoulder with salt and pepper so all sides are seasoned

3. Put the lamb in the cooker and sprinkle the rosemary over the meat.
4. Put the cooker on low heat and cook for 5 hours or until delicate.
5. Leave it to set for 15 minutes, then cut with a sharp blade and serve.
Nutrition Fact: Calories: 134, Fat 7g, Carbs 0.2g, Sugar 0.1g, Protein 15g

ONE-POT BRAISED LAMB WITH CARAMELIZED ONIONS AND ROSEMARY

Prep Time: 30mints, Cooking Time: 2hrs 10mints, Total Time: 2hrs 40mints; Serving: 4

Ingredients
- 2 lbs lamb loin and 3 tbsp olive oil
- 1 1/2 tsp sea salt
- 4-5 large cloves garlic
- 1 1/2 tbsp fresh rosemary
- 1 large sweet onion

Instructions
1. Put the lamb loin on an giant plate and pat dry with a paper towel. Coat the 2 sides with 1 tablespoon of the olive oil.
2. Sprinkle the 2 facets with salt and pat the squashed garlic and fresh rosemary onto both sides as well.
3. Place a tablespoon of olive oil inside the base of an enormous soup pot or Dutch stove.
4. Put half of the onions within the base of the container, and allow the lamb to set on the onions. Shower the top with the final tablespoon of olive oil.
5. Place the pot on the stove over medium-low heat. Cook for 2 hours or till meat is easy to cut with a fork

Nutrition Fact: Calories: 117, Fat 10g, Carbs 4g, Sugar 1g, Protein 6g

SIDE DISHES & SNACKS RECIPES

KETO JALAPENO POPPERS

Prep Time: 10mints, Cook Time: 20mints, Total Time: 30mints, Serving: 16

Ingredients
- 8 oz cream cheese
- 1/2 cup shredded sharp cheddar cheese
- 1 tsp pink Himalayan salt
- 1/2 tsp black pepper
- 8 jalapenos, halved, de-seeded
- 8 slices of bacon, cut in half

Instructions
1. Preheat stove to 375 degrees and line heating sheet with parchment paper.
2. Place bacon cuts on paper towel-lined plate and microwave for 3 minutes. Put aside to cool.
3. In a medium bowl, add cream cheddar, destroyed sharp cheddar, salt, and pepper and microwave for 15 seconds. Mix together
4. Cautiously scoop cream cheddar blend into a plastic baggie
5. Wrap bacon cuts around jalapenos and stick with a toothpick.
6. Put jalapenos on arranged heating sheet and prepare for 15 minutes.
7. Leave stove heat to cook and sear for 2-3 minutes, watching to guarantee cream cheddar doesn't get consumed.
8. Remove from stove and permit cooling marginally before eating.

Nutrition Fact: Calories: 79, Fat 6.6g, Carbs 1g, Sugar 0.4g, Protein 8g

LEMON FRUIT AND NUT BARS

Prep Time: 15mints, Total Time: 15mints, Servings: 10 Bars

INGREDIENTS
- ½ Cup Raw Almonds
- ¾ Cup Raw Cashews
- 1 Cup Deglet Noor Dates
- 1 Lemon – Juice and Zest

Instructions
1. Ground cashews and almonds in a nourishment processor until they are finely cut. Add dates, lemon juice, and lemon pieces. Beat until all ingredients are mixed.
2. Pour blend between two sheets of cling wrap. Utilize your hands to press and frame the blend into a minimized rectangular shape.
3. Fold the saran wrap over it and refrigerate for 2 hours. This will enable it to solidify and make it simpler to cut into bars.
4. Remove from the cooler and cut into 10 bars. Envelop the bars with cling wrap and store them in the ice chest.

Nutrition Fact: Calories 132, Fat 6.5g, Carbs 15g, Sugar 4.2g, Protein 3.2g

CAULIFLOWER FRIED RICE WITH BACON RECIPE

Prep Time: 5mints, Cook Time: 10mints, Total Time: 15mints, Servings: 4

Ingredients:
- 4 slices bacon
- 1 small onion and 1 head cauliflower
- 1 tsp water
- 1 cup frozen mixed vegetables
- 1 tsp Bragg's Liquid Amino

Instructions
1. In a wok or enormous sauté container over medium flame, cook bacon until practically fresh.
2. Add the onions and pan-fried food until translucent.
3. Go heat to high. Add the ground cauliflower and pan-fried food for 1 moment. Add water and blended vegetables, mix well, spread the dish and let the cauliflower blend steam for an additional 3 minutes or until delicate.
4. Reveal and add Bragg's to add. Remove well. Taste and add extra flavoring as wanted.

Nutrition Facts: Calories 315, Fat 25g, Carbs 4g, Sugar 1g, Protein 19g

SPICY KETO DEVILED EGGS

Prep Time: 10mints, Cooking Time: 10mints, Total Time: 20mints; Serving: 6

Ingredients
- 6 eggs
- 1 tbsp red curry paste
- ½ cup mayonnaise
- ¼ tsp salt
- ½ tbsp poppy seeds

Instructions
1. Put the eggs in cool water in a container and pour enough water to cover the eggs. Heat to the point of boiling without a top
2. Give the eggs a chance to stew for around eight minutes. Cool rapidly in super cold water.
3. Remove the eggshells. Cut off the two finishes and split the egg down the middle. Scoop out the egg yolk and put in a little bowl.
4. Put the egg whites on a plate and let sit in the cooler.
5. Blend curry paste, mayonnaise, and egg yolks into a blender. Add salt for taste
6. Draw out the egg whites from the cooler and apply the blend.
7. Sprinkle the seeds on top and serve.

Nutrition Fact: Calories 200, Fat 19g, Carbs 1g, Sugar 3g, Protein 6g

KETO CHEESE OMELET

Prep Time: 5mints, Cooking Time: 10mints, Total Time: 15mints; Serving: 2

Ingredients

- 3 oz. butter
- 6 eggs
- 7 oz. shredded cheddar cheese
- Salt and pepper

Instructions
1. Whisk the eggs until smooth and somewhat foamy. Mix in half of the shredded cheddar. Add salt and pepper for taste
2. Liquefy the butter in a hot skillet. Pour in the egg blend and give it a chance to sit for a couple of moments.
3. Lower the heat and keep on cooking until the egg blend is nearly cooked through. Add the shredded cheddar.
4. Overlap and serve right away.

Nutrition Fact: Calories 897, Fat 80g, Carbs 4g, Sugar 15g, Protein 40g

HALLOUMI CHEESE WITH BUTTER-FRIED EGGPLANT

Prep Time: 5mints, Cooking Time: 10mints, Total Time: 15mints; Serving: 2

Ingredients
- 1 eggplant
- 3 oz. butter
- 10 oz. halloumi cheese
- 10 black olives
- salt and pepper

Instructions
1. Cut the eggplant down the middle, longwise, and cut into cuts which are a big portion of an inch thick.
2. Heat up a healthful dab of butter in an enormous griddle wherein you may shape each cheese and eggplant
3. Add the cheese one side of the dish and eggplant on the other. Season eggplant with salt and pepper
4. Fry over medium-high heat for 5-7mins. Flip the cheese after three minutes, with the aim that it's far darker on the 2 sides.
5. Mix the eggplant now.
6. Present with olives.

Nutrition Fact: Calories 829, Fat 72g, Carbs 11g, Sugar 21g, Protein 32g

KETO BRUNCH SPREAD

Prep Time: 10mints, Cook Time: 20mints, Total Time: 30mints, Serving: 4

Ingredients
- 4 large eggs
- 24 asparagus spears
- 12 slices of pastured, sugar-free bacon

Instructions
1. Pre-warmness your range to 400F
2. At that point, two with the aid of, wrap them with one reduce of bacon. Hold your lances immovably and close to one another with one hand as you wind the reduce of bacon beginning from the base, to the highest factor of the lance.
3. A put in the range set the clock for 20mins.
4. In this time, bring a little pot of water to a fast bubble. Tenderly vicinity 4 big eggs inside the effervescent water, set any other clock for 6mins.
5. At the factor when the 6mins are up, make use of an opened spoon or tongs to unexpectedly move your eggs to the ice shower, let them take a seat for 2mins before stripping the finishes off.
6. Delicately ruin the highest factor of the egg on a hard surface and strip away the shell to discover the tip of the egg.
7. At the point whilst the asparagus is ready, serve on a plate or cutting board. In the occasion that you do not have an egg holder use coffee cups to maintain your eggs up.
8. Dunk your asparagus lances into your eggs. Gala, recognize it!

Nutrition Fact: Calories: 426, Fat 38g, Carbs 3g, Sugar 3g, Protein 17g

BROCCOLI & CHEDDAR KETO BREAD

Prep Time: 5mints, Cook Time: 30mints, Total Time: 35mints, Servings: 10 slices

Ingredients
- 5 eggs beaten
- 1 cup shredded cheddar cheese
- 3/4 cup fresh raw broccoli
- 3 1/2 tbsp coconut flour
- 2 tsp baking powder and 1 tsp salt

Instructions
1. Preheat range to 350. Give a component holder cooking sprinkle.
2. Mix all of the ingredients in a medium bowl.
3. Plan for 30-35mins or till puffed and brilliant. Cut and serve.
4. Microwave or heat in a lubed skillet

Nutrition Facts: Calories 90, Fat 6g, Carbs 2g, Sugars 0.2g, Protein 6g

WIIITE LASAGNA STUFFED PEPPERS

Prep Time: 5mints, Cook Time: 1hr, Total Time: 1hr 5mints, Serving: 4

Ingredients
- 2 large sweet peppers
- 1 tsp garlic salt
- 12 oz ground turkey
- 3/4 cup ricotta cheese
- 1 cup mozzarella

Instructions
1. Preheat stove to 400.
2. Put the split peppers in a heating dish. Sprinkle with 1/4 tsp garlic salt. Gap the ground turkey between the peppers and press into the bottoms. Sprinkle with another 1/4 tsp garlic salt. Prepare for 30 minutes.
3. Partition the ricotta cheddar between the peppers. Sprinkle with the staying 1/2 tsp garlic salt.

Sprinkle the mozzarella on top. Put the cherry tomatoes in the middle of the peppers, if utilizing.
4. Prepare for an extra 30 minutes until the peppers are mollified, the meat is cooked, and the cheddar is brilliant.
Nutrition Facts: Calories 281, Fat 14g, Carbs 7g, Sugars 1g, Protein 32g

EASY TACO CASSEROLE RECIPE

Prep Time: 5mints, Cook Time: 40mints, Total Time: 45mints, Serving: 6
Ingredients
- 2 lb. ground turkey or beef
- 2 tbsp taco seasoning
- 1 cup of salsa
- 16 oz cottage cheese
- 8 oz shredded cheddar cheese

Instructions
1. Preheat range to four hundred.
2. Blend the ground meat and taco flavoring in a massive goulash dish. Heat for 20mins
3. In the interim, combine the curds, salsa, and 1 cup of the cheddar. Put aside.
4. Remove the meal dish from the stove and cautiously channel the cooking fluid from the meat.
5. Separate the beef into little portions. A potato masher works first-rate for this. Spread the curds and salsa mixture over the beef.
6. Return the meal to the stove and heat for a further 15-20 minutes till the meat is cooked all collectively and the cheddar is warm and bubbly.
Nutrition Facts: Calories 367, Fat 18g, Carbs 6g, Sugars 4g, Protein 45g

SPICY KETO CHEESE CHIPS

Prep Time: 5mints, Cook Time: 10mints, Total Time: 15mints; Serving: 12 crisps
INGREDIENTS
- Grass-fed cheddar cheese
- 1 medium-sized jalapeno
- 2 slices of bacon

Instructions
1. Preheat stove to 425°F and line a heating sheet with parchment paper or a silicone preparing mat.
2. Add even stored Tsp of cheddar to the readied oven tray. Put one cut of jalapeno in the focal point of the hill. Sprinkle with disintegrated bacon.
3. Heat on high for 7-10 minutes until cheddar is dissolved and edges are cooked.
4. Remove from stove and let cool totally until fresh.
Nutrition Fact: Calories: 33, Fat 3g, Carbs 0.3g, sugar 1.2g, Protein 2g

BOILED EGGS WITH BUTTER AND THYME

Prep Time: 10mints, Cook Time: 6mints, Total Time: 16mints, Servings: 1
Ingredients
- 3 large eggs
- 1 tbsp good quality unsalted butter
- Freshly ground black pepper
- Salt
- 1/4 tsp thyme leaves

Instructions
7. Fill a medium pan most of the way with water and heat until boiling.
8. When water is bubbling, tenderly put eggs in water and flip using a large spoon.
9. While your eggs are cooking, place one tsp of margarine in a microwave-safe bowl and microwave until dissolved, for around 20 seconds.
10. In the meantime, take the pan and cautiously spill out the excessive temp water carefully.
11. Cautiously strip every egg, wash to remove any shell parts, and add in the softened margarine.
12. Add the thyme leaves as well as the salt and pepper to flavor.
Nutrition Fact: Calories: 159, Fat 18g, Carbs 9g, Sugar 4g, Protein 8g

KETO COOKIE DOUGH (WITH CHOCOLATE CHIPS)

Prep Time: 10mints, Total Time: 10mints, Serving: 6
Ingredients
- 1/2 cup almond flour
- 1/4 cup ghee
- Erythritol or Stevie
- 1 oz 100% chocolate

Instructions
1. Soften the coconut oil or ghee.
2. Blend the almond flour, coconut oil, and sugar in a little bowl to shape a batter.
3. Cautiously overlap in the chocolate pieces.
4. Partition into 6 individual little ramekins or cups
Nutrition Fact: Calories: 151, Fat 15g, Carbs 2g, Sugar 0.4g, Protein 2g

LEMON TURMERIC ROASTED CAULIFLOWER KETO

Prep Time: 5mints, Cook Time: 25mints, Total Time: 30mints, Servings: 4
Ingredients
- 1 head of cauliflower
- 2 tbsp chopped parsley
- 3 tbsp avocado oil
- 2 tbsp lemon juice
- 3 garlic cloves
- 1 tsp turmeric powder
- 1/2 tsp sea salt

Instructions
1. Preheat stove to 425 degrees F.
2. Slash the cauliflower into scaled-down florets, ensuring that the florets are comparative in size.
3. Whisk together all elements for the lemon turmeric dressing.

4. Put the cauliflower florets in an enormous bowl and throw in the dressing.
5. Spread out the cauliflower on a heating sheet in a solitary layer.
6. Cook in the stove for 20-25 minutes until delicate and dark in color, turning the dish half way through.
7. Sprinkle with chopped parsley before serving.
Nutrition Facts: Calories 107, Fat 10g, Carbs 3g, Sugar 5g, Protein 23g

FLUFFY MICROWAVE SCRAMBLED EGGS

Prep Time: 5mints, Cook Time: 5mints, Total Time: 10mints, Serving: 2
Ingredients
- 4 eggs
- 1/4 cup milk
- 1/8 teaspoon salt

Instructions
1. Break the eggs into a microwave-evidence blending bowl. Add drain and salt; blend well.
2. Pop the bowl into the microwave and cook on high control for 30 seconds. Remove the bowl, beat eggs well overall, scratching down the sides of the bowl, and come back to the microwave for an additional 30 seconds.
3. Repeat this example, blending like clockwork for up to 2 1/2 minutes. Stop when eggs have the consistency you want.
Nutrition Facts: Calories 141, Fat 9.3g, Carb 2.1g, Sugar 2.1g, Protein 12.3g

PIZZA EGGS KETO

Prep Time: 10mints, Cooking Time: 20mints, Total Time: 30mints, Serving: 4
Ingredients
- tbsp butter
- Eggs, 2tbsp Pizza, 2tbsp feta cheese
- tbsp mozzarella cheese
- slices pepperoni
- Dash Italian seasoning

Instructions
1. Heat unfolds in an egg skillet over medium-low warm temperature.
2. When the margarine is liquefied and the dish is warmed, smash the eggs into the skillet.
3. When the whites marginally start to set and flip white, spoon the sauce onto the eggs and sprinkle the feta over the pinnacle.
4. Lessen warm temperature to low and maintain cooking. When the whites are totally set, add the mozzarella cheddar, pepperoni, and Italian flavoring on top.
5. Keep cooking on low till the whites are totally set, the pepperoni is cooked and the cheddar is liquefied.
Nutrition Fact: Calories: 397, Fat 31.8g, Carbs 5.5g, Sugar 1.4g, Protein 20.8g

CAESAR SALAD DEVILED EGGS

Prep Time: 120mints, Cooking Time: 10mints, Total Time: 20mints, Serving: 4
Ingredients
- 6 large pastured eggs
- 1/3 cup creamy Caesar dressing
- 1/2 cup Parmesan cheese
- Cracked black pepper
- 1 romaine lettuce leaf

Instructions
1. In a blending bowl, fork crushes the egg yolks. Add Caesar dressing, 1/4 cup of the Parmesan cheddar and half of the destroyed lettuce. Blend until very much joined.
2. Utilize a baked good sack to pipe the blend once more into the eggs.
3. Top each egg with a little Parmesan cheddar, destroyed lettuce and dark pepper.
Nutrition Fact: Calories: 254, Fat 22g, Carbs 2.75g, Sugar 1.3g, Protein 13.5g

CAESAR EGG SALAD LETTUCE WRAPS

Prep Time: 10mints, Cooking Time: 10mints, Total Time: 20mints, Serving: 4
Ingredients
- 6 large hard boiled eggs
- 3 tbsp creamy Caesar and 3 tbsp mayonnaise
- 1/2 cup Parmesan cheese
- Cracked black pepper
- 4 large romaine lettuce leaves

Instructions
1. In a blending bowl, join hacked eggs, velvety Caesar dressing, mayonnaise, 1/4 cup Parmesan cheddar and split dark pepper.
2. Spoon blend onto romaine leaves and top with residual Parmesan cheddar.
Nutrition Fact: Calories: 254, Fat 22g, Carbs 2.75g, Sugar 2g, Protein 13.5g

SOUR CREAM AND CHIVE EGG CLOUDS

Prep Time: 10mints, Cook Time: 6mints, Total Time: 16mints, Serving: 4
Ingredients
- 8 large pastured eggs
- 1/4 cup sharp white cheddar cheese
- 1/4 cup sour cream
- 1 tsp garlic powder
- 2 chives and 2 tsp salted butter

Instructions
1. Preheat stove to 450º Line a rimmed heating sheet with a Silpat or parchment paper.
2. Separate the eggs, emptying the whites into an enormous blending bowl, and the yolks into singular ramekins.
3. Utilizing an electric hand blender, whip the egg whites until they are fleecy and solid pinnacles have begun to frame.

4. Utilizing an elastic spatula, delicately overlap in cheddar, harsh cream, garlic powder, and half of the chives.
5. Spoon blend into 8 separate hills on your Silpat. Make a well in the focal point of each cloud.
6. Heat for 6 minutes or until the mists are brilliant darker on top and the yolks are set.
7. Put a modest quantity of margarine over every yolk. Top with outstanding chives.
8. Serve and Enjoy

Nutrition Fact: Calories: 117, Fat 10g, Carbs 4g, Sugar 1g, Protein 6g

LOW CARB KETO EGG NOODLES

Prep Time: 2mints, Cook Time: 5mints, Total Time: 7mints, Servings: 2

Ingredients
- 1-ounce cream cheese
- 2 eggs
- 1/4 teaspoon wheat gluten

Instructions
1. Preheat the stove to 325F.
2. Add the cream cheddar, eggs, and gluten to the container of a blender.
3. Mix on high for 1 moment, or until smooth.
4. Pour our own on a silicone tangle that is set over a substantial preparing skillet.
5. Smooth out into a square shape, keeping the player exceptionally meager.
6. Heat at 325F for 5 minutes, or until set
7. These are ideal in the event that they are tenderly stewed in a sauce or juices for a couple of moments.

Nutrition Fact: Calories: 111, Fat 9g, Carbs 0.2g, Sugar 0.1g, Protein 6g

EGG FAST RECIPE: EGG PUFFS

Prep Time: 5mints, Cooking Time: 10mints, Total Time: 15mints, Serving: 3

Ingredients:
- 4 eggs
- 1/4 cup grated Dubliner Irish Cheddar
- salt and pepper
- Butter

Instructions
1. Preheat variety to 450 degrees
2. Separate egg whites from yolks, setting the egg whites proper into a mixing bowl and the egg yolks every into a one of a kind little bowl
3. With an electric powered-powered blender, beat egg whites till hardened pinnacles form
4. Tenderly overlap in the floor cheddar
5. Structure four puffs at the making geared up mat with an indent in every puff. Heat for 3mins
6. Remove from the stove, drop one egg yolk into each indented puff, and prepare for 3mins.
7. Remove from the making ready sheet with a spatula, sprinkle with salt and pepper, embody your unfold pinnacle and eat!

Nutrition Fact: Calories: 117, Fat 10g, Carbs 4g, Sugar 1g, Protein 6g

EGG FAST FRIED BOILED EGGS WITH YUM YUM SAUCE

Prep Time: 5mints, Cooking Time: 15mints, Total Time: 20mints, Serving: 1

Ingredients
- 2 eggs, hard-boiled
- 1 tablespoon butter
- 1 tsp Yum Yum Sauce

Instructions
1. Liquefy margarine in a nonstick skillet over medium-high heat.
2. Cut hard-bubbled eggs into thick cuts.
3. Fry in margarine until softly caramelized on the two sides, flipping once.
4. Present with Yum Sauce in a little bowl for plunging.

Nutrition Fact: Calories: 713, Fat 56g, Carbs 0.2g, Sugar 0.3g, Protein 48g

MICROWAVE PALEO BREAD

Prep Time: 3mints, Cook Time: 2mints, Total Time: 5mints, Serving: 4 small round slices

Ingredients
- 1/3 cup almond flour
- 1/2 tsp baking powder
- 1/8 tsp salt
- 1 egg
- 2 and 1/2 Tsp

Instructions
1. Oil a mug.
2. Combine every one of the ingredients with a fork.
3. Empty blend into a mug
4. Microwave for 90 seconds on high
5. Cool for a few moments.
6. Fly out of mug tenderly and cut.

Nutrition Fact: Calories: 132, Fat 13g, Carbs 2g, Sugar 1g, Protein 3.25g

LOW-CARB KETO TUNA PICKLE BOATS

Prep Time: 5mints, Cooking Time: 10mints, Total Time: 15mints, Serving: 2-4

Ingredients
- 5-6 dill pickles
- 1 can light flaked tuna
- 1/4 cup light mayo
- 1 tbsp fresh dill + more for garnish
- Salt & pepper, to taste

Instruction
1. Cut the pickles down the middle.
2. Utilizing a spoon, deseed, and dispose of them.
3. Place the fish in a little bowl, add mayo, dill, salt and pepper. Blend in with a fork.
4. Spoon the fish into the pontoons. Enhancement with dill and enjoy!

Nutrition Fact: Calories: 107, Fat 9g, Carbs 4g, Sugar 2g, Protein 1g

KETO-FRIENDLY BAKED CHEESE CRISPS

Prep Time: 1mints,, Cook Time: 3-5mints, Total Time: 4-6mints, Servings: 16

Ingredients
- 4 cheddar cheese slices, quartered
- Dip of choice

Instruction
1. On a cloth covered heating sheet, place your quartered cheddar cuts approximately an inch separated from one another.
2. Cook on excessive for 3-5mins, or until desired "freshness" is done
3. Remove from stove, and blotch with a paper towel to remove excess oil.
4. Once cool enough, remove from the heating sheet and serve, or allow to cool for later use.

Nutrition Fact: Calories: 313, Fat 16g, Carbs 21g, Sugar 6g, Protein 14g

ONE-MINUTE KETO MUG BREAD

Prep Time: 1mint, Cook Time: 1mint, Total Time: 2mints, Servings: 1

Ingredients
- 4 tbsp almond meal/flour
- 1/2 tsp baking powder
- 1 egg
- 1 tbsp olive oil
- pinch of salt

Instructions
1. Add every one of the ingredients into your mug and blend in with a fork until mixed. The blend will be extremely wet.
2. Microwave on HIGH for 1 moment; tap the top to ensure it's completely cooked through. If it appears half-cooked, place in microwave for another 20-30 seconds.
3. Flip around the mug to discharge the bread-like product and let cool marginally before cutting.
4. Eat promptly, or toast for a crispier surface. Serve alone or as a sandwich bun

Nutrition Facts: Calories 324, Fat 10g, Carbs 15g, Sugar 8g, Protein 28g

KETO CINNAMON CHOCOLATE CHIA PUDDING

Prep Time: 5mints, Total Time: 5mints, Serving: 2

Ingredients
- 2 Tsp unsweetened cacao powder
- 1/2 tsp cinnamon powder
- 2 Tbsp chia seeds
- 1/3 cup of coconut
- 1/8 tsp vanilla extract and Stevie

Instructions
1. Blend the cacao powder, cinnamon powder with the vanilla concentrate and coconut milk.
2. Empty the chia blend into 2 little containers or glasses.
3. Put into your ice chest to set for 4 hours.
4. Enjoy for breakfast or as a brisk snack when in a hurry.

Nutrition Fact: Calories: 77, Fat 5g, Carbs 6g, Sugar 2g, Protein 3g

TURKEY AND CHEESE ROLLS

Prep Time: 15mints, Cooking Time: 15mints, Total Time: 30mints, Serving: 3

Ingredients:
- 6 slices of all-natural turkey breast
- 3 slices all-natural Colby jack cheese

Instructions
1. Lay turkey breast level on a plate then lay a portion of the Colby jack over each bit of turkey.
2. Roll.
3. Pack them up in a compartment as snappy solid snacks for work the following day.

Nutrition Fact: Calories: 104, Fat 3g, Carbs 4g, Sugar 1.2g, Protein 7g

LOW CARB BACON & EGGS

Prep Time: 20mints, Cooking Time: 10mints, Total Time: 30mints, Servings 3

Ingredients
- 3 Hard-Boiled Eggs
- 1-2 pieces bacon
- 3 slices cheese

Instructions
1. Place the hard-bubbled egg in a lengthy manner, and layer on one bit of cheddar, and a huge portion of bacon.
2. Utilize a toothpick to keep it together and serve.

Nutrition Fact: Calories: 197, Fat 15g, Carbs 1g, Sugar 2g, Protein 14g

PORTOBELLO MUSHROOM MINI KETO PIZZAS

Prep Time: 3mints, Cook Time: 25mints, Total Time: 28mints, Servings: 4

Ingredients
- 4 Large Portobello Mushrooms
- 100 g Low carb marinara sauce
- 80 g fresh or grated mozzarella
- 20 slices pepperoni

Instructions
1. Place mushrooms onto the ovenproof plate, gills up. Sprinkle with salt and cook in a stove warmed to 375°F for 20 minutes. Remove from stove and channel away fluid from container and mushrooms.
2. Place mushrooms onto a preparing plate, gill up. Spread 2 tbsp marinara sauce onto each, trailed by 1/4 of the mozzarella. At last, organize 5 cuts of pepperoni onto every pizza

3. Prepare in the stove for 20 minutes at 375°F (190°C) until cheddar starts to turn brilliant and bubbly. Serve right away.
Nutrition Fact: Calories 122, Fats 9g, Carbs 4g, Sugar 2g, Protein 8g

BEST KETO POPCORN CHEESE PUFFS

Prep Time: 5mints, Cook Time: 5mints, Total Time: 10mints, Servings: 4
Ingredients
- 4 ounces cheddar cheese sliced

Instructions
1. Cut the cheddar into little ¼ inch squares.
2. Prior to heating, this formula must be readied 24 hrs in advance
3. Put on a treat sheet fixed with parchment paper and spread with a tea towel.
4. Leave the cheddar to dry out for 24 hours.
5. The following day preheat your stove to 200C/390F and heat the cheddar for 3-5 minutes until it is puffed up.
6. Leave to cool for 10 minutes before serving.
Nutrition Fact: Calories: 114, Fat 9g, Carbs 0.2g, Sugar 0.3g, Protein 7g

KETO LOW CARB TORTILLA CHIPS

Prep Time: 10mints, Cook Time: 7mints, Total Time: 17mints, Servings: 8
Ingredients
- 200 g / 2 cups mozzarella
- 75 g / 3/4 cup almond flour
- 1/4 tsp onion, garlic and paprika
- 2 tbsp psyllium husk
- Pinch salt

Instructions
1. Heat you're stove to 180 Celsius/356°
2. Dissolve the mozzarella in the microwave, heating in a non-stick pot.
3. Add the almond flour/ground almonds and psyllium husk in addition to the salt and flavors, if utilizing. Mix and fold until you have a smooth mixture.
4. Separate the batter into 2 balls and turn out between 2 sheets of preparing/parchment paper. Spread evenly and as much as possible. The more slender, the crispier your tortilla chips will turn out.
5. Cut into triangles and spread out on a sheet of preparing paper so the tortilla chips don't touch.
6. Prepare 6-8 minutes or until sautéed on the edges. Heating time will rely upon the thickness of your tortilla chips. I heated mine in 2 rounds, in addition to a third-round for the off-cuts.
Nutrition Facts: Calories 143, Fat 9.2g, Carbs 4.8g, Sugar 0.6g, Protein 8.3g

CHEDDAR AND EVERYTHING SEASONING FAT BOMBS

Prep Time: 35mints, Cooking Time: 2hrs, Total Time: 2hrs 35mints, Serving: 3

Ingredients
- 1 brick cream cheese
- 1 cup shredded cheddar cheese
- Sesame Seasoning

Instructions
1. Blend the two sorts of cheddar and chill for 2 hours or more.
2. Pick a tsp size ball and move it in the flavoring.
3. Store balls in the ice chest
Nutrition Facts: Calories 324, Fat 12g, Carbs 8g, Sugar 6g, Protein 18g

BACON-WRAPPED AVOCADO FRIES

Prep Time: 10mints, Cook Time: 10mints, Total Time: 20mints, Servings: 20
Ingredients:
- 20 strips of pre-cooked packaged bacon
- 1 large avocado sliced into thin fry-size pieces

Instructions
1. Preheat stove to 425°F. Take one segment of precooked bacon and attempt to tenderly stretch somewhat longer without it breaking.
2. Cautiously fold-over avocado fry, beginning toward one side and attempting to the opposite end, and safely take care of the end piece.
3. Repeat with remaining ingredients and put onto a oven tray. Heat for 5-10 minutes and serve.
Nutrition Facts: Calories 65, Fat 5.1g, Carbs 0.8g, Sugar 0.5g, Protein 4g

KETO STOVE-TOP BONE BROTH

Prep Time: 10mints, Total Time: 6hrs 10mints, Serving: 16
Ingredients
- 2 carrots
- 4 celery stalks
- 1 onion
- 2 lbs beef bones
- Salt

Instructions
1. Add everything to an enormous pot and load up with water.
2. Heat to the point of boiling and afterward lessen to a stew with the top on.
3. Continue stewing for 6 hours on low heat. Top with extra water if necessary.
4. Cool, strainer the fluid out, and store the bone soup in glass containers.
5. Fill the pot with more water and stew for an additional 6 hours.
Nutrition Fact:: Calories: 45, Fat 0.5g, Carbs 1g, Sugar 0.3g, Protein 9g

THE ULTIMATE KETO BUNS

Prep Time: 5mints, Cook Time: 26mints, Total Time: 31mints, Servings: 6
Ingredients

- 4 tbsp lard
- 4 eggs
- 1/2 tsp Himalayan salt and onion flakes
- 100 g blanched almond flour
- 1 tbsp rosemary
- 1 tbsp white and black sesame seed

Instructions
1. Preheat the stove to 220C/430F.
2. Add the softened fat and eggs inside the stick blender measuring utensil. Add the remainder of the ingredients over the fluid and add your stick blender inside the measuring glass. Beat 5-10 times until totally combined.
3. Pour similarly in 6 enormous biscuit molds. Put in the stove. Heat for 26 minutes. Remove from the stove and let totally cool before cutting.

Nutrition Fact: Calories 230, Fat 20.82g, Carbs 3.99g, Sugar 0.91g, Protein 8.45g

CRISPY SWEET POTATO FRIES

Prep Time: 15mints, Cook Time: 10mints, Total Time: 25mints, Serving: 4

Ingredients
- 1 1/2 lbs sweet potatoes
- Sea salt
- Garlic powder
- Onion powder

Instructions
1. In a cast-iron skillet over medium-high to high heat, add 1/2 to 1 inch of oil.
2. When the oil is hot and you can begin to see little air pockets forming, add the sweet potato fries to the container.
3. Fry until they are brilliant darker and marginally firm, around 10 minutes.
4. Remove from oil and move to a paper towel to absorb abundance oil.
5. Add sea salt, garlic powder and onion powder in a little bowl.
6. Sprinkle flavoring over top of the sweet potato fries.

Nutrition Fact: Calories: 102, Fat 8g, Carbs 2g, Sugar 1g, Protein 4g

KETO PIZZA CHIPS

Prep Time: 15mints, Cook Time: 15mints, Total Time: 30mints, Serving: 12 chips

Ingredients
- 1 cup grated parmesan cheese
- 1 teaspoon dried oregano
- 12 slices pepperoni
- Low Carb Pizza Sauce

Instructions
1. Preheat the stove to 400°F. Line tray with parchment paper or a silicone heating mat.
2. Spread the parmesan cheese on top in 12 finger-shaped strips.
3. Remove the plate from the stove and sprinkle the oregano over the cheese.
4. Top with cuts of pepperoni and heat for a further 8 minutes or so.
5. Remove the plate from the stove and utilize a paper towel to remove excess oil.
6. Move the chips to a paper towel-coated cooling rack and enable it to cool.
7. Serve with pizza sauce.

Nutrition Fact: Calories: 104, Fat 7.8g, Carbs 0.7g, Sugar 0.1g, Protein 7.4g

AVOCADO BAKED EGGS

Prep Time: 10mints, Cook Time: 15mints, Total Time: 25mints, Serving: 2

Ingredients
- 1 avocado
- 2 eggs
- Shredded cheddar cheese
- Kosher salt
- Freshly ground black pepper

Instructions
1. Preheat stove to 425°.
2. Cut the avocado fifty-fifty and remove the pit. With a spoon, cut out enough avocado to prepare for the egg
3. Put avocado parts onto the rear of the biscuit dish to settle them while cooking.
4. Air out an egg into every 50% of the avocado, contingent upon the size of your egg, you may have abundance egg white. Season with salt and pepper
5. Sprinkle parts with cheddar and put skillet in the stove for 13-16mins depending on the yolk consistency you want.
6. Serve promptly, top with Sriracha for a little kick of flavor.

Nutrition Fact: Calories: 409, Fat 31g, Carbs 8g, Sugar 5g, Protein 25g

GARLIC DILL BAKED CUCUMBER CHIPS

Prep Time: 15mints, Cook Time: 3hrs, Total Time: 3hrs 15mints, Serving: 8

Ingredients
- 2- large cucumbers
- tbsp dried dill
- tsp onion powder and 1 tsp garlic powder
- tbsp apple cider vinegar
- sea salt

Instructions
1. Meagerly cut the cucumbers in 1/8-inch cuts.
2. In a solitary layer, line cucumbers on a paper towel. Put any other paper towel on top and press into the cucumber cuts to draw out excess dampness. Redo this process two times if necessary. The dryer they are, the crisper they will get as they are heated.
3. Put dry cucumber cuts in an extensive mixing bowl. Preheat stove to 200°F
4. In a big mixing bowl, place the dill, onion powder, garlic powder and apple juice vinegar.

5. Remove cucumbers until absolutely everything is immersed with the herb mixture.
6. Line two significant heating sheets with cloth paper. Line the cucumber cuts on the fabric paper in a solitary layer. Sprinkle with a touch sea salt.
7. Cook for three hours.
8. Turn stove off and allows the plate to chill inside the stove. This will permit them to get notably crispier.

Nutrition Fact: Calories: 15, Fat 0.1g, Carbs 3.7g, Sugar 1.5g, Protein 0.7g

BAKED EGGS AND ASPARAGUS WITH PARMESAN

Prep Time: 7mints, Cook Time: 18mints, Total Time: 25mints, Serving: 2

Ingredients
- thick asparagus spears
- 4- eggs
- 2- tsp. olive oil
- salt and black pepper
- 2- T Parmesan cheese

Instructions
1. Preheat the stove to 400F/200C and shower two gratin dishes with a spray of olive oil.
2. Break each egg into a little dish and give eggs a chance to come to room temperature while you cook the asparagus.
3. Remove the base of every asparagus and dispose of it. Cut the remainder of asparagus into short pieces somewhat under 2 inches in length.
4. Put a large portion of the asparagus pieces into each gratin dish and put gratin dishes into the stove to cook the asparagus, setting a clock for 10 minutes.
5. At the point when the clock goes off following ten minutes, remove gratin dishes from the stove each in turn and cautiously slide two eggs over the asparagus in each dish. Set back in the stove and set the clock for 5 minutes.
6. Following 5 minutes, remove gratin dishes each in turn again and sprinkle each with a tablespoon of coarsely-ground Parmesan.

Nutrition Fact: Calories: 248, Fat 19, Carbs 2g, Sugar 2g, Protein 20g

KETO SAUSAGE BALLS

Prep Time: 10mints, Cook Time: 20mints, Total Time: 30mints, Serving: 24 sausage balls

Ingredients
- 1 pound bulk Italian sausage
- 1 cup blanched almond flour
- 1 cup shredded sharp cheddar cheese
- 1/4 cup grated Parmesan cheese
- 1 large egg and 1 tsp onions
- 2 tsp baking powder

Instructions
1. Preheat the stove to 350°F. Line a rimmed oven tray with a wire cooling rack.
2. Mix the ingredients in a huge bowl and, utilizing your hands, blend until all-around joined.
3. Structure the meat blend into 1/2 – to 2-inch meatballs, making a sum of 24
4. Put the meatballs on the wire rack. Prepare for 20 minutes, or until dark in color on the outside.

Nutrition Fact: Calories: 374, Fat 31g, Carbs 5.5g, Sugar 2g, Protein 22g

EGG & CHORIZO MUFFINS

Prep Time: 5mints, Cook Time: 15mints, Total Time: 20mints , Serving: 4

Ingredients
- 1 lb ground chorizo
- 8 eggs
- 3 oz water
- 2 tbsp coconut oil

Instructions
1. In a huge skillet, add chorizo until cooked completely
2. While chorizo is cooking, liberally oil a biscuit dish with coconut oil.
3. Place onions, asparagus, broccoli, Chile peppers or other veggies with chorizo.
4. Add sautéed chorizo into biscuit skillet.
5. In a huge bowl, whisk eggs and water until feathery and somewhat frothy.
6. Empty eggs into biscuit tins
7. Prepare at 350 for 15 minutes or until totally cooked through
8. Remove and serve and enjoy it!

Nutrition Facts: Calories 110, Fat 7g, Carbs 9g, Sugar 3g, Protein 3g

EGG MUFFINS WITH SAUSAGE, SPINACH, AND CHEESE

Prep Time: 10mints, Cook Time: 20mints, Total Time: 30mints, Serving: 4

Ingredients
- 3 lean breakfast turkey sausage links
- 5 egg whites and 2 whole eggs
- 1/4 cup skim milk and Salt and pepper
- 1/4 cup fresh spinach
- 1/4 cup shredded sharp Cheddar cheese

Instructions
1. Preheat the stove to 350 degrees F. In a medium skillet, place turkey sausages on medium-high heat. Cook until hotdog dark in color. Cut wiener into 1/2-inch pieces and put aside.
2. In a huge blending bowl, whisk together egg whites and eggs. Rush in skim milk and season with salt and pepper, for taste. Mix in the fresh spinach.
3. Oil 6 biscuit tin cups with cooking oil or line cups with paper liners. Empty egg blend equally into the biscuit cups.
4. Add cheddar and turkey sausage similarly between every biscuit cup
5. Heat egg biscuits for 20 minutes or until the biscuits are firm from the inside. Remove from the

stove and tenderly go around each egg with a spread blade. Serve warm.
Nutrition Facts: Calories 110, Fat 7g, Carbs 9g, Sugar 3g, Protein 3g

SPICY SAUSAGE, CHEESE, AND EGG MUFFINS

Prep Time: 5mints, Cook Time: 30mints, Total Time: 35mints, Serving: 9
Ingredients
- 8 eggs
- 1/3 cup milk
- 1/3 cup shredded Jalapeño Havarti cheese
- 2 tbsp cilantro
- 16 oz ground sausage

Instructions
1. Preheat stove to 350 degrees.
2. Shower a biscuit tin altogether with a nonstick spray.
3. In an enormous bowl add milk and eggs, speed until mixed.
4. Add cilantro, frankfurter and cheddar, blend.
5. Spoon blend into the biscuit tin, top with extra cheddar if you desire.
6. Heat 30-35 minutes until done.

Nutrition Facts: Calories 179, Fat 13.2g, Carbs 0.9g, Sugars 0.6g, Protein 13.3g

GHEE AKA CLARIFIED BUTTER

Prep Time: 45mints, Cooking Time: 6hrs, Total Time: 6hrs 45mints, Serving: 3
Ingredients
- oz unsalted grass-fed butter

Instructions
1. Put in the margarine in the bowl simmering pot and cook on LOW for 6-8 hours
2. Pour the margarine through cheesecloth and into a re-sealable container.
3. I store mine in the fridge, however, a few people store theirs on a ledge.

Nutrition Fact: Calories 392; Fat 9g, Carbs 44g, Sugar 6g, Protein 27g

BASIC KETO CHEESE CRISPS

Prep Time: 5mints, Cook Time: 7mints, Total Time: 12mints, Serving: 3
Ingredients
- 1 cup shredded Cheddar cheese

Instructions
1. Preheat stove to 400 degrees F. Line 2 heating trays with parchment paper.
2. Place cheddar in 24 little flat circles on the readied heating sheets.
3. Heat in the preheated stove until brilliant dark-colored, around 7 minutes
4. Cool for 5 to 10 minutes before removing from heating sheets.

Nutrition Facts: Calories 139, Fat 11.4g, Carb 0.4g, Sugar 1.3g, Protein 8.6g

CHEESY KETO BISCUITS

Prep Time: 20mints, Cook Time: 20mints, Total Time: 40mints, Serving: 6
Ingredients
- 2 cups almond flour
- 1 tablespoon baking powder
- 2 1/2 cups shredded Cheddar cheese
- 4 eggs
- 1/4 cup half-and-half

Instructions
1. Preheat the stove to 350 stages F. Line a heating sheet with cooking paper.
2. Join almond flour and baking powder in a huge bowl. Blend in cheddar with hands.
3. Make a hole inside the middle of the bowl; placing eggs and creamer to the center.
4. Utilize a giant fork, spoon, or your palms to mix inside the flour combo until a semi-sticky product forms.
5. Drop nine bits of it onto the pre-heated sheet.
6. Prepare within the preheated stove until cooked, around 20mins.

Nutrition Facts: Calories 329, Fat 27.1g, Carb 7.2g, Sugar 5.1g, Protein 16.7g

OVEN-BAKED BACON

Prep Time: 5mints, Cook Time: 30mints, Total Time: 35mints, Serving: 3
Ingredients
- 16- ounce bacon

Instructions
1. Preheat the stove to 350 degrees F. Line an oven tray with parchment paper.
2. Put bacon cuts next to one another on the oven tray.
3. Heat in the preheated stove for 15 to 20 minutes, remove from the stove. Flip bacon cuts with kitchen tongs and place back to the stove.
4. Prepare until firm, 15 to 20 minutes more. More slender cuts will require less time, around 20 minutes all out. Transfer onto a plate fixed with paper towels.

Nutrition Facts: Calories 134, Fat 10.4g, Carb 10.4g, Sugar 2.4g, Protein 9.2g

CAULIFLOWER-SPINACH SIDE DISH

Prep Time: 10mints, Cook Time: 5mints, Total Time: 15mints, Serving: 7
Ingredients
- 2 3/4 cups cauliflower florets
- 2 cups spinach leaves
- 2 tablespoons butter
- 1 teaspoon of sea salt
- 2 spreadable cheese wedges

Instructions

1. Run cauliflower through a nourishment processor to get 2 cups of cauliflower grounds somewhat bigger than the consistency of cornmeal.
2. Add cauliflower, spinach, margarine, and salt in a huge pot over low heat.
3. Cover and cook until cauliflower is delicate and spinach has withered, 5 to 7 minutes. Mix in cheddar wedges until the cauliflower and spinach are covered and no cheddar bunches remain.
Nutrition Facts: Calories 180, Fat 14g, Carb 9.1g, Sugar 3.2, Protein 7.4g

LOW-CARB KETO CHEESE TACO SHELLS
Prep Time: 10mints, Cook Time: 6mints, Total Time: 16mints, Serving: 5
Ingredients
- 2 cups shredded Cheddar cheese

Instructions
1. Preheat stove to 400°F. Line 2 trays with parchment paper or silicone mats.
2. Spread cheddar at the readied heating sheets into 4 6-inch circles set 2 inches apart.
3. Heat inside the preheated stove till cheddar liquefies and is slightly darker, 6 to 8mins
4. Cool for 2 to 3 minutes. Lift with a spatula; cool till set, round 10 minutes.
Nutrition Facts: Calories 288, Fat 18.7g, Carb 0.7g, Sugar 1.4g, Protein 14.3g

KETO GARLIC CHEESE 'BREAD'
Prep Time: 5mints, Cook Time: 10mints, Total Time: 15mints, Serving: 3
Ingredients
- 1 cup shredded mozzarella cheese
- 1/4 cup grated Parmesan cheese
- 1 large egg
- 1/2 teaspoon garlic powder

Instructions
1. Line the air fryer crate with a bit of parchment paper.
2. Add mozzarella, Parmesan, egg and garlic powder in a bowl; blend until merged. Press into a round oven dish.
3. Heat the air fryer to 350 degrees F. Leave bread to bake for 10 minutes
4. Remove. Serve garlic cheddar bread warm..
Nutrition Facts: Calories 255, Fat 14.3g, Carb 2.7g, Sugar 5.3g, Protein 20.8g

SAVORY SALMON FAT BOMBS
Prep Time: 10mints, Total Time: 1hrs 40mints, Serving: 6
Ingredients
- 1/2 cup full-fat cream cheese
- 1/3 cup butter
- 1/2 package smoked salmon
- 1 tbsp fresh lemon juice
- 1-2 tbsp freshly chopped dill

Instructions
1. Put the cream cheese, butter and smoked salmon into a nourishment processor.
2. Add lemon juice and dill and beat until smooth. I'm utilizing my Kenwood blender with a nourishment processor connection.
3. Line a plate with parchment paper and make little fat bombs utilizing around 2 1/2 tablespoons of the blend per piece. Trimming with more dill and put in the cooler for 1-2 hours or until firm
Nutrition Fact:: Calories 300, Fat 30g Carbs 14g, Sugar 2g, Protein 3g

BACON-WRAPPED MOZZARELLA STICKS
Prep Time: 10mints, Cook Time: 3mints, Total Time: 13mints, Serves: 2
Ingredients
- 1 Frigo cheese heads mozzarella cheese stick
- 2 slices of bacon
- Coconut oil for frying
- Low sugar pizza sauce for dipping
- Toothpicks

Instructions
1. Preheat your coconut oil in a fryer to 350°.
2. Enclose your cut cheese sticks with the bacon, covering as you go so the bacon remains on. Toward the finish of the wrapping, secure with a toothpick.
3. Drop the bacon-enveloped cheddar in the hot oil and cook until the bacon is very dark colored, around 2-3 minutes.
4. Move to a paper towel to soak and cool for a couple of moments. Remove the toothpick and enjoy with your pizza sauce dip.
Nutrition Facts: Calories 148, Fat 11g, Carbs 13g, Sugar 2g, Protein 2g

BACON ONION BUTTER
Prep Time: 15mints, Cooking Time: 35mints, Total Time: 50mints, Serving: 6
Ingredients
- 9 tablespoons butter
- 4 strips bacon sliced into small strips
- 90 grams onion
- 2 teaspoon spicy brown mustard
- 1/2 teaspoon black pepper

Instructions
1. Dissolve 1 tablespoon of margarine in a skillet on medium heat and add bacon pieces.
2. When the bacon fat begins to cook, add diced onion and fry until onion and bacon are done but not overcooked.
3. Put aside bacon/onion blend in a bowl and cool to room temp.
4. Add 8 tablespoons of margarine to an enormous blending bowl.
5. Add bacon and onions, yellow mustard, and pepper.

6. Mix together ingredients or utilize an electric blender.
7. Spoon into a smaller than normal biscuit tin, place in cooler until margarine is firm again for about 30mins.
Nutrition Facts: Calories 1130, Fat 117g, Carbs 10g, Sugars 4g, Protein 15g

BACON & EGG FAT BOMBS

Prep Time: 10mints, Cooking Time: 40mints, Total Time: 50mints, Serving: 3

Ingredients
- 2 large eggs, free-range or organic
- 1/4 cup butter or ghee
- 2 tbsp mayonnaise
- Freshly ground black pepper
- 1/4 tsp salt or more
- 4 large slices of bacon

Instructions
1. Preheat the eggs to one 190 °C/375 °F. Line a heating plate with parchment paper.
2. Lay the bacon strips out on the paper, leaving space between them so as not to touch. Put the plate within the range and cook for round 10-15 minutes until darker in color.
3. Heat up the eggs. Fill a little pan with water up to 75%. Add salt. Utilizing a spoon or hand, dunk each egg into the bubbling water. To get the eggs hard-boiled, leave for about 10mins.
4. Add the mayonnaise, season with salt and pepper and mix nicely. Add the bacon oil.
5. Put in the fridge for 20-30 minutes or until it's solidified and easy to shape fat bombs.
6. Crumble the bacon into little pieces for "breading." Remove the egg combination from the fridge and start making 6 balls.
Nutrition Fact: Calories 268, Fat 17.2g, Carbs 8.3g, sugar 4.5g, Protein 22g

JALAPENO POPPER DEVILED EGGS WITH BACON

Prep Time: 15mints, Cooking Time: 25mints, Total Time: 40mints, Serving: 4

Ingredients
- 6 large eggs
- 6 slices bacon
- 16 sliced pickled jalapenos
- 4 to 6 tablespoons mayonnaise
- 2 ounces cream cheese
- 1/4 teaspoon smoked paprika

Instructions
1. Put the eggs in an enormous pot with cold water.
2. Over high heat, wait for the water to boil. When the water has reached boiling point, remove the skillet from the heat, cover and let sit for 12 minutes.
3. Cut 4 of the jalapenos and put them aside.
4. Strip the eggs and cut into equal parts, the long way. Remove yolks and fork pound them in a medium blending bowl. Blend until all ingredients are all around mixed.
5. Spoon the blend into a plastic pack. Utilize this to pipe the filling into the egg parts.
Nutrition Fact: Calories: 733, Fat 56g, Carbs 10g, Sugar 1g, Protein 42g

EGGPLANT FRENCH TOAST

Prep Time: 20mints, Cooking Time: 15mints, Total Time: 35mints, Serving: 2

Ingredients
- 1 eggplant
- Celtic sea salt
- 2 eggs and 1 tsp vanilla
- Stevie glycerite
- Butter/coconut oil

Instructions
1. Strip eggplant and cut into strips. Sprinkle a limited quantity of salt on the eggplant. Turn eggplant pieces over and sprinkle a modest quantity on the opposite side.
2. Give eggplant a chance to rest for two minutes. Blend eggs, vanilla, cinnamon, and Stevie glycerite in a bowl. Liquefy spread in a griddle on medium heat.
3. Put your eggplant in the egg blend and jab openings into it with a blade or fork. This enables the blend to penetrate the eggplant. Cook "French toast" until dark in color.
4. At that point flip and do likewise on the opposite side. Top up with syrup for flavor.
Nutrition Fact: Calories 229, Fat 6.1g, Carbs 31g, Sugar 2g, Protein 10g

MOCK FRENCH TOAST

Prep Time: 15mints, Cooking Time: 20mints, Total Time: 35mints, Serving: 4

Ingredients
- 2 ounces pork rinds
- 2 eggs and 1/4 cup heavy cream
- 2 tablespoons granulated Splendor
- 1/2 tsp cinnamon
- 1/2 tsp vanilla

Instructions
1. Put the pork skins in a quart-length Ziploc sack, removing any difficult portions. Smash with a meat hammer till finely squashed
2. In a bowl, beat the eggs, blend in the meat except for pork skins.
3. Add the red meat skins and leave for 5-10 minutes till it thickens and becomes "gloppy".
4. Heat a bit of oil in a nonstick skillet, spoon inside the participant, partitioning into 4 medium size hotcakes
5. Cook till pleasantly seared on the bottom; turn and cook until darker. Present with sugar syrup, if necessary.

Nutrition Fact: Calories 124, Fat 10g, Carbs 2g, Sugar 3g, Protein 8g

GARLIC PARMESAN BAKED TORTILLA CHIPS

Prep Time: 10mints, Cook Time: 20mins, Total Time: 30mints, Serving: 2

Ingredients
- 2 large low carb tortillas
- ¼ cup parmesan cheese
- 3 tbsp salted butter
- 1 tbsp garlic powder
- 1 tbsp Italian seasoning

Instructions
1. Preheat stove to 350°
2. Brush softened margarine on one side of tortillas. Blend garlic powder and Italian flavoring together and sprinkle liberally over the buttered side of the two tortillas.
3. Utilizing a pizza shaper, cut the tortillas into triangles, or any other shape you like.
4. On an oiled heating sheet, place the chips in a solitary layer, dry side down. Prepare for 10 minutes.
5. Remove plate from the stove, flip the chips over and brush the opposite side with margarine and coat with parmesan cheddar. Heat 10-12 minutes longer

Nutrition Fact: Calories: 287, Fat 24g, Carbs 6.5g, Sugar 5g, Protein 13g

CRISPY CHEDDAR CRISPS

Prep Time: 5mints, Cook Time: 40mints, Total Time: 45mints, Servings: 1

Ingredients
- 3 cheddar cheese slices
- Salt

Instructions
1. Preheat oven to 250°F.
2. Cut cheddar into quarters and spread out on a material lined heating sheet.
3. Sprinkle with salt.
4. Put into stove and heat for around 30-40 minutes or until dark in color.
5. Remove from stove and let cool for 10-15 minutes.
6. Serve and enjoy

Nutrition Fact: Calories: 130, Fat 11g, Carbs 1g, Sugar, Protein 8g

GRAIN-FREE "WHOLE GRAIN" CRACKERS

Prep Time: 30mints, Cooking Time: 1hrs, Total Time: 1hr 30mints, Serving: 4

Ingredients
- 2 cups unblanched organic almonds
- 1 teaspoon unrefined sea salt
- 1/4 cup unflavored whey protein
- 2 large organic eggs
- 3 tablespoons organic extra virgin olive oil

Instruction
1. Preheat the stove to 250 °F or marginally lower (100 °C).
2. In a nourishment processor, process the almonds and the salt until coarsely ground.
3. Add the whey protein and blend until smooth. Add the eggs and the oil and blend until smooth.
4. Put the mixture on a heating sheet fixed with parchment paper and put another parchment paper on the batter.
5. Utilizing a moving pin, reveal the mixture between the two parchment papers as flimsy as possible.
6. Cut the batter with a blade or pizza shaper into squares, or into rectangular or triangular shapes. Put in the stove and heat for 50min to an hour.
7. Remove from the stove, cool totally and break along the pre-cut lines.
8. Store at room temperature to safeguard the crunchiness. Use within a couple of days.

Nutrition Fact: Calories 165, Fat 14g, Carbs 11g, Sugar 2g, Protein 2g

SOUR CREAM AND CHIVE CRACKERS

Prep Time: 30mints, Cooking Time: 1hrs, Total Time: 1hr 30mints, Serving: 4

Ingredients
- 230g almond flour
- 20g fresh organic chives
- 70g full-fat sour cream
- 1 tsp unrefined sea salt

Instructions
1. Preheat the stove to 250 °F or marginally lower (100 °C).
2. Chop the chives into little pieces.
3. In a medium bowl, blend every one of the ingredients by hand until smooth.
4. Put the batter on a heating sheet fixed with parchment paper. Put another parchment paper on the batter. Utilizing a moving pin, roll the mixture between the two parchment papers as slim as possible.
5. Evacuate the highest parchment paper. Cut the mixture with a blade or pizza shaper into squares.
6. Put in the stove and heat for 50mintunes to an hour. Check as often as possible with the goal that the wafers don't get excessively dull or consume.
7. Cool totally and break into squares.

Nutrition Facts: Calories 268, Fat 17.2g, Carbs 8.3g, sugar 4.5g, Protein 22g

SALT AND VINEGAR ZUCCHINI CHIPS

Prep Time: 15mints, Cook Time: 12hrs, Serving: 8

Ingredients
- 4- cups zucchini
- 2- tsp extra virgin olive oil
- 2- tsp white balsamic vinegar
- 2- tsp coarse sea salt

Instructions

1. Cut zucchini as small as could be expected under the circumstances.
2. In a little bowl whisk olive oil and vinegar together.
3. Put zucchini in the bowl.
4. Add zucchini in even layers to dehydrator then sprinkle with coarse ocean salt.
5. Depending on how small you cut the zucchini, leave to dry out somewhere in the range of 8-14 hours. My temperature setting was 135 degrees F.
6. Line a treat sheet with parchment paper. Lay zucchini uniformly. Heat at 200 degrees F for 2-3 hours. Turn over most of the way during cooking time.

Nutrition Facts: Calories 40, Fat 3.6g, Carbs 2.9g, Sugar 2g, Protein 0.7g

BRUSSELS SPROUTS CHIPS

Prep Time: 20mints, Cooking Time: 20mints, Total Time: 40mints, Serving: 4

Ingredients
- 1 pound brussels sprouts washed and dried
- 2 tablespoons extra virgin olive oil
- 1 teaspoon kosher salt

Instructions
1. Preheat stove to 400 degrees F.
2. To set up the Brussels sprouts, trim off the stock and dispose of the external leaves. Keep stripping off the leaves individually adding them to an enormous bowl. In case you're having trouble getting them off, simply trim the stalk some more.
3. Add the oil to the leaves of the sprouts, making sure to rub the oil everywhere throughout the leaves with your fingers to guarantee they're all around covered. Add the salt.
4. Spread uniformly on 1 or 2 heating sheets, spreading the leaves separated so they're not stacked on one another. You need a lot of room around them.
5. Heat for 10-15 minutes until dark in color and firm. Remove from the stove, permit to cool. If necessary, sprinkle with salt and serve.

Nutrition Fact: Calories 104; Fat 7g, Carbs 9g, Sugar 2g, Protein 3g

SESAME MIRIN KALE CHIPS

Prep Time: 10mints, Cooking Time: 15mints, Total Time: 25mints, Serving: 4

Ingredients
- 170g kale leaves
- 2 tsp melted extra virgin coconut oil
- 1 tsp mirin or rice vinegar
- 1/2 tsp unrefined sea salt
- 4 tsp hulled sesame seeds

Instructions
1. Preheat stove to 350 °F. Wash the kale leaves and pat dry with towel or paper.
2. Tear the leaves into scaled-down pieces. Dispose of the thick stem in the center.
3. Take the greatest bowl you have and put the bits of kale leaves in there.
4. Add the remainder of the ingredients to the bowl and blend and back rub altogether so the bits of leaves are secured wherever with oil and flavors.
5. Spread the bits of leaves on an oven tray fixed with parchment paper so they contact each other as little as possible.
6. Prepare for 10-13 minutes, or until firm and not very dark-colored. Let cool and serve.

Nutrition Facts: Calories 442, Fat 45g, Carbs 11g, Sugar 2g, Protein 4g

SPICY CHEDDAR CRISPS

Prep Time: 5mints, Cooking Time: 3mints, Total Time: 8mints, Serving: 8

Ingredients
- 1 cup finely shredded Cheddar cheese
- 1/2 tsp Tabasco

Instructions
1. In a little bowl, remove shredded Cheddar with Tabasco sauce until all around covered.
2. Heat bread press (toaster) to medium.
3. Utilizing a large portion of the cheddar, spoon four circles of cheddar around 3 inches in distance onto the hot press.
4. Close cover and let cook 1 to 2 minutes, until sautéed and firm. You can look and check whether they are finished.
5. Utilize an elastic spatula to strip crisps off press. Repeat with residual cheddar.

Nutrition Fact: Calories 114, Fat 9g, Carbs 0.3g, Sugar 2.1g, Protein 7g

CRISPY GREEN BEAN CHIPS

Prep Time: 1hr 30mints, Cooking Time: 10hrs 20mints, Total Time: 11hrs 40mints, Serving: 4

Ingredients
- 5 pounds green beans
- 1/3 cup oil
- 4 tsp salt
- 1/4 cup nutritional yeast

Instructions
1. Put green beans in an enormous bowl. On the off chance that you're utilizing frozen green beans, leave them to defrost in a bowl.
2. Pour oil over beans. In the case of utilizing coconut oil, liquefy the oil first and work quickly as the oils cement rapidly if your room or beans are cold.
3. Sprinkle seasonings over covered beans and mix well.
4. Dry in a dehydrator until dried out. This takes roughly 10 - 12 hours at 125 degrees or 8 hours at 135 degrees.
5. Store in a airtight compartment

Nutrition Facts: Calories 148, Fat 11g, Carbs 13g, Sugar 2g, Protein 2g

CARROT CHIPS

Prep Time: 10mints, Cooking Time: 20mints, Total time: 30mints, Serving: 4
Ingredients
- 2 large carrots
- 1/2 teaspoon olive oil
- 1/8 teaspoon sea salt

Instructions
1. Preheat grill to 350°F.
2. Wash and strip the carrots.
3. Using a mandolin slicer or a cutting edge, tilt the carrot, and cut out oval-formed bits.
4. Place the carrot cuts in a bowl and add olive oil and salt.
5. Lay the carrots in a singular layer on a treat sheet fixed with textured paper.
6. Heat for 15 to 20 minutes, or till the carrots are dry and shimmering.

Nutrition Facts: Calories 328, Fat 6g, Carbs 17g, Sugar 3g, Protein 25g

TOMATO CHIPS

Prep Time: 1hr, Cooking Time: 8hrs 20mints, Total Time: 9hrs 20mint, Serving: 4
Ingredients
- Roma Tomatoes Can use others
- Kosher or Sea Salt
- Dried Basil

Instructions
1. Cut tomatoes into 1/4 inch cuts. Organize on the dehydrator plate.
2. Sprinkle gently with salt and basil.
3. Dry out the vegetable setting for 8-12 hours, or until crispy.

Nutrition Facts: Calories 148, Fat 11g, Carbs 13g, Sugar 2g, Protein 2g

KETO CURRY CANDIED BACON RECIPE

Prep Time: 5mints, Cook Time: 20mints, Total Time: 25mints, Serving: 4
Ingredients
- 8 slices of bacon
- 2 Tsp erythritol
- 1 Tsp curry powder

Instructions
1. Preheat stove to 400°F (200°C).
2. Lay the bacon cuts on a preparing rack.
3. Blend the curry powder with the erythritol and rub over the bacon cuts.
4. Cook the bacon until firm.
5. Serve and enjoy as whole cuts or cut into little pieces for a snack.

Nutrition Fact: Calories: 261, Fat 26g, Carbs 1g, Sugar 0.3g, Protein 6g

PARMESAN CRISPS BAKED WITH ZUCCHINI AND CARROTS

Prep Time: 10mints, Cook Time: 8mints, Total Time: 18mints, Servings: 6
Ingredients
- 1 cup Parmesan cheese freshly shredded
- 1/2 cup shredded zucchini

Instructions
1. Preheat stove to 375°F.
2. Utilizing a paper towel, remove excessive dampness from chopped zucchini and carrots.
3. Add shredded Parmesan.
4. Put Tablespoon length drops of the cheddar and vegetable mixture on a parchment sheet
5. Delicately straighten combo with the back of a spoon.
6. Heat for round 8mins or till the cheddar crisps are scorching and the rims are beginning to darken.
7. Crisps will maintain on cooling.

Nutrition Fact: Calories: 67, Fat 4g, Carbs 2g, Sugar 1.2g, Protein 6g

PUMPKIN SPICE APPLE CHIPS

Prep Time: 15mints, Cook Time: 3hrs, Total Time: 3hrs 15mints, Serving: 6
Ingredients
- 2 medium apples
- 2 tablespoons Pumpkin Pie Spice
- 2 tablespoons confectioners' erythritol

Instructions
1. Preheat the stove to 200°F.
2. Utilizing a mandolin, cut the apples as daintily as could be expected under the circumstances, you can center the apples first however I simply cut the entire apple and afterward evacuate the seeds.
3. Line 2 heating sheets with parchment paper. Put the apple cuts in a solitary layer over the parchment paper.
4. Add the pumpkin pie spices and erythritol and sprinkle liberally over the apple cuts. Put the plate in the stove on the top and base racks. Prepare for 2.5 to 3 hours.

Nutrition Fact: Calories: 24, Fat 0.2g, Carbs 5.2, Sugar 2.1g, Protein 0.2g

KETO SALT AND PEPPER CRACKERS

Prep Time: 15mints, Cooking Time: 10mints, Total Time: 25mints, Serves: 20 crackers
Ingredients
- 2 cups blanched almond flour
- 1 large egg
- ½ teaspoon Celtic sea salt
- ½ teaspoon ground black pepper

Instructions
1. Put almond flour, egg, salt, and pepper in a nourishment processor
2. Beat until batter structures
3. Separate batter into equal parts
4. Put 50% of batter between two bits of parchment paper
5. Turn out the batter to 1/16-inch thick, at that point evacuate the top bit of parchment paper

6. Move base bit of parchment paper with turned out batter onto a heating sheet
7. Cut into 2-inch squares utilizing a pizza shaper or a blade. Sprinkle with additional salt and pepper if necessary.
8. Prepare at 350°F for 6-10 minutes

Nutrition Facts: Calories 268, Fat 17.2g, Carbs 8.3g, sugar 4.5g, Protein 22g

ROSEMARY AND SEA SALT CRACKERS

Prep Time: 10mints, Cooking Time: 15mints, Total Time: 25mints, Serving: 36 crackers

Ingredients
- 1 1/2 cups almond flour
- 1/2 tsp Celtic sea salt
- 2 Tbsp coconut oil
- 1 egg and 1 Tbsp rosemary
- 1/4 tsp black pepper

Instructions
1. Preheat stove to 350 F
2. In a huge bowl, join the almond flour and ocean salt.
3. In a different little bowl, add the coconut oil, egg, rosemary, and dark pepper.
4. Add the wet ingredients to the dry and blend to add.
5. Roll the batter between two bits of parchment paper until around 1/4" thick
6. Cut the batter into even vertical strips and repeat with even flat stripes.
7. Put the pieces on a parchment paper-lined oven tray and heat for 10-15 minutes or until brilliant dark-colored.

Nutrition Fact: Calories 176, Fat 16g, Carbs 10g, Sugar 6g, Protein 3g

HOMEMADE BAKED BANANA CHIPS

Prep Time: 5mints, Cook Time: 2hrs, Total Time: 2hrs 5mints, Serving: 4

Ingredients
- 2 Bananas
- Lemon juice
- Water
- Kosher salt

Instructions
1. In a little bowl, join 3/4 section lemon juice with 1/4 section water
2. Cut bananas neatly, around 1/8" thick coins, brush with lemon squeeze and water blend. Sprinkle with salt.
3. Prepare at 250F for around 1/2 to 2 hours or until they are firm, trying to flip them over half way through the cooking process.
4. Remove them from the stove and allow them to cool.

Nutrition Fact: Calories: 110, Fat 0.4g, Carbs 28.5g, Sugar 2g, Protein 1.4g

ROSEMARY & SEA SALT FLAX CRACKERS

Prep Time: 15mints, Cooking Time: 20mints, Total Time: 35mints, Serving: 4

Ingredients
- cup ground flax seeds
- eggs
- 1/2- cup grated parmesan
- tsp minced fresh rosemary
- Sea salt or kosher salt

Instructions
1. Preheat stove to 350 degrees F and bathe a treat sheet with a nonstick oil.
2. Add the ingredients into a medium bowl. Mix until completely blended. Let sit down for round 5mins
3. Shower a big cutting board with a nonstick spray.
4. Utilize a bread cutter or sharp blade to cut a pattern of one inch-ash rectangular.
5. Use a spatula or pie server to transport the squares onto your box.
6. Keep rerolling and slicing your pieces until the batter is altogether long gone.
7. Sprinkle with salt. Heat for 10mins, remove and flip, prepare an additional three minutes.
8. Present with your selected cheddar or dip!

Nutrition Facts: Calories 108, Fat 8.9g, Carbs 2.5g, Sugar 0.3g, Protein 4.6g

CAULIFLOWER MAC AND CHEESE IN 4 MINUTES

Prep Time: 2mints, Cook Time: 2mints, Total Time: 4mints, Servings: 4

Ingredients
- 3/4 cup frozen cauliflower florets
- 1-ounce cheddar cheese
- 1 tablespoon heavy cream

Instructions
1. In a little microwavable dish with top, microwave cauliflower secured for about a moment.
2. Remove from microwave and cleave cauliflower into little pieces.
3. Microwave for an additional 50 seconds or thereabouts, at that point adds shredded cheddar.
4. Microwave for an additional 10 seconds or something like that
5. Mix liquefied cheddar in and then add substantial cream until sauce structures.
6. Serve and enjoy!

Nutrition Fact: Calories: 191, Fat 14.9g, Carbs 4.8g, Sugar 4.3g, Protein 9.4g

EASY LOW CARB CAULIFLOWER PIZZA CRUST RECIPE

Prep Time: 15mints, Cook Time: 30mints, Total Time: 45mints, Serving: 8

Ingredients
- 1 1/2 lb Cauliflower
- 1 1/2 cup grated parmesan cheese
- 1 large Egg

- 1/2 tbsp Italian seasoning
- 1/2 tsp Garlic powder

Instructions
1. Preheat the range to 400°F. Put a bit of cloth paper onto a pizza strip on the off threat that you intend to make use of a pizza stone.
2. Beat the cauliflower florets in a nourishment processor until they're the consistency of rice
3. In a pan sauté the cauliflower for round 10mins.
4. Put the cauliflower rice right into a kitchen towel and press over the sink.
5. Place on the pizza tray and leave to cool for 5-10 minutes at room temperature to solidify more.
6. Add wanted ingredients. Bring to the stove for round 5-10 minutes, until cheese melts.

Nutrition Fact: Calories: 80, Fat 8g, Carbs 5g, Sugar 3g, Protein 14g

KETO DEVILED EGGS

Prep Time: 5mints, Cooking Time: 10mints, Total Time: 15mints; Serving: 4

Ingredients
- 4 eggs
- 1 tsp tabasco and fresh dill
- ¼ cup mayonnaise
- 1 pinch herbal salt
- 8 cooked and peeled shrimp
- fresh dill

Instructions
1. Start by heating up the eggs by setting them in a pot and covering them with water. Put the pot over medium heat and bring it to a light boil.
2. Boil for 8-10 minutes to ensure the eggs are hardboiled.
3. Remove the eggs from the pot and put them in an ice shower for a couple of moments before stripping.
4. Split the eggs down the middle and scoop out the yolks. Put the egg whites on a plate.
5. Crush the yolks with a fork and add Tabasco, herbal salt and custom made mayonnaise.
6. Add the blend, utilizing two spoons, to the egg whites and top with a shrimp on each, or a bit of smoked salmon.
7. Sprinkle with dill and serve.

Nutrition Fact: Calories 163, Fat 15g, Carbs 0.5g, Sugar 10g, Protein 7g

SPICY KETO DEVILED EGGS

Prep Time: 10mints, Cooking Time: 10mints, Total Time: 20mints; Serving: 6

Ingredients
- 6 eggs
- 1 tbsp red curry paste
- ½ cup mayonnaise
- ¼ tsp salt
- ½ tbsp poppy seeds

Instructions
1. Put the eggs in cool water in a dish, simply enough water to cover the eggs. Heat to the point of boiling without a placing the cover on the pot.
2. Give the eggs a chance to stew for around eight minutes. Cool rapidly in super cold water.
3. Remove the eggshells. Cut off the two closures and split the egg into equal parts. Scoop out the egg yolk and put in a little bowl.
4. Put the egg whites on a plate and let sit in the fridge.
5. Blend curry paste, mayonnaise and egg yolks into a smooth batter. Salt to taste
6. Draw out the egg whites from the fridge and apply the batter.
7. Sprinkle the seeds on top and serve.

Nutrition Fact: Calories 200, Fat 19g, Carbs 1g, Sugar 7g, Protein 6g

ITALIAN KETO PLATE

Prep Time: 5mints, Total Time: 5mints; Serving: 2

Ingredients
- 7 oz. fresh mozzarella cheese
- 7 oz. prosciutto
- 2 tomatoes and salt and pepper
- 1/3 cup olive oil
- 10 green olives

Instructions
1. Put tomatoes, prosciutto, cheddar, and olives on a plate. Present with olive oil and season with salt and pepper to taste.

Nutrition Fact: Calories 822, Fat 69g, Carbs 8g, Sugar 21g, Protein 40g

MEAT-LOVER PIZZA CUPS

Prep Time: 15mints, Cook Time: 11mints, Total Time: 26mints, Serving: 4

Ingredients
- 12 deli ham slices
- 1 lb. bulk Italian sausage
- 12 Tbsp sugar-free pizza sauce
- 3 cups grated mozzarella cheese
- 24 pepperoni
- 1 cup bacon

Instructions
1. Preheat stove to 375 F. Place peperoni in a skillet, removing excess oil.
2. Line 12-cup biscuit tins with ham cuts. Gap hotdog, pizza sauce, mozzarella cheddar, pepperoni cuts, and bacon separated equally between each cup, in a specific order.
3. Heat at 375-degree F for 10 minutes. Sear for 1 minute until cheese forms air pockets and tans and the edges of the meat ingredients look firm.
4. Remove pizza cups from biscuit tin and set on paper towels to keep the bottoms from getting wet. Serve and enjoy quickly or refrigerate and warm in toaster/stove or microwave.

Nutrition Facts: Calories 401, Fat 24g, Carbs 2g, Sugar 1g, Protein 42g

TACO SAUCE – LOW CARB, GLUTEN-FREE

Prep Time: 10mints, Cooking Time: 10mints, Total Time: 20mints, Serving: 4

Ingredients
- 8 oz can Organic Tomato Sauce
- ¼ cup of water
- 3 Tbs. Taco Seasoning
- 1 tbsp white vinegar
- 1 tbsp dried onion flakes

Instructions
1. In a medium pot, over medium warm temperature, add all ingredients.
2. Heat to the factor of boiling over medium, lessen to low, and stew.
3. Stew for 5-10mins, stiring at times.

Nutrition Fact: Calories: 33, Fat 3g, Carbs 0.3g, sugar 1.2g, Protein 2g

FATHEAD PIZZA DOUGH- KETO

Prep Time: 2mints, Cook Time: 14mints, Total Time: 16mints , Serving: 2

Ingredients
- 2 oz cream cheese
- 3/4 cup shredded mozzarella
- 1 egg, beaten
- 1/4 tsp garlic powder
- 1/3 cup almond flour

Instructions
1. Preheat the stove to 425°F
2. In a little bowl, add cream cheese and mozzarella. Microwave on high for 20 seconds one after another until softened
3. Add remaining ingredients to the liquefied cheese.
4. Blend.
5. Oil a pizza dish, spread mixture out into a 1/2" thick circle.
6. Cook for 12-14 minutes or until darker in color.
7. Top with your preferred ingredients or try out the White Keto Pizza.

Nutrition Fact: Calories: 280, Fat 31g, Carbs 2.8g, Sugar 2.2g, Protein 1g

BACON, BRAUNSCHWEIGER, & PISTACHIO TRUFFLES

Prep Time: 20mints, Cooking Time: 35mints, Total Time: 55mints, Serving: 4

Ingredients
- 8 oz Braunschweiger
- 1/4 cup chopped pistachio kernels
- 6 oz cream cheese
- 1 tsp dijon mustard
- 8 slices bacon

Instructions
1. Combine the Braunschweiger and pistachios in a little nourishment processor and mix.
2. In a different little bowl, whip the mellowed cream cheese and mustard together until smooth.
3. Fold the Braunschweiger into 12 little balls.
4. At that point take each ball and structure around a 1/4 inch thick layer of cream cheddar with your fingers.
5. When you have done every one of them, chill for around 30 minutes
6. Roll each ball in the finely cut bacon bits and put it on a serving dish.
7. Serve cold, or at room temperature.

Nutrition Fact: Calories 145, Fat 12g, Carbs 1.5g, Sugar 2.1g, Protein 7g

COCONUT FLOUR PIZZA CRUST RECIPE

Prep Time: 15mints, Cooking Time: 25mints, Total Time: 40mints, Serving: 4

Ingredients
- 4 eggs
- 1/4 cup coconut flour
- 1/2 tsp garlic powder
- 1/2 tsp onion powder and 2 Tsp water
- 1/3 cup parmesan cheese

Instructions
1. Preheat stove to 400º
2. Beat eggs and water together. Add dry ingredients and mix into the egg blend.
3. Generously oil a 12" pizza skillet, or 9×13 preparing dish with oil
4. Spread pizza blend onto the container.
5. Heat for 10-15 minutes until the edges start to darken.
6. Remove from stove and add your pizza ingredients.
7. Put back in the stove for another 8-10 mins until cheese is bubbly and somewhat toasted on top. Remove from the stove and let cool five minutes before cutting.
8. Serve and enjoy

Nutrition Fact: Calories: 86, Fat 5g, Carbs 3g, Sugar 2g, Protein 6g

BETTER THAN FAT HEAD PIZZA – PIZZA CRUST

Prep Time: 15mints, Cook Time: 20mints, Total Time: 35mints, Serving: 2

Ingredients
- 1 cup pork rinds
- cups cheddar cheese
- 2 tbsp cream cheese
- 1 egg

Instructions
1. Place pork rinds in blender or nourishment processor until finely grounded.
2. In a microwaveable bowl, heat shredded cheddar and cream cheese until smooth ~ 45 seconds

3. Mix cheeses and egg. Work rapidly, if cheddar turns out to be hard, microwave for 10 sec
4. Add grounded pork rinds and mix until blended.
5. Press batter out onto the material secured heating sheet. ~1/4-inch-thick, or wanted thickness
6. Prepare at 350 degrees F for 5 minutes
7. Remove and top with wanted garnishes and heat for extra 10-15 minutes or until cheese melts.
Nutrition Fact: Calories: 469, Fat 38.5g, Carbs 1.9g, Sugar 2.4g, Protein 28.4g

EASY CROCKPOT BONE BROTH

Prep Time: 30mints, Cooking Time: 45mints, Total Time: 1hr 15mints, Serving: 3
Ingredients
- A mixing bowl of chicken bones and cartilage
- Coarsely chopped carrots
- 2 tbsp raw apple cider vinegar
- Filtered Water
- Salt and pepper

Instructions
1. Add vegetables and chicken bones and cartilage.
2. Add inlet leaves if utilizing
3. Load up with filtered water
4. Add 2 tbsp apple juice vinegar
5. Cook on low for about 24 hours
6. Strain and store or serve

Nutritional Fact: Calories 388, Fat 14g, Carbs 2g, Sugar 1g, Protein 60g

SPINACH PIZZA CRUST

Prep Time: 10mints, Cook Time: 15mints, Total Time: 16mints, Serving: 4
Ingredients
- 4 cup baby spinach leaves
- 1 cup grated cheese
- 2 eggs and 1/4 tsp salt
- 1/4 teaspoon garlic powder
- 1 tablespoon dried oregano

Instructions
1. Preheat stove to 200°C (400°F).
2. Line a heating tray with a bit of parchment paper. Spray some olive oil to maintain a strategic distance from the hull to adhere to the paper. Put aside.
3. Wash the baby spinach leaves. You can pat dry. Or use pre-washed baby spinach leaves to stay away from this progression. Mix for 30 seconds or until smooth.
4. Pour the spinach blend onto the readied heating sheet. Utilizing a spatula spread the blend into a square shape that covers the entire oven tray or uses two heating sheets and makes two round pizza bases of 10 inches.
5. Cook the spinach pizza blend for 15-20 minutes or until the sides are darker and firm.
6. Remove from the stove and add your preferred low carb ingredients like a tomato pizza base.

Nutrition Facts: Calories 59, Fat 3.8g, Carbs 2.4g, Sugar 0.9g, Protein 4.6g

STEAMED ARTICHOKE

Prep Time: 5mints, Cook Time: 20mints, Total Time: 25mints, Serving: 4
INGREDIENTS
- 2 medium artichokes
- 1 lemon
- 2 tablespoons mayonnaise
- 1 teaspoon Dijon mustard
- 1 pinch paprika

INSTRUCTIONS
1. Wash properly and remove the tarnished leaves. Trim the spines off the encompassing leaves if present.
2. Wipe any reduce edges with a lemon - this will protect them from oxidizing.
3. In the occasion that your artichoke has a stem, cut it off to make a base for the artichoke. (Boil the stem together with the artichoke in pressure cooker.)
4. Add one cup of water to the pressure cooker base and lower the steamer bin inside.
5. When time is up, open the pressure cooker through the Natural discharge method - flow the cooker off the burner and accept as true with that the weight will descend in my view.
6. Blend mayonnaise in with mustard and put in the little dip compartment and sprinkle with paprika.
7. Serve warm.

Nutritional Fact: Calories: 77.5, Fat 5g, Carbs 3.5g, Sugar 0.2g, Protein 2gù

FAT HEAD PIZZA - THE HOLY GRAIL

Prep Time: 10mints, Cook Time: 20mints, Total Time: 30mints; Serving: 6
Ingredients
- 170 g pre shredded/grated cheese mozzarella
- 85 g almond meal/flour
- 2 tbsp cream cheese
- 1 egg
- pinch salt to taste

Instructions
1. Blend the shredded/ground cheddar and almond flour/meal in a microwaveable bowl. Add the cream cheddar. Microwave on HIGH for 1 minute.
2. Mix and microwave on HIGH for an additional 30 seconds.
3. Add the egg, salt, rosemary and some other flavorings, blend carefully.
4. Put in the middle of 2 bits of heating material/paper and fold into a round pizza shape.
5. Make fork gaps everywhere throughout the pizza base to guarantee it cooks uniformly.

6. To make the base extremely firm and tough, flip the pizza over once the top has cooked.
7. When cooked, remove from the stove and add toppings of your choice. Ensure any meat is as of now cooked and return to stove just to warm up the garnishes and liquefy the cheese.
Nutrition Facts: Calories 203, Fat 16.8g, Carbs 4g, Sugar 1g, Protein 11g

ASPARAGUS + GOAT CHEESE FRITTATA

Prep Time: 10mints, Cooking Time: 25mints, Total Time: 35mints; Serving: 4
Ingredients:
- 1/2 pound asparagus
- 12 eggs
- 2 Tablespoons milk or cream
- 2 to 4 ounces soft goat cheese
- Olive oil, black pepper, and 1/2 tsp salt

Instructions:
1 Beat the eggs and trim and reduce the asparagus into scaled-down pieces.
2 Toss the asparagus into the solid iron with some olive oil, season it with salt and pepper, and prepare dinner until softly roasted and soft, around 12-15 mins.
3 Empty the eggs into the cast iron, spreading them equally. Cook them until they may be set round the rims.
Asparagus and Goat Cheese Frittata Camping Recipe
4 Sprinkle little bits of the goat cheese round the very best factor of the frittata.
5 Spread with tinfoil and prepare dinner for 15-20mins. Evacuate the tinfoil and permit the frittata sit down for round 5mins before slicing and serving.
Nutrition Fact: Calories: 321, Fat 9g, Carbs 14g, Sugar 4.1g, Protein 24g

FANCY AF EGG CLOUDS RECIPE

Prep Time: 15mints, Cooking Time: 20mints, Total Time: 35mints; Serving: 1
Ingredients:
- 3 eggs
- 3 Tsps crumbled bacon
- 3 Tsps grated Parmesan cheese
- 1/8 tsp salt and Black pepper
- 2 Tsps parsley

Instructions:
1 Line an oven tray with cloth paper and preheat the stove to 375ºF. Utilizing your fingers, carefully separate the whites from the egg yolks, allowing the whites to drop in a huge bowl. Beat egg whites with a stand blender or hand-held blender on medium-high.
2 Utilizing an elastic spatula, delicately overlap in bacon pieces, Parmesan, salt, and 1 Tablespoon of parsley.
3 Partition the egg white combo onto the fabric paper, shaping 3 even "mists," dispersing them 1-inch separated.

4 With the spatula, make a well inside the focal point of every cloud; at that factor cautiously drop in egg yolks to the focal point of the wells.
5 Heat for 8-10 minutes for runny yolks, or 14-16 minutes for properly done yolks, or till yolks have set and whites emerge as caramelized. Embellishment with black pepper and cut parsley, serve on toasted.
Nutrition Fact: Calories 264, Fat 9g, Carbs 8g, Sugar 5g, Protein 27g

EGG NEST RECIPE WITH BRAISED CABBAGE

Prep Time: 2mints, Cook Time: 7mints, Total Time: 9mints; Serving: 2
Ingredients
- 1 teaspoon ghee
- 4 cups cabbage shredded
- 1/8 teaspoon salt
- 1 tablespoon apple cider vinegar
- Pepper and 2 eggs

Instructions
1 Soften ghee in a huge griddle that has a fitted top over medium-high heat.
2 Add cabbage and salt. Remove with the liquefied ghee.
3 Keep cooking over medium-high heat until the cabbage tans, around 3-4 minutes. Blend in apple juice vinegar and pepper.
4 Accumulate cabbage into two little hills. Utilizing the back of a spoon, structure a well in each hill to make space for the eggs
5 Break an egg into every space in the cabbage.
6 Decrease the heat to low-medium and cook until whites of egg firm and yolk arrive at wanted consistency.
7 Season with salt and pepper to taste
Nutrition Fact: Calories: 121, Fat 6g, Carbs 8g, Sugar 4g, Protein 7g

EGGS EN COCOTTE RECIPE

Prep Time: 10mints, Cook Time: 15mints, Total Time: 25mints; Serving: 3
Ingredients
- 1 tablespoon ghee
- 2 cups mushrooms
- salt and 3 eggs
- 1 tablespoon chives
- 3 tablespoons heavy cream

Instructions
1 Utilizing a multi-cooker, dissolve ghee, and at the same time sauté mushrooms together, until delicate, caramelized, and reduced to 3/4 cup. Season with salt for taste
2 In the meantime, oil the ramekins. Whilst mushrooms are cooked, separate into ramekins. Top with a teaspoon of chives, a crisply cut up egg, and a tablespoon of cream
3 The multi-cooker pots are nonstick; Essentially add 2 cups of water to the bottom of the Instant Pot.

4 Get a stand and put the egg-crammed ramekins on top. Verify and lock the duvet of the multi-cooker. Cook on low for 1-2mins
5 Discharge quick and remove the ramekins. They'll be hot, so use heatproof stove gloves.
6 Present with newly toasted bread.
Nutrition Fact:: Calories: 113, Fat 6.9g, Carbs 6.8g, Sugar 4.3g, Protein 7.9g

CLOUD EGGS

Prep Time: 10mints, Cook Time: 6mints, Total Time: 16mints; Servings: 4
Ingredients
- 4 large eggs
- 1/2 cup grated parmesan cheese
- 1/2 tbsp chopped garlic chives
- 2 green scallions
- 2 crispy bacon crumbled

Instructions
1. Preheat stove to 450°F. Line a massive heating tray with fabric paper.
2. Separate egg whites from egg yolks. Put egg whites into the mixing bowl and beat. Be cautious while separating that you don't contaminate the egg whites.
3. Heat for round 4-5mins or until egg whites begins to turn darkish in color. Add egg yolk and cook 1-3 minutes greater, contingent upon the amount you need to cook your egg yolk.
4. Add bacon and scallions.
5. Serve right away as the eggs will shrivel as they start to cool.
Nutrition Facts: Calories 173, Fat 12g, Carbs 1g, Sugar 4g, Protein 12g

HUEVOS PERICOS COLOMBIAN SCRAMBLED EGGS

Prep Time: 10mints, Cook Time: 10mints, Total Time: 20mints; Serving: 2
Ingredients
- 2 teaspoons olive oil
- 3 to 4 medium scallions
- 1 medium tomato
- 6 large eggs
- Kosher salt or adobo seasoning salt

Instructions
1. Cook the scallions.
2. In the meantime, season tomato with selected salt
3. Allow liquid from the tomato evaporates, around 3 to four minutes.
4. Add the squashed eggs to the skillet with more salt.
5. Cook over medium heat, blending two or multiple times till certainly cooked.
Instructions: Calories: 272, Fat 19g, Carbs 5g, Sugar 6g, Protein 19.5g

CAESAR EGG SALAD LETTUCE WRAPS

Prep Time: 10mints, Cooking Time: 15mints, Total Time: 25mints; Serving: 3
Ingredients
- 6 large hard-boiled eggs
- 3 tbsp creamy Caesar dressing
- 3 tbsp mayonnaise
- 1/2 cup Parmesan cheese
- Cracked black pepper
- 4 large romaine lettuce leaves

Instructions
1. In a blending bowl, mix hard-boiled eggs, velvety Caesar dressing, mayonnaise, 1/4 cup Parmesan and cracked dark pepper.
2. Spoon blend onto romaine leaves and top with left over cheese.
Nutrition Fact: Calories: 254, Fat 22g, Carbs 2.75g, Sugar 1.3g, Protein 13.5g

LOW CARB CHEESE ENCHILADAS

Prep Time: 2mints, Cook Time: 3mints, Total Time: 5mints; Servings: 1
Ingredients
- 2 eggs
- 1 ounce shredded sharp cheddar
- 1 ounce Pepper Jack shredded
- 1-ounce grass-fed butter
- Salt, Pepper, Cumin, and Smoked paprika

Instructions
1. Mix the eggs and cheddar in a blender until smooth.
2. Liquefy the spread in an omelet dish.
3. Pour in the egg blend.
4. Cook until cooked on the base then lifting the egg up with a spatula and giving the uncooked egg a chance to stream underneath.
5. Top with the Pepper Jack, salt, pepper and cumin.
6. Overlay in thirds and scoop out onto a plate.
7. Sprinkle with smoked paprika and any leftover shredded cheddar.
Nutrition Fact: Calories: 321, Fat 9g, Carbs 14g, Sugar 4.1g, Protein 24g

KETO 2 MINUTE AVOCADO OIL MAYO

Prep Time: 2mints, Total Time: 2mints; Serving: 2
Ingredients
- 2 teaspoons lemon juice
- 1 large egg
- 1/2 teaspoon dry mustard powder
- 1/2 teaspoon sea salt
- 1 cup avocado oil

Instructions
1. In a tall, wide-mouth container, add the lemon squeeze juice, a large egg, seasonings and lastly the oil. Give the ingredients a chance to rest for 20 seconds or so.
2. Put the blender right at the base of the container. Turn it on rapid and leave it at the base of the container for around 20 seconds. The

mayonnaise will promptly start to set up and fill the container.
3. After the mayonnaise is practically set, gradually pull the blender towards the highest point of the container without removing the cutting edges from the mayonnaise. Gradually drive it back towards the base of the container. Repeat this stage a few times until the ingredients are mixed well.
4. Taste and add salt if needed.

Nutrition Fact: Calories: 134, Fat 14.9g, Carbs 0.1g, Sugar 1.2g, Protein 0.4g

TACO SAUCE

Prep Time: 10mints, Cooking Time: 10mints, Total Time: 20mints; Serving: 2

Ingredients
- 8 oz can Organic Tomato Sauce
- ¼ cup water
- 3 Tbs. Taco Seasoning
- 1 tbsp white vinegar
- 1 tbsp dried onion flakes

Instructions
1. In a medium pot, over medium warm temperature, add all ingredients.
2. Heat until boiling then decrease heat to low and stew
3. Stew for 5-10mins, mixing from time to time.

Nutrition Fact: Calories: 261, Fat 23g, Carbs 3.6g, Sugar 0.8g, Protein 13.6g

BACON-WRAPPED SCALLOPS

Prep Time: 10mints, Cook Time: 15mints, Total Time: 25mints; Serving: 4

Ingredients
- 16 sea scallops
- 8 slices bacon
- 16 toothpicks
- olive oil for drizzling
- Black pepper and kosher salt to taste

Instructions
1. Preheat stove to 425°F.
2. Line a heating sheet with parchment paper. Put aside.
3. Envelop one scallop by using half a piece of bacon and hold with a toothpick.
4. Shower olive oil over every scallop and season with pepper and salt.
5. Place scallops in a solitary layer on a readied oven tray, giving every scallop some space to permit the bacon to cook.
6. Heat 12 to 15mins until scallop and bacon are cooked thoroughly.
7. Serve warm.

Nutrition Fact: Calories: 224, Fat 17g, Carbs 2g, Sugar 3g, Protein 12g

LOW CARB FRIED MAC & CHEESE

Prep Time: 10mints, Cooking Time: 15mints, Total Time: 25mints; Serving: 4

Ingredients
- 1 ½ cups shredded cheddar cheese
- 3 large eggs
- 2 teaspoons paprika
- 1 teaspoon turmeric and 1 medium cauliflower
- ¾ teaspoon rosemary

Instructions
1. Rice the cauliflower in a nourishment processor.
2. Cook it in the microwave for 5 minutes.
3. Dry it out by wringing it in a kitchen towel or paper towels. You need as little dampness as possible.
4. Add your eggs, cheese and flavors to the cauliflower and combine.
5. Heat olive oil and coconut oil in a skillet, on high
6. Structure little patties out of the cauliflower blend
7. Fry on the two sides until done and serve warm.

Nutrition Fact: Calories: 40, Fat 2.4g, Carbs 1.5g, Sugar 1g, Protein 3.2g

CAPRESE GRILLED EGGPLANT ROLL-UPS

Prep Time: 5mints, Cook Time: 8mints, Total Time: 13mints; Servings: 8 bites

Ingredients
- 1 eggplant
- 4 oz mozzarella 115g
- 1 tomato large
- 2 basil leaves
- Good quality olive oil

Instructions
1. Ensure your blade is sharp before beginning. Cut the end of the eggplant into slim cuts, around 0.1in/0.25cm thick the long way. Dispose of the smaller pieces that are mostly skin and not as long from either side.
2. Cut the mozzarella and tomato daintily too. Shred the basil leaves.
3. Warm a frying pan and gently brush the eggplant cuts with olive oil. Put the eggplant cuts on the skillet and cook for two or three minutes on each side.
4. Top it with a cut of tomato and add a little bit of mozzarella at the slenderer end. Sprinkle over two or three bits of basil and shower a little olive oil and two or three toils of dark pepper.
5. Roll the eggplant from the slenderer end, which has just the cheese.

Nutrition Fact: Calories: 59, Fat 3g, Carbs 4g, Sugar 2g, Protein 3g

ROASTED SQUASH, POMEGRANATE SEEDS AND SPICED WALNUT SALAD

Prep Time: 20mints, Cooking Time: 35mints, Total Time: 55mints; Serving: 8

Ingredients
- 1 bunch of purple kale
- 1/2 cup Cinnamon and Walnut Oil Dressing
- 1/2 cup pomegranate seeds
- Roasted Butternut Squash
- Spiced walnuts

Instruction
1. Cut kale leaves from stem, wash, rinse and dry.
2. Cut leaves daintily and puts in a big bowl. Pour dressing over the leaves and with fingers, "knead" dressing into leaves
3. Blend within the roasted squash, pomegranate seeds, and spiced walnuts and serve.
4. Add more dressing or salt for taste.

Nutrition Facts: Calories 467, Fat 27g, Carbs 2g, Sugar 2g, Protein 36g

ROASTED BUTTERNUT SQUASH CUBES

Prep Time: 20mints, Cooking Time: 25mints, Total Time: 45mints; Serving: 4

Ingredients
- 1 butternut squash
- 2 tablespoon coconut oil
- 1 teaspoon cinnamon
- 1/4 teaspoon sea salt

Instructions
1. Preheat stove to 400F.
2. Strip the skin of the butternut squash utilizing a y-peeler. Cut down the middle and dispose of seeds. Cut into pieces then into 1-inch solid shapes.
3. Remove squash shapes and with remaining ingredients, put on a material lined sheet skillet in a solitary layer.
4. Cook squash for 45 minutes, or until edges begin to darken.

Nutrition Facts: Calories 276.4, Fat 14.5g, Carbs 1.8g, Sugars 0.3g, Protein 35.5g

WILTED ORGANIC KALE & BACON

Prep Time: 5mints, Cook Time: 5mints, Total Time: 10mints; Serving: about 4 cups

Ingredients
- 8 cups of packed kale leaves
- 2 slices of country thick bacon
- Sea salt and pepper

Instructions
1. Rinse kale and chop the kale into huge scaled-down pieces.
2. In a huge sauté skillet, cook the bacon over medium heat.
3. When the bacon is done, remove and put aside, leaving the bacon oil in the dish.
4. Put the kale into the dish with the bacon oil, season with salt and pepper and enable the kale to shrink over medium heat.
5. Keep on mixing until done. The kale is done when it is delicate.
6. Cut bacon into little pieces and mix in with kale.
7. Serve right away.

Nutrition Fact: Calories: 213, Fat 15g, Carbs 3g, Sugar 5g, Protein 28g

90-SECOND KETO BREAD IN A MUG

Prep Time: 5mints, Cook Time: 2mints, Total Time: 7mints; Serving: 4

Ingredients
- 1 tablespoon butter
- 1/3 cup blanched almond flour
- 1 egg
- 1/2 teaspoon baking powder
- 1 pinch salt

Instructions
1. Put spread in a microwave-safe mug. Microwave until liquefied, around 15 seconds.
2. Add almond flour, egg, baking powder and salt in the mug; stir until smooth.
3. Microwave at most extreme power until set, around 90 seconds
4. Let cool for 2 minutes before cutting.

Nutrition Facts: Calories 408, Fat 36.4g, Carbs 9.8, Sugar 16g, Protein 14.5g

GRAIN-FREE BUTTER BREAD

Prep Time: 20mints, Total Time: 50mints; Serving: 4

Ingredients
- eggs
- 1 1/2- cups almond flour
- tsp salt
- 2 tsp baking powder
- 1/4- cup butter
- 1/8- tsp cream tartar

Instructions
1. Preheat the range to 375 degrees F.
2. Put almond flour in a nourishment processor. Add salt, baking powder and egg yolks. Pour in liquefied margarine.
3. Sprinkle cream of tartar into the egg whites. Mix until sensitive tops shape. Move around 1/3 of the combination into the nourishment processor.
4. Beat, scratching the sides of container with a spatula as required, until all-around combined.
5. Scratch mixture into the bowl with the egg whites. Mix till uniform.
6. Heat within the preheated stove till darker in color and a knife cut through the middle comes out clean.
7. Run a flimsy blade alongside the edge of bread and leave to rest for 10mins.

Nutrition Facts: Calories 241, Fat 21g, Carb 5.6g, Sugar 4.2g, Protein 9.7g

PUMPKIN SPICE ROASTED PECANS

Prep Time: 5mints, Cook Time: 12mints, Total Time: 17mints; Serving: 2
Ingredients
- 2 cups raw pecans
- 3 tablespoons salted butter
- 1 teaspoon pure vanilla extract
- 2 tablespoons Pumpkin Pie Spice
- 2 tablespoons confectioners erythritol

Instructions
1. Preheat the stove to 350°F. Line a rimmed heating sheet with a silicone preparing mat or parchment paper.
2. Add the walnuts, margarine, and vanilla to a blending bowl. Utilize an elastic spatula to remove the nuts and coat them equally in the softened spread.
3. Sprinkle the pumpkin pie flavor and erythritol over top. Move about to equally coat the nuts.
4. Spread the nuts over the oven tray in a solitary layer.
5. Heat for 12 minutes.

Nutrition Fact: Calories: 215, Fat 22.3g, Carbs 4.7g, Sugar 1g, Protein 2.4g

KETO HOLLANDAISE

Prep Time: 5mints, Cook Time: 10mints, Total Time: 15mints; Serving: 2
Ingredients
- 4 egg yolks
- 2 tablespoons fresh lemon juice
- 1/2 cup butter
- dash hot sauce
- Cayenne pepper and sea salt

Instructions
1. In a tempered steel blending bowl, whisk the egg yolks and lemon squeeze together. The blend ought to get thicker and increment in volume.
2. Heat a pot with water in it over medium heat until the water is boiling. Lower the heat to medium-low. Put the bowl over the highest point of the pan, ensuring that the water isn't contacting the base of the bowl
3. Gradually, race in the softened margarine until the sauce has thickened and is light and cushy.
4. Remove from heat and delicately race in hot sauce, cayenne pepper, and ocean salt.

Nutrition Fact: Calories: 132, Fat 14g, Carbs 4g, Sugar 3g, Protein 2g

KETO BACON WRAPPED ASPARAGUS WITH A SECRET SAUCE

Prep Time: 10mints, Cook Time: 20mints, Total Time: 30mints; Serving: 4
Ingredients
- 1 bundle of Asparagus
- 1 package sugar-free bacon
- 1 teaspoon Coconut Amino
- 4 oz butter
- 1 tbs ChocZero Honest Maple Syrup
- 1 tsp pepper

Instructions
1. Wash and set up the crisp asparagus by removing the stems. Pat dry.
2. Fold a bit of bacon over every asparagus.
3. Lay the prepared asparagus strips on a heating sheet fixed with parchment paper.
4. Utilize a treating brush and cover each piece of asparagus with the syrup blend.
5. Cook at 400 degrees F for around 20 minutes or until the bacon gets dark-colored just as you would prefer.

Nutrition Fact: Calories: 149, Fat 11.9g, Carbs 3.5g, Sugar 0.9g, Protein 7g

KETO HONEY MUSTARD DRESSING

Prep Time: 5mints, Total Time: 5mints; Serving: 1
Ingredients
- 1/2 cup full-fat sour cream
- 1/4 cup water
- 1/4 cup Dijon mustard
- 1 tablespoon apple cider vinegar
- 1 tablespoon granular erythritol

Instructions
1. Add all ingredients in a blending bowl and mix to blend them.
2. Can be stored in the cooler for as long as about fourteen days

Nutrition Fact: Calories: 38, Fat 2.5g, Carbs 0.5g, Sugar 0.3g, Protein .4g

PARMESAN CHIVE AND GARLIC KETO CRACKERS

Prep Time: 10mints, Cook Time: 30mints, Total Time: 40mints; Serving: 100 crackers
Ingredients
- 1 3/4 cups blanched almond flour
- 2 cups finely grated Parmesan cheese
- 1 tsp garlic powder
- 2 tsp fresh chives
- 2 tsp butter and 2 large eggs

Instructions
1. Preheat the stove to 340°F. Line two huge rimmed oven trays with parchment paper.
2. In an enormous blending bowl, add the almond flour, parmesan cheese, garlic powder and chives. Blend until all ingredients are very much mixed.
3. Empty the wet ingredients into the dry ingredients and blend well.
4. Utilize a baked good shaper or a sharp blade to cut each sheet of batter into 50 equivalent estimated shapes.
5. Move the heating sheets to the stove and cook for 15 minutes.
6. Remove the trays from the stove and cautiously re-cut the crackers anyplace they may be in contact with one another and separate them only marginally to enable them to cool.

7. With the stove off, set the plate back into the stove and leave them there as the stove cools. This will yield superbly crunchy crackers.
Nutrition Fact: Calories: 104, Fat 8.6g, Carbs 2.1g, Sugar 0.9g, Protein 5.8g

SPINACH-MOZZRELLA STUFFED BURGERS

Prep Time: 15mints, Cooking Time: 20mints, Total Time: 35mints; Serving: 4

Ingredients
- 1½ lbs ground chuck
- 1 teaspoon salt
- ¾ tsp black pepper and 2 cups fresh spinach
- ½ cup shredded mozzarella cheese
- 2 tsps grated Parmesan cheese

Instructions

1. In a medium bowl, add ground meat, salt and pepper.
2. Put spinach in a pan over medium-high heat. Cover and cook for 2 minutes, until shriveled.
3. Drain and let cool. With your hands press the spinach to drain further. Move to a cutting board, cut the spinach and put it in a bowl. Mix in mozzarella and Parmesan.
4. Scoop about ¼ cup of blend into 4 patties and seal the edges by squeezing hard together.
5. Cup every patty with your hands to balance the edges, and push on the top to straighten somewhat into a solitary thick patty.
6. Heat a barbecue to medium-high. Flame broil burgers for 5 to 6 minutes on each side.

Nutrition facts: Calories 414g, Fat 29g, Carbs 1g, Sugar 3g, Protein 36g

DESSERTS

MACADAMIA NUT FAT BOMB

Prep Time: 20mints, Cook Time: 20mints, Total Time: 40mints, Serving: 6

Ingredients
- 1/3 cup unrefined coconut oil
- 2 tbsp. unsweetened cocoa powder
- 2 tbsp. Monk fruit or Stevia
- 1 tsp vanilla extract
- 12 macadamia nuts
- Pinch salt

Instructions
1. In a little container whisk collectively the coconut oil, vanilla, sugar, and vanilla concentrate till creamy.
2. Line a little holder with parchment paper.
3. Pour in the chocolate blend, utilize a spatula to extended it far and equally along the base.
4. Put macadamia nuts in the chocolate blend.
5. Sprinkle salt gently everywhere.
6. Put the compartment in the cooler for 20 minutes.
7. Store in the cooler for a fast-sweet treat or fat bomb

Nutrition Fact: Calories: 99, Fat 16.9g, Carbs 1.9g, Sugar 1g, Protein 0.8g

SUGAR-FREE LOW CARB DRIED CRANBERRIES

Prep Time: 15mints, Cook Time: 4hrs, Total Time: 4hrs 15mints, Serving: about 3 cups

Ingredients
- 2 – 12-ounce bags fresh cranberries
- 1 cup granular erythritol
- 3 tablespoons avocado oil
- 1/2 teaspoon pure orange extract

Instructions
1. Preheat the stove to 200°F. Line two rimmed oven trays with parchment paper or silicone heating mats.
2. Wash and dry the cranberries and remove any seared or delicate berries. Cut the cranberries down the middle and add them to a blending bowl.
3. Add the sugar, avocado oil, and orange concentrate, if utilizing. Remove to equitably cover the entirety of the berries.
4. Line the berries in single layers over the oven trays.
5. Leave to cook for 3 to 4 hours.

Nutrition Fact: Calories: 61, Fat 3.5g, Carbs 7g, Sugar 2g, Protein 15g

STRAWBERRY ICE CREAM

Prep Time: 25mints, Cooking Time: 2hrs, Total Time: 2hrs 25mints, Serving: 4

Ingredients
- 13.5 oz coconut milk
- 16 oz frozen strawberries
- 1/2-3/4 cup equivalent sweetener
- 1/2 cup chopped fresh strawberries

Instructions
1. In a blender add every one of the ingredients, except for the new strawberries, and mix until smooth.
2. Add the strawberries directly before the frozen yogurt is solid.
3. Serve promptly or place the dessert in the cooler for 1-2 hours to solidify further.

Nutrition Fact: Calories 264, Fat 9g, Carbs 8g, Sugar 5g, Protein 27g

MALTED MILK ICE CREAM

Prep Time: 4mints, Total Time: 4mints, Serving: 5

Ingredients
- 5 egg yolks
- 1/2 cup Swerve confectioners
- 1 cup heavy whipping cream
- 1 cup unsweetened cashew milk
- 2-3 tsp organic MACA powder
- 1/4 tsp sea salt

Instructions
1. In a medium pan place the egg yolks and sugars in to blend on high with a hand blender. Whip yolks until light in shading and twofold in size. Mix in the whipping cream.
2. Mix until thickened into a custard. Remove from heat and mix in the almond milk, MACA powder, and salt. Let cool totally.
3. Put into your frozen yogurt machine and watch the enchantment occur inside 10 minutes or as per your dessert producer's bearings.
4. Stop until set for frozen yogurt or mix in your preferred whirl flavor to blend it up.

Nutrition Fact: Calories 230, Fat 13.9g, Carbs 23g, Sugar 8g, Protein 4g

LOW CARB CHOCOLATE MASON JAR ICE CREAM

Prep Time: 8mints, Total Time: 8mints, Serving: 2

INGREDIENTS
- 1 cup heavy cream
- 2 tablespoons granular erythritol
- 1 tablespoon unsweetened cocoa powder
- 1 teaspoon pure vanilla extract
- 2 tablespoons sugar-free chocolate chips

Instructions
1. Add all ingredients in a wide mouth smallish artisan container. Screw the cover on and shake overwhelmingly for 5 minutes.
2. The fluid inside should twofold in volume, filling the artisan container.
3. Leave in cooler for 3 to 24 hours.
4. Scoop, serve and enjoy it!

Nutrition Fact: Calories: 206, Fat 22g, Carbs 18g, Sugar 7g, Protein 1g

SUGAR-FREE COCONUT ICE CREAM

Prep Time: 20mints, Total Time: 20mints, Serving: 5
Ingredients
- 5 egg yolks
- 500 ml coconut cream full fat
- 250 ml double/heavy cream
- 4 tbsp powdered sweetener or more
- 1 tsp vanilla

Instructions
1. Whisk the egg yolks in a widespread heatproof bowl. Put aside.
2. In a pan, add coconut cream, cream and sugar. Delicately heat on the stovetop blending until the sugar is broken down.
3. Start delicately whisking the egg yolks once more and add a spoon of heavy cream to the egg yolks. Proceed till all the cream has been mixed.
4. Mix in the vanilla into the pot and heat again whilst mixing, to thicken to a custard consistency.
5. Remove from the heat and permit to chill completely. Mix in the toasted coconut, saving 2 tablespoons to beautify the finished dessert while serving.
6. Cool the frozen yogurt mixture inside the cooler as soon as made.
7. Add the left-over coconut shavings when serving.

Nutrition Facts: Calories 413, Fat 41g, Carbs 6.5g, Sugar 3g, Protein 5.5g

CHOCOLATE CHIP ICE CREAM

Prep Time: 10mints, Cook Time: 25mints, Total Time: 35mints, Serving: 8
Ingredients
- 16 ounces heavy whipping cream
- 1/2 cup granulated stevia/erythritol blend
- 2 teaspoons vanilla extract unsweetened
- 1-2 tsps peppermint extract
- 1 cup unsweetened almond milk
- 3 ounces stevia-sweetened dark chocolate

Instructions
1. Empty heavy cream into a medium bowl. Utilizing a hand blender, beat cream fast until firm pinnacles structure
2. Step by step add a couple of tablespoons of sugar one after another, continuously beating during the process.
3. Beat in vanilla and peppermint next.
4. Bit by bit add the almond milk, a couple of tablespoons one after another, beating after every addition.
5. Empty blend into the dessert cooler and stop as indicated by the product's directions.
6. Move to a hermetically sealed compartment and enable it to solidify in the cooler for a couple of hours before serving.

Nutrition Fact: Calories: 255, Fat 26g, Carbs 6g, Sugar 3g, Protein 2g

KETO CRÈME BRULE

Prep Time: 10mints, Cook Time: 34mints, Total Time: 44mints, Serving: 3
Ingredients
- 4 egg yolks
- 1 teaspoon vanilla extract
- 2 cups heavy whipping cream
- 5 tsp low-calorie natural sweetener

Instructions
1. Preheat stove to 325 degrees F.
2. Whisk egg yolks and vanilla extract in a bowl.
3. Pour whipping cream and 1 tablespoon sugar into a pot over medium heat. Whisk continually until it begins to stew. Remove from heat; add yolk blend gradually, whisking continually, until very much mixed.
4. Separation equally between 4 ramekins and put them in a glass preparing dish; pour in enough bubbling water to come 1 inch up the sides of the ramekins.
5. Prepare in the preheated stove on the center rack until set, around 30 minutes.
6. Sprinkle 1 tablespoon sugar over each crème Brule. Utilize a culinary light to warm sugar until liquefied and burnt like.

Nutrition Facts: Calories 466, Fat 48.4g, Carb 16.9g, Sugar 4.3g, Protein 5.1g

KETO PEANUT BUTTER FUDGE FAT BOMB

Prep Time: 10mints, Total Time: 2hrs 10mints, Serving: 7
Ingredients
- 1 cup unsweetened peanut butter
- 1 cup of coconut oil
- 1/4 cup vanilla-f almond milk
- 2 teaspoons vanilla liquid Stevie

Instructions
1. Line a component dish with textured paper.
2. Place peanut butter and coconut oil in a microwave secure dish.
3. Microwave 30 seconds till possibly broken down
4. Pour into a separating dish and refrigerate till set, around 2 hours.

Nutrition Facts: Calories 341, Fat 34.9g, Carb 5.3g, Sugar 4.2g, Protein 4.5g

LOW CARB JELLO POPS

Prep Time: 5mints, Cook Time: 5mints, Total Time: 10mints, Serving: 6
Ingredients:
- 1 - (0.3 oz) box of sugar free Jello gelatin
- ½ - cup boiling water
- Cup heavy whipping cream

Instructions:
1. In a bowl, place your gelatin and bubbling water.
2. Blend until the gelatin is broken down.

3. Add this blend to a blender and add your cream.
4. Mix on high until it's liquified.
5. Immerse your Popsicle and place in freezer until solid.
Nutrition Fact: Calories: 51, Fat 0.4g, Carbs 11g, Sugar 2g, Protein 3g

STRAWBERRY CHEESECAKE FAT BOMBS

Prep Time: 1hr 10mints, Cooking Time: 3hrs, Total Time: 4hrs 10mints, Serving: 4
Ingredients
- 70g strawberries
- 150g cream cheese
- 60g butter or coconut oil
- 20g powdered erythritol
- 1 vanilla bean

Instructions
1. Put the cream cheddar and spread cut into little pieces into a blending bowl. Leave at room temperature for 30–an hour until mollified. Ensure the spread is relaxed; else it will be hard to blend and accomplish a smooth surface.
2. In the meantime, wash the strawberries and remove the green parts. Put them into a bowl and crush utilizing a fork or put in a blender for a smooth surface.
3. Before you blend the strawberries in with the rest of the ingredients, ensure they have arrived at room temperature.
4. Utilize a hand whisk or nourishment processor and blend until all-around joined.
5. Spoon the blend into little biscuit silicon forms or treat molds. Put in the cooler for around 2 hours or until set.
6. At the point when done, unmold the fat bombs and put them into a holder. Keep in the cooler and serve and enjoy it whenever!
Nutrition Fact: Calories 432.2, Fat 8.3g, Carbs 10.4g, Sugar 1.4g, Protein 42g

ENGLISH TOFFEE FAT BOMBS

Prep Time: 15mints, Cooking Time: 20mints, Total Time: 35mints, Serving: 4
Ingredients:
- 1 cup of coconut oil
- 2 tbs butter
- 4 oz cream cheese
- 3/4 Tbs cocoa powder
- 1/2 cup of Natural Peanut Butter
- 3 Tbs Davinci Gourmet Sugar

Instructions
1. Put the entirety of your ingredients in a pot on the stovetop on medium/low heat.
2. Mix until everything liquefies together and is smooth.
3. Empty them into a shape or something to that effect. Pop those suckers in the cooler for a couple of hours.
4. Following a couple of hours, they'll be a great idea to go. Pop them out and do whatever it takes not to eat them all! They store well in the cooler.
Nutrition Facts: Calories 315, Fat 25g, Carbs 4g, Sugar 1g, Protein 19g

LOW CARB ROLLS

Prep Time: 5mints, Cook Time: 25mints, Total Time: 30mints, Servings: 10 rolls
Ingredients
- 1/2 cup Coconut flour
- 2 tbsp psyllium husk powder
- 1/4 tsp Pink Himalayan Salt and 3/4 cup Water
- 4 large eggs
- 4 tbsp Butter

Instructions
1. Start by mixing all the dry ingredients and blending completely.
2. In a different bowl start beating the eggs with a hand blender. Add melted margarine and water and keep on blending until merged.
3. Empty the dry ingredients into the wet and keep blending until the mixture turns out to be thick and very much blended. On the off chance that mixture isn't effectively shapeable by hand keep including more psyllium husk powder until it is less clingy.
4. Structure into 10 supper rolls and put on a lubed oven tray or silicone heating mat. Bigger rolls can be made whenever wanted, simply add a few moments onto the preparing time.
5. Heat for 30-35 minutes at 350 degrees. Serve and enjoy!
Nutrition Facts: Calories 102, Fat 7g, Carbs 5.8g, Sugar 4.5g, Protein 3g

CINNAMON BUN FAT BOMB BARS

Prep Time: 10mints, Cook Time: 5mints, Total Time: 15mints, Serving: 2
Ingredients
- Base
- 1/2 cup creamed coconut
- 1/8 tsp ground cinnamon
- First Icing:
- 1 tbsp extra virgin coconut oil
- 1 tbsp almond butter
- Second Icing:
- 1 tbsp extra virgin coconut oil
- 1/2 tsp ground cinnamon

Instructions
1. Line a dish or a smaller than expected portion container, biscuit skillet, and so on with proper liners.
2. In a bowl, utilizing your hands, blend the coconut cream and cinnamon.
3. First Icing: In another bowl utilizing a whisk, whisk together the coconut oil and almond

spread. Spread this over the creamed coconut. Put the bars in the cooler for around 5 minutes or more.
4. Second Icing: Using a whisk, combine the icing in a bowl. Shower the icing over the bars and either solidify again or expend.
Nutrition Fact: Calories: 170, Fat 18.7g, Carbs 3g, Sugar 2.3g, Protein 1.1g

LEMON CHEESECAKE FAT BOMBS WITH CREAM CHEESE

Prep Time: 15mints, Cooking Time: 15mints, Total Time: 30mints, Servings 16 fat bombs
Ingredients
- 6 oz wt. cream cheese
- 4 tbsp salted butter
- 3 tbsp granular swerve sweetener
- 2 tbsp fresh lemon juice
- 1 tbsp finely grated lemon zest

Instructions
1. Allow cream cheddar to sit at room temperature before proceeding.
2. In a bowl, join sugar, lemon juice, and lemon get-up-and-go, blending until well-blended.
3. In a different bowl, microwave the cream cheddar for around 10 seconds until delicate and flexible.
4. Add cream cheddar and margarine to the bowl with the lemon juice blend. Utilize an electric hand blender on low speed to beat until well-blended.
5. Separation into 16 round silicone molds and leave for a few hours until solid, before serving. Store remains in the cooler.

Nutrition Facts: Calories 60, Fat 7g, Carb 0.5g, Sugars 0.1g, Protein 1g

FAT BOMBS

Prep Time: 15mints, Cooking Time: 25mints, Total Time: 40mints, Serving: 5
Ingredients
- 3/4 cup melted coconut oil
- Tbs. almond butter
- 60 drops liquid Stevie
- 3 Tbs. cocoa
- 9 Tbs. melted salted butter

Instructions
1. Pour a sparse 2 Tbs. into every one of 24 sweet or smaller than normal biscuit molds. On the off chance that you like, you can utilize those little paper small scale biscuit cups, arranged on a treat sheet.
2. Put your treat form on a little treat sheet first, and afterward fill it, at that point put it in the cooler. In the event that you attempt to place it in the cooler without first putting it on a treat sheet, you'll be heartbroken.
3. Stop for at any rate 30 minutes, at that point fly out the Fat Bombs and store them in a pack or other compartment in the cooler. You can keep them in the refrigerator, yet when you hold one with your hot little fingers, it will liquefy truly quickly. Solidified, it liquefies slower.

Nutritional Fact: Calories 145, Fat 14.7g, Carbs 1.7g, Sugar 1.53g, Protein 23g

KETO CHOCOLATE NUT CLUSTERS

Prep Time: 5mints, Cook Time: 10mints, Total Time: 15mints, Serving: About 25 nut clusters
Ingredients
- 9 ounces sugar-free dark chocolate chips
- 1/4 cup unrefined coconut oil
- 2 cups salted mixed nuts

Instructions
1. Line a rimmed warming sheet with textured paper.
2. In a microwave-secure bowl, place pieces of the chocolate chips and coconut oil and microwave till the chocolate is condensed.
3. Use a versatile spatula to mix till blended. Let cool.
4. Mix in the nuts inside the chocolate.
5. Drop gigantic spoonfuls of the combo onto the prepared sheet.
6. Store in refrigerator until solid then serve.

Nutrition Fact: Calories: 170, Fat 14.9g, Carbs 2.5, Sugar 0.7g, Protein 3.2g

HAPPY ALMOND BOMBS – KETO FAT BOMBS

Prep Time: 20mints, Cooking Time: 25mints, Total Time: 45mints, Serving: 3
Ingredients
- 4 tbsp coconut butter
- 4 tbsp almond butter
- 1 oz cream cheese
- 1 tbsp cocoa powder
- 2 tbsp sugar-free syrup
- 16 grams dark chocolate

Instructions
1. In the event that you have to improve the hitter, I would likewise add a bundle or two of Splendor or Stevie or utilize a lighter level of dull chocolate
2. Add all ingredients aside from coconut margarine to a microwave-safe dish.
3. Microwave in 15-second interims, blending each time until the chocolate and cream cheddar are softened, and all ingredients are completely mixed.
4. At that point add the coconut margarine and combine everything completely.
5. Spoon player into 12 proportional segments
6. Fly in your cooler. They ought to be set inside 60 minutes, and you can pop them out effectively with a margarine blade.

Nutrition Fact: Calories 165, Fat 14g, Carbs 11g, Sugar 2g, Protein 2g

PALEO VEGAN COCONUT CRANBERRY CRACK BARS

Prep Time: 2miuts, Cook Time: 10mints, Total Time: 12mints, Servings: 20

Ingredients
- 2 1/2 cups shredded unsweetened coconut flakes
- 1/2 cup unsweetened cranberries
- 1 cup coconut oil, melted
- 1/4 cup sticky sweetener of choice

Instructions
1. In a fast blender or nourishment processor, add your coconut and cranberries and heartbeat until mixed and a thick, brittle surface remains.
2. In an enormous blending bowl, add your coconut/cranberry blend, coconut oil and clingy sugar of decision, and blend until completely mixed.
3. Empty player into a lined 8 x 8 inch or 8 x 10-inch heating plate, gently wet your hands at that point press the blend solidly into the right place. Refrigerate until firm. Cut into bars and plunge into any chocolate of your decision.

Nutrition Facts: Calories 98, Fat 9g, Carbs 3g, Sugar 2g, Protein 2g

NO-BAKE KETO BUTTER COOKIES

Prep Time: 10mints, Cook Time: 10mints, Total Time: 20mints, Serving: 6

Ingredients
- 1/2 cup almond flour
- 1/4 cup ghee
- Erythritol or Stevie
- 1 oz chocolate chunks

Instructions
1. Dissolve the ghee.
2. Blend the almond flour, ghee, and sugar in a little bowl to frame a batter.
3. Structure into little treats and top with chocolate pieces.
4. Refrigerate to set the treats more.

Nutrition Fact: Calories: 76, Fat 7g, Carbs 1g, Sugar 0.2g, Protein 1g

3-INGREDIENT KETO NO-BAKE COCONUT COOKIES RECIPE

Prep Time: 10mints, Total Time: 10mints, Serving: 12 cookies

Ingredients
- 1 cup coconut butter
- 1/4 cup chopped or slivered almonds
- Erythritol or Stevie

Instructions
1. Combine each one of the ingredients in a bowl.
2. Structure into treats and place on a plate covered in cloth paper.
3. Heat the coconut oil if the sheet unfolds excessively.
4. If it's too liquidity pour the oil onto the fabric paper and refrigerate to frame extra slim treats.
5. Refrigerate for two+ hours till it's time to serve.

Nutrition Fact: Calories: 151, Fat 14g, Carbs 5g, Sugar 1g, Protein 2g

4 INGREDIENT CHOCOLATE PEANUT BUTTER NO-BAKE COOKIES

Prep Time: 5mints, Cook Time: 15mints, Total Time: 20mints, Servings: 20

Ingredients
- 3/4 cup coconut flour
- 2 cups smooth peanut butter
- 1/2 cup sticky sweetener
- 2-3 cups chocolate chips of choice

Instructions
1. Line an enormous heating plate or platter with parchment paper and put aside.
2. In a microwave-safe bowl or stovetop, add your nutty spread and sweetener and liquefy until mixed. Add your coconut flour and blend until a thick player remains.
3. Utilizing your hands, structure little balls and put them on the lined plate. Flatten with a fork or spoon.
4. When treats are firm, soften your chocolate chips. Utilizing two forks, dunk every treat in the liquefied chocolate until totally joined. Repeat the procedure until all treats are solid. Refrigerate until firm.

Nutrition Facts: Calories 99, Fat 7g, Carbs 4g, Sugar 3g, Protein 4g

4 INGREDIENT LOW CARB HOT CHOCOLATE ICE CREAM

Prep Time: 5mints, Cook Time: 15mints, Total Time: 20mints, Servings: 12

Ingredients
- 13.66 oz canned coconut milk
- 1-4 scoops chocolate protein powder
- 2 tbsp cocoa powder
- 1-2 tbsp granulated sweetener

Instructions
1. Put a profound portion skillet in the cooler.
2. Remove coconut milk from the fridge and separate the cream from the water. In a rapid blender or nourishment processor, add the cream first, trailed by the coconut water. Mix until simply mixed.
3. Add your granulated sugar, protein powder, and cocoa powder and mix until thick and rich Do not over-mix.
4. Move the hot cocoa frozen yogurt to the chilled portion container. To guarantee it doesn't turn out to be excessively frosty, softly blend your dessert ever 20-30 minutes within an hour.

5. Softly wet a frozen yogurt scoop before scooping out into a bowl.
Nutrition Facts: Calories 130, Fat 11g, Carbs 2g, Sugar 1.2g, Protein 7g

HEALTHY 3 INGREDIENTS NO BAKE PALEO VEGAN COCONUT CRACK BARS

Prep Time: 2mints, Cook Time: 3mints, Total Time: 5mints, Servings: 20
Ingredients
- 3 cups shredded unsweetened coconut pieces
- 1 cup of coconut oil
- 1/4 cup organic product improved maple syrup

Instructions
1. Line an 8 x 8-inch container or 8 x 10-inch skillet with parchment paper and put aside. Then again, you can utilize a portion dish.
2. In a huge blending bowl, add your shredded unsweetened coconut. Add your liquefied coconut oil and organic product improved maple syrup and blend until a thick hitter remains. In the event that it is excessively brittle, add some additional syrup or a modest piece of water.
3. Pour the coconut split bar blend into the lined dish. Gently wet your hands and press immovably into the right pla.ce Refrigerate or stop until firm. Cut into bars, serve and enjoy!
Nutrition Facts: Calories 108, Fat 11g, Carbs 2g, Sugar 2g, Protein 2g

EASY STOVETOP SUGAR-FREE CANDIED ALMONDS

Prep Time: 1mint, Cook Time: 5mints, Total Time: 6mints, Servings: 10
Ingredients
- 3 cups raw unsalted almonds
- 1 cup granulated monk fruit sweetener
- 1/4 cup water
- 1 tsp vanilla extract
- Pinch sea salt

Instructions
1. Preheat stove to 250 degrees. Line an enormous heating plate with parchment paper and put aside.
2. Spread out almonds on a solitary layer.
3. Heat for 45 minutes, blending every so often.
4. When almonds have quite recently started to take shape, remove and permit to cool for 1-2 minutes, before blending
5. Permit cooling totally, before covering in an extra tsp or two of organic product sugar.
Nutrition Fact: Calories: 199, Fat 18g, Carbs 7g, Sugar 4g, Protein 7g

HEALTHY NO CHURN WORKOUT PROTEIN ICE CREAM

Prep Time: 5mints, Cook Time: 2mints, Total Time: 7mints, Servings: 16
Ingredients
- 2 14 oz cans coconut milk
- 1-4 scoops vanilla protein powder
- 1-2 tbsp granulated sweetener
- 1 tsp vanilla extract

Instructions
1. Put a huge, profound portion skillet or profound container in the cooler.
2. In a blender or nourishment processor, add your coconut milk and mix until smooth and velvety. Add your protein powder and granulated sugar or dates and mix until a thick and rich surface remains.
3. Move exercise protein frozen yogurt to the portion container. To guarantee it doesn't turn out to be excessively frigid, gently blend your frozen yogurt ever 20-30 minutes for the principal hour.
4. Defrost for 10-15 minutes before eating. Softly wet a dessert scoop before scooping the frozen yogurt into a bowl and serve
Nutrition Fact: Calories: 500, Fat 40g, Carbs 11g, Sugar 1g, Protein 25g

4-INGREDIENT NO-BAKE CHOCOLATE COCONUT CRACK BARS

Prep Time: 1mint, Cook Time: 5mints, Total Time: 6mints, Servings: 22 bars
Ingredients
- 3 cups destroyed unsweetened coconut drops
- 1 cup of coconut oil
- 1/4 cup priest organic product improved maple syrup
- 1-2 cups chocolate chips

Instructions
1. Line an 8 x 10-inch container or enormous portion dish with parchment paper and put aside.
2. In an enormous blending bowl, add every one of your ingredients and blend well. Empty into the lined container; softly wet your hands and press. Put in the cooler to solidify
3. When firm, remove and cut into bars. Put in the cooler.
4. Liquefy your chocolate chips of decision and separately, plunge every coconut bar in the softened chocolate until covered uniformly. Repeat until every one of the bars is equally covered. Refrigerate until chocolate solidifies, serve and enjoy!
Nutrition Facts: Calories 106, Fat 11g, Carbs 3g, Sugar 2g, Protein 2g

3-INGREDIENT KETO PEANUT BUTTER FUDGE

Prep Time: 2mints, Cook Time: 2mints, Total Time: 4mints, Servings: 18 cups
Ingredients
- 1/2 cup peanut butter
- 1/2 cup coconut oil

- 1 serving sweetener of choice liquid Stevie

Instructions
1. Line a component dish with biscuit liners and set aside.
2. In a microwave-secure bowl, add peanut butter with coconut oil and dissolve together.
3. Add your sugar of choice, tasting it to guarantee it has enough sweetness.
4. Separate the fudge into cups and leave to cool.
5. Top with shredded softened chocolate.

Nutrition Facts: Calories 89, Fat 8g, Carbs 1g, Sugar 1g, Protein 2g

EASY KETO GARLIC ROASTED BOK CHOY

Prep Time: 10mints, Cook Time: 20mints, Total Time: 30mints, Serving: 4

Ingredients
- 1 large head Bok choy
- 1/4 cup Avocado oil
- 1 tsp Sea salt
- 1/2 tsp Black pepper
- 4 cloves Garlic

Instructions
1. Preheat the stove to 425 stages F
2. Place the Bok choy in a solitary layer on a massive heating sheet
3. Sprinkle with 2 tbsp avocado oil. Sprinkle with 1/2 of the salt and pepper. Repeat oil, salt, and pepper on the opposite side.
4. Flip returned finished, with the intention that the reduce side is up.
5. Spread the minced garlic anywhere at some stage on the Bok choy.
6. Cook the Bok choy in the stove for 10mins on the rack.
7. Rotate the dish and cook for 10 additional minutes

Nutrition Facts: Calories 152, Fat 14g, Carbs 5g, Sugar 2g, Protein 3g

3 INGREDIENT FLOURLESS SUGAR FREE COOKIES

Prep Time: 2mints, Cook Time: 10mints, Total Time: 12mints, Servings: 12 cookies

Ingredients
- 1 cup smooth almond butter
- 3/4 cup granulated sweetener
- 1 large egg

Instructions
1. Preheat oven to 350 degrees Fahrenheit and line a heating plate with parchment paper.
2. In a big mixing bowl, place all your ingredients and mix until all around mixed.
3. Shape little balls on the threatened sheet with fingers or utensil; spread 3-4 inches apart
4. Press every ball right into a treat form and press down with a fork. Prepare for 8-10mins

5. Remove from the stove and permit cooling until delicate, firm but slightly chewy.

Nutrition Fact: Calories: 101, Fat 9g, Carbs 3g, Sugar 2g, Protein 5g

4 INGREDIENT KETO VEGAN CHOCOLATE COCONUT COOKIES

Prep Time: 5mints, Cook Time: 5mints, Total Time: 10mints, Servings: 30 cookies

Ingredients
- 4 cups unsweetened shredded coconut
- 1/4 cup granulated sweetener
- 1/2 cup coconut milk
- 2-3 cups chocolate chips

Instructions
1. Line a huge heating plate or platter with parchment paper and put aside.
2. In a rapid blender or nourishment processor, add your unsweetened coconut and mix until a fine consistency remains. Add your granulated sugar of decision and mix for an additional moment.
3. Add your coconut milk and keep mixing, scratching down the sides. When a thick batter remains, remove and place in a huge blending bowl. Softly wet your hands and structure little balls. Put on the lined heating plate and press each ball into a treat shape. Put treats in the cooler to solidify.
4. When treats are firm, dissolve your chocolate chips. Utilizing two forks, dunk every treat in the softened chocolate until totally mixed. Repeat the procedure until all treats are secured. Refrigerate until firm.

Nutrition Facts: Calories 43, Fat 4g, Carbs 3g, Sugar 2g, Protein 1g

3 INGREDIENT KETO ALMOND BUTTER CUPS

Prep Time: 2mints, Cook Time: 3mints, Total Time: 5mints, Servings: 18 cups

Ingredients
- 1/2 cup almond butter
- 1/2 cup coconut oil
- 1 serving sweetener Liquid Stevie
- 1/2 cup chocolate of choice Optional

Instructions
1. Line a normal biscuit tin with parchment paper and put aside. Then again, cover a little portion skillet with parchment paper.
2. In a microwave-safe bowl or stovetop, join your almond spread and coconut oil. On low heat/low power, soften until thick and velvety. Add your sugar of decision and blend well.
3. Equitably appropriate the almond margarine blend among the biscuit liners. Refrigerate until firm.

Nutrition Facts: Calories 91, Fat 9g, Carbs 1g, Sugar 0.1g Protein 2g

4 INGREDIENT KETO VEGAN CHOCOLATE SNOWBALL COOKIES

Prep Time: 5mints, Cook Time: 5mints, Total Time: 10mints, Servings: 40 cookies

Ingredients
- 4 cups shredded unsweetened coconut
- 1/4 cup cocoa powder
- 2 tbsp granulated sweetener
- 1 cup coconut cream

Instructions
1. In an enormous blending bowl or fast blender, add the shredded coconut, cocoa powder and granulated sugar of decision and blend or mix until joined.
2. Add your chilled coconut cream and blend or mix until a thick player remains. Refrigerate for 30 minutes or until chilled.
3. Utilizing your hands, structure the mixture into little balls. When every one of the balls is shaped, place them on a lined plate. Press down on each ball to frame a treat shape. If you wish, roll every treat in extra shredded coconut.

Nutrition Facts: Calories 42, Fat 4g, Carbs 2g, Sugar 2g, Protein 1g

NO-BAKE KETO VEGAN PEANUT BUTTER COOKIES

Prep Time: 2mints, Cook Time: 3mints, Total Time: 5mints, Servings: 20 cookies

Ingredients
- 3/4 cup coconut flour
- 2 cups smooth peanut butter
- 1/2 cup sticky sweetener

Instructions
1. Line a huge plate with parchment paper and put in a safe place.
2. In a microwave-safe bowl or stovetop, add your nutty spread and sticky sugar and soften until mixed.
3. Utilizing your hands, structure little balls and put them on the lined plate or plate.
4. Press each ball into a level treat shape, utilizing a fork. Refrigerate until firm but slightly fudgy.

Nutrition Facts: Calories 113, Fat 8g, Carbs 5g, Sugar 3g, Protein 4g

KETO CHOCOLATE PEANUT BUTTER COOKIES

Prep Time: 10mints, Cook Time: 12mints, Total Time: 22mints, Serving: 3

Ingredients
- 1 cup unsalted peanut butter fresh
- 1/4 cup coconut flour sifted
- 2 tablespoons unsweetened cocoa powder
- 1/4 cup sugar-free natural liquid sweetener or maple syrup

Instructions
1. Preheat stove to 180°C (356°F).
2. Set up a treat rack secured with parchment paper. Put aside.
3. In nourishment processor with the S sharp edge connection, add every one of the ingredients, on medium speed for around 1 minute or until all the ingredients meet up into a ball.
4. Split into 8 even pieces.
5. Fold each piece into a treat ball, place each ball on the readied treat rack leaving half thumb space between every treat. The treats won't spread so don't leave excess of room, heat for 10-12 minutes.
6. Remove from treat rack and allow to chill.
7. When chilling off, enhance with sugar-free syrup, cocoa powder and unsalted peanut butter. Put the treats in the cooler for a couple of minutes to allow toppings to set if necessary.

Nutrition Facts: Calories 218, Fat 15.6g, Carbs 10.6g, Sugar 2.6g, Protein 9.3g

KETO VEGAN CHOCOLATES

Prep Time: 10mints, Cooking Time: 15mints, Total Time: 25mints, Serving: 8

Ingredients
- 3/4 cup coconut oil
- 9 Tbsp cocoa powder
- 3 Tbsp Lakanto Sugar-Free Maple Syrup
- 2 tsp vanilla extract
- 12 drops liquid stevia extract

Instructions
1. Liquefy coconut oil in a little bowl: microwave for 30 to 45 seconds till liquified.
2. Add cacao, agave, vanilla concentrate, and stevia to coconut oil and blend completely.
3. Utilize a spoon to painstakingly placed chocolate right into a coronary heart shape.
4. Put coronary heart form, chocolate bar shape or heating dish inside the cooler for at any fee 10mins to permit the chocolate to solidify.
5. Make the most of your delightfully chocolaty treat!

Nutrition Fact: Calories: 454, Fat 31g, Carbs 26g, Sugars 4.4g, Protein 22g

FRESH STRAWBERRY LIME POPSICLES

Prep Time: 5mints, Total Time: 3hrs, Serving: 4

Ingredients
- 10 medium to large strawberries
- Zest of 1 lime
- 2 tbsp water

Instructions
1. Remove any stems from strawberries
2. Add lime zest
3. Mix together
4. Pour into your decision of Popsicle cylinders, freeze, serve and enjoy!

Nutrition Fact: Calories: 10, Fat 0.1g, Carbs 2g, Sugar 1g, Protein 3g

STRAWBERRY LOW CARB POPSICLES FREEZER POPS

Prep Time: 10mints, Cook Time: 10mints, Total Time: 20mints, Servings: 12 freezer pops

Ingredients
- 1/2 cup low carb sugar substitute
- 2 cups strawberries
- 2 Tsp lemon juice
- 4 cups of water

Instructions
1. In a pot, heat sugar and strawberries on medium-low until a sauce is formed.
2. Put warm strawberry sauce and lemon juice in a blender until smooth.
3. Place in an enormous bowl with some water.
4. Empty fluid into Popsicle molds or cooler pop packs.
5. Freeze and serve.

Nutrition Fact: Calories: 18, Fat 0.1g, Carbs 2.1g, Sugar 0.4g, Protein 0.2g

3-INGREDIENT KETO RASPBERRY LEMON POPSICLES

Prep Time: 5mints, Total Time: 6hrs 5mints, Servings: 10 Popsicles

Ingredients
- 1cuplemon juice
- 2cupswater
- 3 to 5 drops of Stevie more or less
- 1/2cupfrozen raspberries

Instructions
1. Cut the raspberries and partition them equally between Popsicle molds.
2. Whisk collectively the lemon juice, water and Stevie.
3. Fill the Popsicle shape.
4. Secure the top and add Popsicle sticks.
5. Freeze for 4 hours or so.
6. Serve and enjoy!

Nutrition Fact: Calories: 500, Fat 40g, Carbs 11g, Sugar 1g, Protein 25g

PEANUT BUTTER CHOCOLATE COOKIES

Prep Time: 10mints, Cook Time: 10mints, Total Time: 20mints, Serving: 6

Ingredients
- 1 cup creamy peanut butter
- 1 egg
- 1/4 cup Stevie sweetener
- 2 tsps unsweetened cocoa powder
- 1 tablespoon vanilla extract

Instruction
1. Preheat stove to 350 degrees F.
2. Add peanut butter, egg, stevia sugar, cocoa powder, and vanilla extract together with a blender.
3. Fold mixture into 1-inch balls. Put 1 to 2 inches separated on an ungreased baking sheet. Smooth balls with a fork.
4. Heat in the preheated stove until edges are set, around 10 minutes, let cool on the heating sheet for 10 minutes.
5. Line a plate with waxed paper. Move treats to plate until cooled to room temperature, around 15 minutes, at that point refrigerate for 30 minutes.

Nutrition Facts: Calories 105, Fat 8.5g, Carb 5.8g, Sugar 3.2g, Protein 5.6g

FUDGY MACADAMIA CHOCOLATE FAT BOMB

Prep Time: 20mints, Cooking Time: 15mints, Total Time: 35mints, Serving: 4

Ingredients
- 2- oz Cocoa Butter
- 2 Tbs unsweetened cocoa powder
- 2 Tbs Swerve
- 4- oz macadamias
- ¼ cup Heavy cream

Instructions
1. Soften cocoa margarine in a little pan in a shower of water.
2. Add cocoa powder to the pan.
3. Presently add the Swerve and blend well until all ingredients are very much mixed and softened.
4. Add macadamias and mix them in well. Add cream, blend well and take back to heat.
5. Presently pour in molds or paper tray cups.
6. Let cool, and place in fridge to solidify.
7. Keep at room temperature, with a somewhat gentler consistency than chocolate

Nutrition Fact: Calories: 267, Fat 28g, Carbs 3g, Sugar 2g, Protein 3g

JELLO CREAM CHEESE FAT BOMB

Prep Time: 20mints, Cooking Time: 25mints, Total Time: 45mints, Serving: 3

Ingredients
- oz of Kraft Philadelphia Cream Cheese
- 1 package of sugar-free jello or pudding mix

Instructions
1. Take the bundle of Cream cheddar and cut it into 16 squares.
2. Put the sans sugar jello or pudding blend in a sandwich baggie.
3. Take each square and shake until secured with jello or pudding blend on all sides.
4. At that point fold into a ball in your hands.
5. Keep with saran wrap in the cooler.

Nutrition Fact: Calories 165, Fat 14g, Carbs 11g, Sugar 2g, Protein 2g

LOW CARB CHOCOLATE COCONUT FAT BOMBS

Prep Time: 1hr 30mints, Cook Time: 5mints, Total Time: 1hr 35mints, Servings: 10 balls

Ingredients
- 1 cup coconut butter almond

- 1 cup coconut milk full fat
- 1 teaspoon vanilla extract gluten-free
- 4 Tbsp quality cocoa powder
- 1 teaspoon stevia powder
- 1 cup coconut shreds

Instructions
1. Put every one of the ingredients apart from shredded coconut in medium warm temperature bowl with water
2. Blend the ingredients.
3. Put the bowl inside the ice chest until it's far hard enough to fold into balls, around half-hour.
4. Fold the substance into one-inch balls and flow them through the coconut shreds.
5. Put the balls on a plate and refrigerate for 60mins.
6. Serve and enjoy.

Nutrition Facts: Calories 251, Fat 21.7g, Carbs 12.8g, Sugar 4.4g, Protein 2.8g

KETO PEANUT BUTTER COOKIES

Prep Time: 10mints, Cook Time: 15mints, Total Time: 25mints, Serving: 7

Ingredients
- 1 cup peanut butter
- 1/2 cup natural sweetener
- 1 egg
- 1 teaspoon sugar-free vanilla extract

Instructions
1. Preheat stove to 350 degrees F. Line a oven tray with parchment paper.
2. Add peanut butter, sugar, egg, and vanilla extract in a bowl; blend well until a batter is shaped.
3. Fold batter into 1-inch balls. Put on the parchment paper and press down twice with a fork in a jumbled design.
4. Place in the preheated stove until edges are done, 12 to 15 minutes. Cool on the heating sheet for 1 minute before removing to a wire rack to cool totally.

Nutrition Facts: Calories 133, Fat 11.2g, Carb 12.4g, Sugar 8.3g, Protein 5.8g

PUMPKIN SEED BARK AND DARK CHOCOLATE & SEA SALT

Prep Time: 5mints, Cook Time: 5mints, Total Time: 10mints, Servings: 10

Ingredients
- 3 oz dark chocolate Lily's
- 1/4 cup roasted pumpkin seeds
- 1/2 tbsp sea salt

Instructions
1. Soften dark chocolate in a microwave-safe bowl for 30 seconds.
2. Repeat until the chocolate has absolutely dissolved.
3. Save a confined amount of the cooked pumpkin seeds to sprinkle on top. Add the rest of the seeds with the softened chocolate.
4. Pour chocolate pumpkin seed combo into an eight x 4-inch preparing dish fixed with parchment paper.
5. Use an elastic spatula to help circulate the blend into the compartment and easy it into an even layer.
6. Sprinkle the sea salt and saved toasted pumpkin seeds over the combo.
7. Leave the combination to remain at room temperature till set or place in the fridge for 10 to 15 minutes to speed the process.
8. Cut chocolate into 10 portions.

Nutrition Fact: Calories: 37, Fat 3g, Carbs 5g, Sugar 4g, Protein 1g

LOW CARB CHOCOLATE BARK

Prep time: 3mints, Cook time: 15mints, Total time: 18mints, Serves: 1

Ingredients
- ¼ cup of melted extra virgin coconut oil
- 2 tbsp of unsweetened cocoa
- 2 tsp – 1 tbsp of raw honey

Instructions
1. In the event that your coconut oil is strong, you can blend it in with the cocoa powder and sugar.
2. In large container, blend the coconut oil with the cocoa powder and sugar until smooth.
3. Taste for sweetness
4. Let it set for around 10-15 minutes then place in the cooler.
5. Serve and enjoy!

Nutrition Fact: Calories: 82, Fat 8g, Carbs 2g, Sugar 2g, Protein 2g

CHOCOLATE COCONUT GUMMES

Prep Time: 10mints, Cooking Time: 20mints, Total Time: 30mints, Serving: 5

Ingredients
- can full-fat coconut milk
- tbsp gelatin
- 1/4- tsp vanilla bean powder or 1 tsp vanilla extract
- 2-3- tsp cacao powder
- a couple of sea salt and Stevie

Instructions
1. Put all ingredients in a blender and blend until very much joined
2. Fill a treat shape or glass dish and refrigerate until firm
3. Cut into wanted measure and store in the fridge

Nutrition Fact: Calories: 107, Fat 9g, Carbs 4g, Sugar 2g, Protein 1g

3 INGREDIENT KETO CHOCOLATE COCONUT CUPS

Prep Time: 2mints, Cook Time: 3mints, Total Time: 5mints, Servings: 18 cups

Ingredients

- 1/2 cup coconut butter, melted
- 1/2 cup cocoa powder
- 1/2 cup coconut oil
- 1 serving sweetener

Instructions
1. Line an 18-tally small scale biscuit tin with smaller than expected biscuit liners and put aside.
2. In a microwave-safe bowl, soften your coconut oil. Add your cocoa powder and blend until completely joined and no bunches remain. In the event that you use alternatives to sweeteners, add at this point.
3. Moving rapidly, coat the base and sides of the biscuit liners with liquefied chocolate.
4. When firm, partition the coconut margarine among the cups. Top with the rest of the chocolate and leave to set until firm.

Nutrition Fact: Calories: 43, Fat 4.2g, Carbs 1g, Sugar 0.3g, Protein 0.5g

KETO VANILLA ALMOND FAT BOMB

Prep Time: 5mints, Total Time: 5mints, Serving: 6
Ingredients
- 6 Tsp coconut butter, warmed
- 1 tsp vanilla extract
- 6 almonds
- Stevie or erythritol

Instructions
1. Blend the coconut spread with the vanilla concentrate and sugar.
2. Fill ice solid shape plate.
3. Place an almond into each.
4. Set in the cooler for 2-3 hours.

Nutrition Fact: Calories: 216, Fat 20g, Carbs 7g, Sugar 2g, Protein 2g

KETO ALMOND BUTTER FAT BOMB SANDWICHES RECIPE

Prep Time: 5mints, Total Time: 5mints, Serving: 4
Ingredients
- 1 bar of dark chocolate
- 2 Tsp almond butter
- Stevie or erythritol
- Dash of cinnamon powder

Instructions
1. Break the dark chocolate into 8 squares.
2. Blend the sugar and cinnamon powder with the almond spread.
3. Utilize a blade to spread the almond margarine on 4 of the squares.
4. Put other squares on top to shape sandwiches.

Nutrition Fact: Calories: 190, Fat 12g, Carbs 3g, Sugar 1g, Protein 4g

KETO COCONUT FAT BOMB SANDWICHES RECIPE

Prep Time: 5mints, Total Time: 5mints, Serving: 4
Ingredients
- 1 bar of dark chocolate
- 2 Tsp coconut butter
- 1 tsp vanilla extract
- Stevie or erythritol, to taste

Instructions
1. Break the dark chocolate into 8 squares.
2. Blend the sugar and vanilla concentrate in with the coconut margarine. You may need let the coconut spread set.
3. Utilize a blade to spread the coconut margarine on 4 of the squares.
4. Put different squares on top to shape sandwiches.

Nutrition Fact: Calories: 192, Fat 12g, Carbs 4g, Sugar 1g, Protein 4g

WHITE CHOCOLATE FAT BOMBS

Prep Time: 5mints, Cook Time: 10mints, Total Time: 15mints, Servings: 8
Ingredients
- 1/4 cup cocoa butter
- 1/4 cup coconut oil
- 10 drops vanilla Stevie drops

Instructions
1. Soften together cocoa margarine and coconut oil over low heat or in a twofold heater.
2. Remove from heat and mix in vanilla-seasoned Stevie drops.
3. Fill molds.
4. Chill until solidified.
5. Remove from molds or keep in the icebox if not eaten immediately.

Nutrition Fact: Calories: 125, Fat 10g, Carbs 3g, Sugar 0.2g, Protein 12g

NUTELLA FAT BOMBS

Prep Time: 5mints, Total Time: 5mints, Serving: 12
Ingredients
- 100 g Hazelnuts
- 150 g Coconut Oil
- 2 Scoops Keto Chocolate Collagen
- 1 Pinch Salt

Instructions
1. Put all ingredients into a rapid blender, mix until smooth
2. Gap the blend equitably between your molds.
3. Chill in the cooler until firm

Nutrition Fact: Calories: 173, Fat 18g, Carbs 1g, Sugar 1g, Protein 2g

RASPBERRY FAT BOMBS - CREAM HEART JELLIES

Prep Time: 10mints, Cook Time: 1mint, Total Time: 11mints, Servings: 26 Jellies
Ingredients
- 1 pk Raspberry Sugar Free Jello 9g packet
- 15 g Gelatin Powder
- 1/2 cup water boiling

- 1/2 cup Heavy Cream

Instructions
1. Break up gelatin and jello in boiling water.
2. Add the cream gradually while mixing and keep on blending. In the event that you add the cream at the same time and it doesn't blend, the jams will part making a layered impact.
3. Empty the blend into sweet shapes and set in the cooler for about 30 minutes.
4. Serve and enjoy!

Nutrition Fact: Calories: 21, Fat 2g, Carbs 0.1g, Sugar 0.005g, Protein 0.4g

KETO FAT BOMBS | COOKIES AND CREAM

Prep Time: 10mints, Total Time: 1hr 10mints, Servings: 10 fat bombs

Ingredients
- 1/2 cup coconut oil
- 2 scoops Protein Powder
- 1/4 cup macadamia nuts
- Fat Bomb Mold

Instructions
1. Heat a pan to low heat
2. Add the coconut oil and protein powder. Utilizing a spatula, mix the ingredients together until you get a smooth white consistency.
3. Fill a silicone shape to make ten fat bombs. Pour and fill up to about 80% of the shape for each fat bomb.
4. Crush the macadamia nuts and circulate over the 10 fat bombs uniformly. Note: Any nut will work!
5. Discretionary: sprinkle the fat bombs with a little ocean salt to increase the flavor!
6. Put the fat bombs in the cooler and permit sitting for about 2 hours.
7. These can be put away in a zip lock sack in the cooler for as long as 2 months.

Nutrition Facts: Calories 141, Fat 13g, Carbs 0.5g, Sugar 0.3g, Protein 5.3g

KETO AVOCADO DESSERT

Prep Time: 10mints, Total Time: 1hr 10mints, Serving: 7

Ingredients
- 1 ripe avocado
- 1/4 cup heavy whipping cream
- 1/2 teaspoon liquid stevia
- 1/4 teaspoon vanilla extract
- 1/4 teaspoon ground cinnamon

Instructions
1. Pound avocado in a bowl. Add substantial cream, Stevie, vanilla, and cinnamon; blend completely.
2. Refrigerate avocado blend for 1 hour before serving.

Nutrition Facts: Calories 266, Fat 25.7g, Carb 9.7g, Sugar 1.4g, Protein 26g

LOW CARB PUMPKIN CHEESECAKE MOUSSE

Prep Time: 15mints, Total Time: 15mints, Serving: Makes 10

Ingredients
- 12 ounces cream cheese
- 15 ounces pumpkin puree
- 1/2 cup confectioner's erythritol
- 2 teaspoons pure vanilla extract
- 2 tablespoons Pumpkin Pie Spice
- 3/4 cup heavy cream

Instructions
1. In a huge blending bowl, join the cream cheese and pumpkin puree. Utilizing a hand blender until there are no noticeable lumpss and the blend is smooth and velvety.
2. Add the erythritol, vanilla concentrate, pumpkin pie flavor, and substantial cream. Blend until all ingredients are very much mixed.
3. Refrigerate for an hour before serving.

Nutrition Fact: Calories: 215, Fat 18g, Carbs 3g, Sugar 1g, Protein 3g

STRAWBERRY DOLE WHIP RECIPE

Prep Time: 10mints, Cooking Time: 15mints, Total Time: 25mints; Serving: 4-5

Ingredients
- 1 cup sliced frozen strawberries
- 1 cup frozen raspberries
- Level 1/4 cup milk of choice
- 1 1/2 tsp sugar and 1/16 tsp salt
- 2 tsp lemon juice

Instructions
1. Strawberry Dole Whip Recipe: Combine all ingredients in a blender and mix until smooth.

Nutrition Facts: Calories 427, Fat 35g, Carbs 6.6g, Sugar 1.6g, Protein 25g

EASY KETO HAM AND CHEESE ROLLS RECIPE

Prep Time: 5mints, Total Time: 20mints; Serving: 6

Ingredients
- 3/4 cup shredded mozzarella cheese.
- 1/2 cup shredded cheddar cheese.
- 1/2 cup grated parmesan
- 1 cup diced ham
- 2 eggs

Instructions
1. Preheat grill to 375 degrees F.
2. Set out a lubricated heating sheet.
3. Partition the mixture further into six to eight sections and structure into spherical rolls.
4. Heat at 375 degrees F for around 15 to 20mins till the cheese has completely softened and made a slight darker hull
5. Don't hesitate to stir up your cheese

Nutrition Fact: Calories 198, Fat 13g, Carbs 3g, Sugar 1g, Protein 17g

KETO BAGELS RECIPE WITH FATHEAD DOUGH

Prep Time: 15mints, Cook Time: 12mints, Total Time: 27mints; Serving: 6

Ingredients
- 1 1/2 cup Blanched almond flour
- 1 tbsp Gluten-free baking powder
- 2 1/2 cup Mozzarella cheese
- 2 oz Cream cheese
- 2 large Egg

Instructions
1. Preheat the stove to 400 degrees F. Line a oven tray with parchment paper.
2. Mix collectively the almond flour and baking powder. Put in a secure place.
3. Join the destroyed mozzarella and cubed cream cheddar in a big bowl.
4. Microwave for two minutes, mixing throughout.
5. Mix the flour combination and eggs into the softened cheese combination. Working swiftly at the same time as the cheddar is still warm, ply together with your palms until structure combines.
6. On the off chance that the mixture turns out to be tough before completely blended, you could microwave/warm for 15-20 seconds more. Then ply all over again.

Nutrition Facts: Calories 314, Fat 18.5g, Carbs 5.8g, Sugar 2.3g, Protein 33.4g

PROTEIN PUDDING - CHOCOLATE OR VANILLA

Prep Time: 5mints, Total Time: 5mints; Servings: 1

Ingredients
- 3/4 cup Water or Almond milk
- 1 Prima Fuel Protein Powder
- Tsp Chia Seeds and 1 Tsp Cocoa powder
- 1 Tablespoon Sugar-free chocolate chips
- Flaked sea salt

Instructions
1. Add all ingredients to a blender container, try to add the fluid first. Mix for 30 seconds.
2. Serve promptly or let chill in the cooler for 60 minutes.
3. Top with chocolate chips and flaked sea salt

Nutrition Facts: Calories 423, Fat 18g, Carbs 8g, Sugar 3g, Protein 24g

CREAM CHEESE PANCAKES – LOW CARB & KETO

Prep Time: 3mints, Cook Time: 9mints, Total Time: 12mints, Serving: 4 pancakes

Ingredients
- 2 oz cream cheese
- 2 eggs
- 1 tsp granulated sugar substitute
- 1/2 tsp cinnamon

Instructions
1. Put all ingredients in a blender. Mix until smooth.
2. Leave to rest for 2 minutes so the air pockets can settle.
3. Pour 1/4 of the batter into a hot skillet lubed with spread or oil.
4. Cook for 2 minutes then flip and cook on the opposite side.
5. Repeat with the remainders of the batter.
6. Present with sugar-free syrup.

Nutrition Fact: Calories: 344, Fat 29g, Carbs 3g, Sugar 6g, Protein 17g

KATHLEEN'S COTTAGE PANCAKES

Prep Time: 20mints, Cooking Time: 25mints, Total Time: 45mints, Serving: 4

Ingredients
- 6 eggs
- 1 1/2 cups cottage cheese
- 1/2 teaspoon kosher or sea salt
- 1/2 cup flour
- 1/4 teaspoon baking soda

Instructions
1. Beat eggs until light.
2. Add the rest of the ingredients. Drop, using tablespoons, onto a delicately lubed frying pan and cook over medium heat until seared on the two sides and cooked thoroughly.
3. Top with maple syrup.

Nutrition Fact: Calories 176, Fat 16g, Carbs 10g, Sugar 6g, Protein 3g

CHOCOLATE PROTEIN PANCAKES

Prep Time: 10mints, Cooking Time: 20mints, Total Time: 30mints, Serving: 8

Ingredients
- 1 1/2 cups almond flour
- 1/4 cup chocolate protein powder
- 1 tsp baking powder
- 1/4 tsp salt and 2 eggs
- 3/4 cup unsweetened almond milk
- 1 tsp vanilla extract

Instructions
1. Combine the ingredients - eggs, almond milk and vanilla concentrate.
2. Gradually blend in the flour, protein, heating powder and salt. Combine until the product is smooth and free of lumps.
3. Heat a skillet on medium and coat with your preferred oil
4. Pour around 1/4 of a cup of the batter onto the skillet.
5. Cook until bubbles start forming.
6. Flip the flapjacks and cook for about one more minute or two.
7. When the pancakes have cooked on both sides, remove them from the skillet, stack them up, serve and enjoy.

Nutrition Fact: Calories 321, Fat 5g, Carbs 21g, Sugar 3g, Protein 23g

LOW-CARB WAFFLES

Prep Time: 10mints, Cooking Time: 15mints, Total Time: 25mints, Serving: 1

Ingredients
- 2- egg whites
- 1 1/2- scoops vanilla protein powder
- A sprinkle of cinnamon

Instruction
1. Whisk or mix two egg whites and 1/2 scoop of protein powder in a little bowl.
2. Spray your waffle iron with cooking oil and give it a chance to warm up.
3. Pour your batter onto the waffle creator and make your waffles. I generally get 2-3 waffles for every formula.
4. Utilize a spatula to remove from the waffle maker.
5. Top with your preferred garnishes and enjoy your low-carb breakfast!

Nutrition Facts: Calories 275, Fat 28g, Carbs 3g, Sugar 0.4g, Protein 1g

ALMOND JOY FRUIT AND NUT BARS

Prep Time: 15mints, Total Time: 15mints; Serving: Makes 8 Bars

Ingredients
- 1 cup almonds
- 1 cup Deglet Noor dates
- ¼ cup unsweetened coconut
- 2 tbsp unsweetened cocoa powder

Instructions
1. Pound the almonds in a nourishment processor until they are finely crushed. Add dates, coconut and cocoa powder. Beat until all ingredients are mixed and equally measured.
2. Pour blend between two sheets of saran wrap. Utilize your hands to press and frame the blend into a smaller rectangular shape. Firmly fold the cling wrap over it and refrigerate for 60 minutes. This will enable it to solidify and make it simpler to cut into bars.
3. Remove from the cooler and cut into 8 bars.
4. Separately envelop the bars with cling wrap and store them in the ice chest.

Nutrition Fact: Calories: 162, Fat 9g, Carbs 17g, Sugar 7g, Protein 4g

PUMPKIN PIE FRUIT AND NUT BARS

Prep Time: 15mints, Total Time: 15mints; Serving: Makes 10 Bars

Ingredients
- ½ cup raw cashews
- ½ cup raw pepitas
- 1 cup Deglet Noor dates
- ½ cup dried apricots
- 2 tablespoons Pumpkin Pie Spice

Instructions
1. Granulate cashews and pepitas in a nourishment processor until they are finely hacked. Add dates, apricots, and pumpkin pie flavor. Beat until all ingredients are mixed.
2. Pour blend between two sheets of cling wrap. Utilize your hands to press and frame the blend into a reduced rectangular shape. Wrap the cling wrap firmly around it and refrigerate for 60 minutes. This will enable it to solidify and make it simpler to cut into bars.
3. Remove from the ice chest and cut into 10 bars.
4. Independently envelop the bars by saran wrap and store them in the refrigerator.

Nutrition Fact: Calories: 140, Fat 5.6g, Carbs 18g, Sugar 6g, Protein 3.5g

LOW CARB KETO BANANA NUT PROTEIN PANCAKES

Prep Time: 5mints, Cook Time: 25mints, Total Time: 30mints; Serving: 8 Pancakes

Ingredients
- 2 scoops Banana Nut Protein Powder
- 2 ounces cream cheese
- 4 large pastured eggs
- 1 teaspoon pure vanilla extract
- 2 teaspoons baking powder and Butter
- 1 tsp confectioner's erythritol

Instructions
1. Blend all ingredients in a powerful blender. You may need to scratch down the sides with an elastic spatula and beat again to ensure everything is totally blended.
2. Brush a huge non-stick skillet or frying pan container with margarine and heat over medium-low heat.
3. When the skillet is hot, add 1/4 cup of the blend and cook until it is bubbly on top and dark colored on the base, around 3 minutes. Flip and cook the opposite side until it cooked as well, around 2-3 minutes.
4. Repeat this procedure until all the batter is used up.

Nutrition Fact: Calories: 85, Fat 5.4g, Carbs 1.8g, Sugar 1g, Protein 7.4g

KETO CHOCOLATE MASON JAR ICE CREAM

Prep Time: 8mints, Total Time: 8mints; Serving: 2

Ingredients
- 1 cup heavy cream
- 2 tablespoons granular erythritol
- 1 tablespoon unsweetened cocoa powder
- 1 teaspoon pure vanilla extract
- 2 tablespoons sugar-free chocolate chips

Instructions
1. Mix all ingredients in a container and close with cover to be shaken vigorously for 5 minutes.

The fluid inside should twofold in volume, filling the container.
2. Leave to set for 3-24hours.
3. Scoop, serve and enjoy it!
Nutrition Fact: Calories: 206, Fat 22g, Carbs 10g, Sugar 6g, Protein 1g

CHOCOLATE PEANUT BUTTER BALLS

Prep Time: 10mints, Cooking Time: 5mints, Total Time: 15mints; Serving: 3
Ingredients
- 4 oz. Cream Cheese
- 8 oz. Milk Chocolate Delight Atkins Shake
- 1 box Sugar-Free Chocolate Pudding
- 4 Tbs. Peanut Butter

Instructions
1. Blend cream cheese and Atkins shake in an enormous blending bowl in with a blender on low speed until cream cheese is all around mixed and there are no lumps left. Add the sugar-free pudding and the peanut spread.
2. Blend until thoroughly mixed. It will turn out to be thick. Line a plate with wax paper. Fold the blend into little balls and put them on the wax paper. Put them in the cooler to set.
3. Store in the cooler in a holder with a top, serve and enjoy!!
Nutrition Fact: Calories: 118, Fat 7g, Carbs 1.5g, Sugar 0.2g, Protein 11g

KETO CHEESECAKE CUPCAKES

Prep Time: 10mints, Cook Time: 15mints, Total Time; Serving: 3
Ingredients
- 1/2 cup almond meal
- 1/4 cup butter and 2 eggs
- ounce cream cheese
- 3/4 cup granular no-calorie sucralose sweetener
- 1 teaspoon vanilla extract

Instructions
1. Preheat stove to 350 degrees F. Line 12 biscuit cups with paper liners.
2. Combine almond meal and margarine in a bowl; spoon into the bottom of the paper liners and press into a level outside layer.
3. Beat cream cheese, eggs, sugar and vanilla concentrate together in a bowl with an electric blender set to medium until smooth; spoon over to the paper liners.
4. Prepare in the preheated stove until the cream cheese blend is about set in the center, 15 to 17 minutes.
5. Give cupcakes a chance to cool at room temperature until cool enough to handle. Refrigerate 8 hours before serving.
Nutrition Facts: Calories 204, Fat 20g, Carb 2.1g, Sugar 2.3, Protein 4.9g

EASY KETO FUDGE RECIPE WITH COCOA POWDER

Prep Time: 10mints, Cook Time: 45mints, Total Time: 55mints; Serving: 12
Ingredients
- 1 cup Coconut oil
- 1/4 cup Powdered erythritol
- 1/4 cup Cocoa powder
- 1 tsp Vanilla extract
- 1/8 tsp Sea salt

Instructions
1. Line a 28 oz. Square glass holder with cloth paper, so the material hangs out over the sides.
2. Utilizing a hand blender at LOW velocity, beat the coconut oil and sugar collectively, till smooth and mixed.
3. Beat within the cocoa powder, vanilla and ocean salt to flavor.
4. Move the mixture into a container and refrigerate the keto fudge for around 45-60mins till robust.
5. Sprinkle the best factor of the fudge with ocean salt pieces and press tenderly.
6. Run a blade alongside the brink and take out utilizing the rims of the cloth paper.
7. Keep the fudge refrigerated and convey it to room temperature at once before serving.
Nutrition Facts: Calories 161, Fat 18g, Carbs 1g, Sugar 0.3g, Protein 12g

KETO MUFFINS

Prep Time: 5mints, Cook Time: 26mints, Total Time: 31mints; Serving: 12
Ingredients
- 8 oz Cream Cheese
- 8 large eggs
- 4 tbsp Butter
- 2 scoops Whey Protein

Instructions
1. In a blending bowl liquefy butter and cream cheese.
2. Add whey protein and eggs, cautious not to cook the eggs from the heat of the butter.
3. Join with a hands until totally blended.
4. Fill biscuit preparing plate and heat at 350 degrees for 26 minutes.
5. Serve and enjoy!
Nutrition Facts: Calories 165.1, Fat 13.6g, Carbs 1.5g, Sugar 4g, Protein 9.6g

DRINKS RECIPES

KETO TRADITIONAL COFFEE RECIPE
Prep Time: 2mints, Total Time: 2mints, Serving: 1 mug
Ingredients
- 1 cup black coffee
- 1/2 tsp MCT oil
- 1 Tspghee

Instructions
1. Blend really well.

Nutrition Fact: Calories: 143, Fat 17g, Carbs 2g, Sugar 0.4g, Protein 4g

VANILLA LATTE MARTINI
Prep Time: 5mints, Total Time: 5mints, Servings: 2
Ingredients
- 3 ounces vanilla vodka
- 2 ounces homemade coffee liqueur
- 1 tbsp cream

Instructions
1. Fill a mixed drink shaker with ice. Add espresso alcohol, vanilla vodka and cream. Shake well and pour into two chilled martini glasses.

Nutrition Fact: Calories: 454, Fat 31g, Carbs 26g, Sugars 4.4g, Protein 22g

KETO BOOSTED COFFEE RECIPE
Prep Time: 2mints, Total Time: 2mints, Serving: 16 ounces
Ingredients
- 2 cups freshly brewed hot coffee
- 2 tablespoons grass-fed butter
- 1 scoop Perfect Keto Powder
- 1 teaspoon Ceylon cinnamon

Instructions
1. Add the entirety of the ingredients in a blender.
2. Utilizing a submersion blender or frothier, mix on low bringing the accelerate to high for 30 seconds or until foamy.
3. Serve, taste, and serve and enjoy.

Nutrition Fact: Calories: 280, Fat 31g, Carbs 2.8g, Sugar 2.2g, Protein: 1g

KETO COCONUT COFFEE RECIPE
Prep Time: 2mints, Total Time: 2mints, Serving: 1 mug
Ingredients
- 1 cup of black coffee
- 1/2 Tsp coconut oil
- 1 Tsp ghee

Instructions
1. Blend really well.

Nutrition Fact: Calories: 179, Fat 21g, Carbs 3g, Sugar 1.1g, Protein 5g

KETO FROTHY COFFEE RECIPE
Prep Time: 2mints, Total Time: 2mints, Serving: 1 mug
Ingredient
- 1 cup of black coffee
- 1/2 Tsp coconut oil
- 1 Tsp ghee
- 2 Tsp unsweetened coconut

Instructions
1. Blend really well.

Nutrition Fact: Calories: 190, Fat 22g, Carbs 2g, Sugar 0.3g, Protein 9g

KETO COLLAGEN BOOSTED COFFEE
Prep Time: 2mints, Total Time: 2mints, Serving: 1 mug
INGREDIENT
- 1 cup of black coffee
- 1 Tsp ghee
- 1/2 scoop unflavored hydrolyzed collagen powder

Instructions
1. Blend really well.

Nutrition Fact: Calories 160, Fat 14g, Carbs 2g, Sugar 3g, Protein 5g

KETO ICED LEMON COFFEE RECIPE
Prep Time: 5mints, Total Time: 5mints, Serving: 1 cup
Ingredients
- 1 cup cold brew coffee
- 1/4 cup ice cubes
- 1/4 cup freshly squeezed lemon juice
- Stevie to taste
- 1 slice of lemon for garnish

Instructions
1. Add everything into a glass and mix. Toss in a cut of lemon for decoration.

Nutrition Fact: Calories: 16, Fat 3g, Carbs 4g, Sugar 4g, Protein 5g

LOW CARB BLUEBERRY MOJITOS
Prep Time: 10mints, Total Time: 10mints, Serving: 4
Ingredients
- 3/4 cup fresh blueberries
- 3 to 4 tbsp powdered Swerve Sweetener
- 1/4 cup packed mint leaves
- 1 cup white rum
- 1/3 cup fresh lime juice
- 1/2-liter club soda

Instructions
1. In a blender, add blueberries and powdered sugar. Mix to a thick puree. Move to a pitcher.
2. Tear mint leaves by way of hand and upload to a tumbler that holds, in any occasion, one liter.
3. Pound with a muddle or the end of a wooden spoon to discharge the oils

4. Add blueberry puree, white rum, lime juice, and dad and blend to join.
5. Fill four highball or basin glasses with squashed ice. Empty mojitos into glasses, embellish with blueberries and mint leaves and serve.
Nutrition Facts: Calories 153, Fat 0.1g, Carbs 6g, Sugar 1g, Protein 0.4g

APPLE MARTINI

Prep Time: 5mints, Total Time: 5mints, Serving: 2
Ingredients
- Apple slice
- 1 teaspoon of low carb sugar syrup
- 2 ounces plain vodka
- 2 ounces of apple-flavored vodka

Instructions
1. Finely dice the apple cut and put in a mixed drink shaker. Add the sugar syrup and crush them together.
2. Add the two kinds of vodka and ice. Shake well. Strain into a martini glass. The aggregate of 2 grams of carb
Nutrition Facts: Calories 300, Fat 19g, Carbs 6g, Sugar 1g, Protein 25g

BLUEBERRY MARTINI

Prep Time: 5mints, Total Time: 5mints, Serving: 3
Ingredients
- 6-7 good-sized fresh blueberries
- 1 teaspoon of low carb sugar syrup
- 2 ounces plain vodka
- 2 ounces blueberry flavored vodka

Instructions
1. Put the blueberries in a mixed drink shaker. Add the sugar syrup and squash them together.
2. Add the two kinds of vodka and ice. Shake well. Strain into a martini glass. Aggregate of 2 grams of carb
Nutrition Fact: Calories 368, Fat 38.85g, Carbs 3.7g, Sugar 1.28g, Protein 1.69g

CRANBERRY GINGER MULLED WINE

Prep Time: 10mints, Cooking Time: 30mints, Total Time: 40mints, Serving: 4
Ingredients
- 1 bottle full-bodied red wine
- 1 cup fresh cranberries
- 1/2 cup granulated erythritol
- juice of half a lemon
- 1 cinnamon stick and 1 inch of ginger root

Instructions
1. Join all ingredients in an enormous pan and bring it to a stew. Stew tenderly over low heat for 30 minutes.
2. Fill mugs and embellishment with cranberries and lemon.
Nutrition Fact: Calories 168, Fat 15g, Carbs 5g, Sugar 2g, Protein 4g

BLACK BEAUTY – LOW CARB VODKA DRINK

Prep Time: 5mints, Total Time: 5mints, Serving: 1
Ingredients
- 2 ounces vodka
- 5 fresh blackberries
- ¾ ounce fresh lemon juice
- 2 tsp powdered erythritol
- ¼ tsp black pepper, 5 fresh mint leaves, and Soda water

Instructions
1. Fill an enormous rocks glass with ice.
2. Join the vodka, blackberries, lemon juice, erythritol, dark pepper, and mint leaves in a mixed drink shaker. Jumble until the foods grown from the ground are squashed and have discharged their juices.
3. Strain the substance of the mixed drink shaker over top of the ice.
4. Top with soft drink water and embellishment with blackberries and a new mint leaf
Nutrition Fact: Calories: 180, Fat 0.2g, Carbs 5g, Sugar 2g, Protein 1g

LOW CARB STRAWBERRY MARGARITA GUMMY WORMS

Prep Time: 10mints, Cook Time: 5mints, Total Time: 45mints , Serving: 6
Ingredients
- 10 hulled strawberries
- 2 ounces silver tequila
- 3 tsps gelatin collagen protein
- 2 tablespoons powdered erythritol
- 1 ½ ounces fresh lime juice

Instructions
2. Put the strawberries and tequila in a blender and heartbeat till clean.
3. Pour the strawberry-and-tequila mixture right into a medium pan and set over low heat.
4. Add the gelatin, erythritol, and lime squeeze and rush to interrupt up the gelatin and be part of the ingredients. Keep on warming for round 10 minutes, whisking habitually, until the combo is pourable.
5. Move the mixture to a cup or a bowl.
6. Refrigerate for 10 to 15 minutes, till set. Pop the sticky worms out of the shape and serve and enjoy it! Store leftovers inside the icebox for so long as seven days
Nutrition Fact: Calories: 50, Fat 0.3g, Carbs 2.2g, Sugar 0.4g, Protein 3.2g

DAIRY-FREE BOOSTED KETO COFFEE

Prep Time: 20mints, Cooking Time: 15mints, Total Time: 35mints, Serving: 4
Ingredients
- 8 ounces dark roast coffee
- 1 tablespoon butter flavored coconut oil
- 1 scoop Keto Zone French Vanilla

- 1 scoop Collagen Peptides
- 2 teaspoons monk fruit sweetened caramel syrup
- Almond milk

Instructions
1. Join all ingredients in a blender or milk frothier. Mix until smooth and rich
2. Serve and enjoy

Nutrition Fact: Calories: 440, Fat 48g, Carbs 0.2g Sugar 0.4g, Protein 4g

CACAO COFFEE RECIPE

Prep Time: 20mints, Cook Time: 10mints, Total Time: 30mints, Serving: 2

Ingredients
- 1 cup Cacao nibs
- Boiling water
- 1/2 tsp gelatin
- Coconut oil
- Cinnamon powder

Instructions
1. Preheat your stove to 350 degrees. Put the cacao nibs in a slim layer on a heating sheet.
2. Put in the stove and let cook for 15 - 18 minutes.
3. Remove from the stove and let cool.
4. To make some Cacao espresso, you will require 1 tsp of Cacao nibs per 1 cup of bubbling water.
5. Put the cacao nibs in your espresso processor and beat multiple times for 2 seconds each. On the off chance that you hold the conservative you will get a powder. Evacuate and put in your French press and add bubbling water.
6. In your cup add your gelatin and some cold water and mix with spoon.
7. Pour in your cacao espresso and add coconut oil and cinnamon.

Nutrition Fact: Calories: 335, Fat 19g, Carbs 10g, Sugar 7g, Protein 8g

COCONUT MILK LATTE

Prep Time: 5mints, Cook Time: 5mints, Total Time: 10mints, Servings: 2

Ingredients
- 3 cups prepared hot coffee
- 1/2 cup coconut cream
- Dash of cinnamon

Instructions
1. Empty the espresso into a blender alongside the coconut milk.
2. Mix on medium-high for about a moment, or until the coconut milk is totally fused.
3. Fill a mug or serve over ice. You can spoon the foamed coconut milk on top for some "froth".
4. Change the measure of coconut milk to your taste buds… you may need pretty much.

Nutrition Facts: Calories 114, Fat 12g, Carbs 1g, Sugar 2g, Protein 1g

CHAMOMILE MINT TEA RECIPE

Prep Time: 5mints Total Time: 5mints, Serving: 1

Ingredients
- 1 tsp chamomile flowers
- 1 tsp peppermint leaves
- 1 cup (240 ml) boiling water

Instructions
1. Combine the chamomile and peppermint to a tea kettle
2. Mix for 4-5mins, discharges the herbs and drink.

Nutrition Fact: Calories: 159, Fat 18g, Carbs 9g, Sugar 4g, Protein 8g

KETO ICED APPLE GREEN TEA

Prep Time: 5mints, Total Time: 5mints, Serving: 2

Ingredients
- 1 cup of brewed green tea
- 1 cup ice
- 1 tsp apple cider vinegar
- Stevie

Instructions
1. Mix the green tea with high temp water for 2-3 minutes.
2. Add every one of the ingredients to a blender and mix well.

Nutrition Fact: Calories 190, Fat 17g, Carbs 10g, Sugar 1g, Protein 3g

TURMERIC GINGER LIME TEA RECIPE

Prep Time: 5mints, Total Time: 5mints, Serving: 1

Ingredients
- 1 lime
- 1 small turmeric root
- 1 piece of ginger

Instructions
1. Put 1 lime cut alongside all the turmeric and ginger pieces into a huge tea kettle.
2. Fill the tea kettle with bubbling high temp water.
3. Give the tea a chance to brew for 5 minutes.
4. Serve and enjoy hot or let it cool.

Nutrition Fact: Calories: 500, Fat 40g, Carbs 11g, Sugar 1g, Protein 25g

ZINGY SALTED LIME SODA

Prep Time: 2mints, Total Time: 2mints, Serving: 1

Ingredients
- 1 lime
- 1 1/4 cups seltzer water
- 1/8 to 1/4 tsp salt

Instructions
1. Juice 1 lime and add the chilled seltzer water and salt to the lime juice.
2. Mix tenderly to disintegrate the salt.
3. Serve chilled.

Nutrition Fact: Calories: 159, Fat 18g, Carbs 9g, Sugar 4g, Protein 8g

CUCUMBER BASIL ICE CUBES RECIPE
Prep Time: 15mints, Total Time: 15mints, Serving: 3
Ingredients
- 1 cucumber
- 5 small basil leaves
- Juice from 1/4 lime
- 1/4 cup water

Instructions
1. Put everything into the blender and mix well.
2. Strain the puree and empty the subsequent fluid into a huge ice shape plate or forms. Spare the subsequent cucumber solids to make this formula.
3. Leave to freeze for 4-5 hours.
4. Make beverages utilizing the ice 3D squares e.g., add them to water to enhance the taste or to vodka for a simple cucumber basil seasoned chilled vodka drink!

Nutrition Fact: Calories: 45, Fat 0.5g, Carbs 1g, Sugar 0.3g, Protein 9g

CUCUMBER LIME WATER
Prep Time: 4mints, Total Time: 4mints, Serving: 1
Ingredients
- 1 cucumber
- 1 lime
- 50 fl oz of water

Instructions
1. Strip the cucumber and afterward cut it up into 1/4-inch-thick cuts. Add to container
2. Press in juice from 1 lime.
3. Add the water and blend.
4. Sit in refrigerator medium-term.

Nutrition Fact: Calories 140, Fat 12g, Carbs 5g, Sugar 2.1g, Protein 8g

HONEYSUCKLE TEA
Prep Time: 6hrs, Total Time: 6hrs, Serving: 4
Ingredients
- 1 part honeysuckle flowers
- 2 parts water
- Ice for serving

Instructions
1. Delicately break down your honeysuckle flowers. You can do that by hand or tenderly with a wooden spoon.
2. Add honeysuckle blossoms to a pitcher or cup.
3. Top with water and mix. Spread.
4. Put the pitcher in the cooler for about 6-15 hours.
5. Strain the blossoms out and make the most of your honeysuckle tea over ice.

An alternative method:
6. Add the broken-down honeysuckle blossoms to a pitcher or cup. Add water and blend. Spread.
7. Put the pitcher in full sun for 3-4 hours.
8. Strain the blooms out and serve and enjoy over ice.

Nutrition Fact: Calories: 214, Fat 6g, Carbs 4g, Sugar 6g, Protein 18g

KETO TURMERIC BONE BROTH
Prep Time: 5mints, Cook Time: 10mints, Total time: 15mints; Serving: 1
Ingredients
- 1 cup of Keto bone broth
- 1 tsp turmeric powder
- 1 tsp ginger powder
- Dash of cumin powder
- Dash of pepper and salt to taste

Instructions
1. Heat up the bone soup and speed in different ingredients

Nutrition Fact: Calories: 20, Fat 1g, Carbs 0.1g, Sugar 0.2g, Protein 2g

KAMIKAZE SHOT SUGAR-FREE
Prep Time: 1mint, Total Time: 1mint, Serving: 2
Ingredients
- 3/4 shaker Ice
- 2 tbsp Lime Juice
- 2 g Granulated Stevia or Erythritol
- 1 shot Vodka

Instructions
1. Put ice in a shaker.
2. Add lime juice, sugar, and vodka.
3. Cover and shake.
4. Serve in a chilled rocks glass or short tumbler.

Nutrition Fact: Calories: 109, Fat 3g, Carbs 2g, Sugar 1g, Protein 12g

LOW CARB PINA COLADA
Prep Time: 5mints, Total Time: 5mints, Serving: 2
Ingredients
- 3 ounces of rum
- 2/3 cup coconut milk
- 1/2 cup sugar-free pineapple syrup
- 2 cups crushed ice

Instructions
1. Add ingredients to a blender and blend until slushy. Makes two beverages
2. Check 5 grams of carb per serving.

Nutrition Facts: Calories 215, Fat 10g, Carbs 7g, Sugar 3g, Protein 23g

DIRTY CHAI
Prep Time: 5mints, Cook Time: 5mints, Total Time: 10mints, Serving: 2
Ingredients
- 1/2 tbsp of entire espresso beans
- 1/2 tsp peppercorn
- 1 stick of cinnamon
- 2 cardamom cases
- 1 bit of ginger

- 3 cups of bubbling water

Instructions
1. Add the ground espresso and flavors to a French press. Pour 3 cups of bubbling water over the flavors and close your press.
2. Allow to soak for 5 minutes and afterward a chance to serve and enjoy with coconut milk or whipped cream.

Nutrition Fact: Calories: 143, Fat 17g, Carbs 2g, Sugar 0.4g, Protein 4g

LOW CARB MARGARITAS

Prep Time: 5mints, Total Time: 5mints; Serving: 2
Ingredients
- 3 ounces good tequila white
- 2 ounces freshly squeezed lime juice
- 1/2 tsp orange extract
- Crushed ice
- Kosher salt for rimming

Instructions
1. In a mixed drink shaker or an estimating cup, add tequila, lime juice, orange concentrate, and sugar, if utilizing.
2. Fill two margarita glasses or antiquated glasses most of the way with squashed ice.
3. Gap blend equitably between glasses
4. On the off chance that you like a salted edge, run a wedge of lime around the outside of the glass before loading up with ice and plunge in a plate of fit salt.

Nutrition Facts: Calories 140, Fat 2.3g, Carbs 3g, Sugar 1.2g, Protein 3g

SPIKED ROOT BEER FLOAT

Prep Time: 3mints, Total Time: 3; Serving: 1
Ingredients
- 1 cup diet Root Beer
- 1-ounce spiced rum
- 2 tsps heavy whipping cream
- Handful ice

Instructions
1. Put the two ingredients into a martini shaker with ice and shake intensely for around 30 seconds.
2. Pout into a glass, serve and enjoy

Nutrition Fact: Calories: 713, Fat 56g, Carbs 0.2g, Sugar 0.3g, Protein 48g

THE SPLENDIDO

Prep Time: 15mints, Total Time: 15mints; Serving: 4
Ingredients
- 1 lime
- 8 fresh mint leaves
- 1/4 cup white rum
- 1 packet Splendor
- 1 cup ice cubes and Soda

Instructions
1. Join lime wedges and mint in the base of a huge mixed drink glass. Utilize a meddler or the base of a wooden spoon to squash the mint and lime together, discharging the juices and oils.
2. Pour in the rum, ice and Splendor and utilize a spoon to mix.
3. Finish off with soft drink water and serve with an extra leaf of mint.

Nutrition Fact: Calories 327, Fat 33g, Carbs 7g, Sugar 1g, Protein 5g

LOW CARB MARGARITA

Prep Time: 5mints, Total Time: 5mints; Serving: 2
Ingredients
- ounces of tequila
- 2 ounces lime juice
- 1/4 teaspoon of orange extract
- 1/4 cup prepared lemon-lime Crystal Light
- Crushed ice

Instruction
1. Put all ingredients and blender and blend until slushy.
2. Present with lime wedges.

Nutrition Fact: Calories: 100, Fat: 9.5g, Carbs 2g, Sugar 5g, Protein 1g

LOW CARB MOJITO

Prep Time: 5mints, Total Time: 5mints; Serving: 2
Ingredients
- 7-8 Mint leaves with stems attached
- 1 tablespoon of low carb sugar syrup
- ounces light rum
- 1 lime

Instructions
1. Finely dice the mint leaves and blend in with low carb sugar syrup in a tall glass.
2. Cut the lime down the middle and dispose of the seeds. Crush the juice from the two parts into the glass. Add the rum and mix.
3. Add ice and club soft drinks to taste.

Nutrition Fact: Calories: 70, Fat 5g, Carbs 2g, Sugar 2g, Protein 2g

COSMOPOLITAN COCKTAIL RECIPE

Prep Time: 5mints, Total Time: 5mints; Servings: 1
Ingredients
- 1 jigger vodka
- 2 tsp low-calorie cranberry juice
- 1 tablespoon lime juice
- 2 to 3 drops orange extract
- 1 drop liquid stevia and Lime wedge

Instructions
1. Put 1 jigger standard vodka, 1-ounce low-calorie cranberry juice or 2 teaspoons unsweetened cranberry juice and 2 tablespoons water, 1 tablespoon crisp lime juice, 2 to 3 drops orange concentrate and sugar in a drink shaker half-brimming with ice. Shake well.
2. Taste for sweetness if utilizing unsweetened cranberry juice. You may need to add

more sugar. Strain into a martini glass. Enhancement with a little lime wedge or twist of a lime strip.
Nutrition Fact: Calories 103, Fat 0.2g, Carbs 1g, Sugar 0.1g, Protein 7g

TRADITIONAL LIME MOJITO RECIPE WITH HONEY

Prep Time: 5mints, Total Time: 5mints; Servings: 1
Ingredients
- 8 mint leaves
- 1 tsp honey
- 2 tsp lime juice
- 1 jigger and Club soda
- Garnish: fresh mint sprig

Instructions
1. Put mint, a sprinkle of club pop, and the honey into the base of a highball glass or Tom Collins glass. Crush the ingredients together. Customarily, a muddler, which resembles a smaller than normal wooden slugging stick, is utilized to achieve this. Be that as it may, the handle of a wooden spoon or spatula works fine.
2. Press the juice of the lime into the glass. Add the rum and mix.
3. Fill the glass around 3/4 of the way full of ice. Finish off with club pop. Mix and serve and enjoy it.
4. In the event that serving in a Collins glass, including a tall mixed drink straw makes a pleasant and helpful touch.

Nutrition Fact: Calories 169, Fat 0.5g, Carbs 20g, Sugar 2g, Protein 20g

PUMPKIN SPICE BOOSTED KETO COFFEE

Prep Time: 3mints, Total Time: 3mints; Serving: 1
Ingredients
- 12 ounces dark roast coffee
- 1 tablespoon grass-fed butter
- 2 tsp sugar-free caramel syrup syrup
- 2 tsps grass-fed collagen peptides
- Spray almond or coconut milk
- 1 teaspoon Pumpkin Pie Spice

Instructions
1. Add all ingredients in a blender or milk frother and mix until smooth.

Nutrition Fact: Calories: 261, Fat 23g, Carbs 3.6g, Sugar 0.8g, Protein 13.6g

ALMOND COCONUT MILK CREAMER

Prep Time: 10mints, Cooking Time: 20mints, Total Time: 30mints; Serving: 4
Ingredients
- 2 cups of raw almonds
- 2 cups of filtered water
- 14.5 ounce organic coconut cream
- 2 teaspoons pure vanilla extract

Instructions
1. Soak the raw almond with filtered water then dispose of the water.
2. Put the almonds in a powerful blender with 2 cups of water, coconut cream and vanilla concentrate. Mix on high for 2 minutes.
3. Put a working strainer over a bowl or an enormous estimating cup. Put a huge nut sack over the sifter. Empty the almond blend into the nut sack and give it a chance to strain through into the bowl.
4. Close the nut sack and curve around the almond mash and press. Press strainer to extract as much of the milk as possible.
5. Store in the cooler for as long as seven days.

Nutrition Fact: Calories: 138, Fat 12.2g, Carbs 2.8g, Sugar 0.7g, Protein 4.2g

THE GARDEN SURPRISE – KETO GIN COCKTAIL

Prep Time: 5mints, Total Time: 5mints; Serving: 1
Ingredients
- 4 blueberries and 5 fresh mint leaves
- 2 ounces dry gin
- 1/2 ounce fresh lime juice
- 1 tsp powdered erythritol
- Club soda

Instructions
1. To a mixed drink shaker, add the blueberries and mint. Jumble until the berries have discharged their juices and the mint is squashed.
2. Add the gin, lime juice, erythritol and ice. Close the top and shake.
3. Strain into a martini glass, or mixed drink glass of your choice and top with club pop.
4. Topping with new mint and serve.

Nutrition Fact: Calories: 139, Fat 0.1g, Carbs 2.9g, Sugar 0.4g, Protein 0.2g

KETO BLUEBERRY MOJITO

Prep Time: 10mints, Total Time: 10mints; Serving: 1
Ingredients
- 2 ounces white rum
- Juice of 1/2 lime
- 1 teaspoon powdered erythritol
- 4 fresh mint leaves
- Club soda and 5 blueberries

Instructions
1. Softly tangle the rum, lime juice, erythritol and mint leaves. Pour over ice and top with club pop. Enhance with crisp blueberries.

Nutrition Fact: Calories: 113, Fat 6.9g, Carbs 6.8g, Sugar 4.3g, Protein: 7.9g

SEAFOOD & FISH RECIPES

CURRY-ROASTED SHRIMP WITH ORANGES

Prep Time: 25mints, Cooking Time: 25mints, Total Time: 50mints; Serving: 4

Ingredients
- 2 large seedless oranges
- ½ tsp kosher salt and ½ tsp pepper
- 1½ pounds shrimp
- 1 tsp extra-virgin olive oil
- 1 tsp curry powder

Instruction
1. Preheat stove to 400°F. Line an oven tray with parchment paper. Finely grind the skin of 1 orange; put aside.
2. Daintily cut the oranges across, cut into quarters. Spread the orange cuts on the readied heating sheet and sprinkle with ¼ teaspoon salt.
3. Broil until the oranges are somewhat dry, around 12 minutes.
4. In the meantime, cover shrimp with oil, curry powder, pepper, the orange left over and the remaining ¼ teaspoon salt in a huge bowl. Move the shrimp to the heating sheet with the oranges and cook until pink and twisted, around 6 minutes.
5. Distribute the oranges and the shrimp among 4 plates and serve.

Nutrition Fact: Calories 188; Fat 5g, Carbs 10g, Sugar 6g, Protein 24g

SEARED SALMON WITH GREEN PEPPERCORN SAUCE

Prep Time: 15mints, Cooking Time: 15mints, Total Time: 30mints; Serving: 4

Ingredients
- 1¼ pounds wild salmon fillet
- 2 tsp canola oil
- ¼ cup lemon juice
- 4 tsp unsalted butter
- 1 tsp green peppercorns and ¼ pinch of salt

Instructions
1. Sprinkle salmon portions with ¼ teaspoon salt. Heat oil in a sizable nonstick skillet over medium-high heat.
2. Add the salmon and cook until darker in the interior, delicately turning midway, 4 to 7mins all out.
3. Wild salmon from the Pacific is preferred.

Nutrition Fact: Calories 266; Fat 11g, Carbs 1g, Sugar 0.1g, Protein 28g

FIVE-SPICE TILAPIA

Prep Time: 15mints, Cooking Time: 15mints, Total Time: 30mints; Serving: 4

Ingredients
- 1 pound tilapia fillets
- 1 tsp Chinese five-spice powder
- ¼ cup reduced-sodium soy sauce
- 3 tsp light brown sugar
- 1 tsp canola oil and 3 scallions

Instructions
1. Sprinkle the two sides of tilapia fillets with Chinese five-spice powder.
2. Add soy sauce and brown sugar in a little bowl.
3. Heat oil in a huge nonstick skillet over medium-high heat, add the tilapia and cook for around 2 minutes.
4. Decrease heat to medium, turn the fish over, mixing in the soy blend. Heat the sauce to the point of boiling and cook until the fish is cooked thoroughly, and the sauce has thickened somewhat, around 2 minutes more.
5. Add scallions and remove from the heat.
6. Serve the fish covered with the fish sauce.

Nutrition Fact: Calories 180; Fat 6g, Carbs 9g, Sugar 7g, Protein 24g

SHRIMP STACKS

Prep Time: 5mints, Cook Time: 10mints, Total Time: 15mints; Serving: 4

Ingredients
- 9–12 tail-on shrimp
- Coconut oil spray
- 3 ripe but firm Hass avocado
- 4 large basil leaves
- 1 tsp pink salt and 2 limes
- Biscuit cutter

Instructions
1. Put a cooling rack over a sheet dish. Spray with coconut oil.
2. Place your shrimps next to each other on the rack. Sprinkle with salt.
3. Set your stove rack to the top row. Set your stove on 500°F.
4. Put the shrimp under the grill. Set the clock for 5 minutes.
5. Utilizing a cutout on a plate, spoon a portion of the avocado blends into the circle and delicately push down, cautiously slide up the treat spread to uncover a pounded avocado.
6. Put 3-4 shrimp on every avocado round, tails up.
7. Cautiously cut the basil, roll sparsely, making basil chiffonier. Sprinkle over your shrimp.

Nutrition Fact: Calories: 289, Fat 21.8g, Carbs 14.2g, Sugar 4.2g, Protein 12.3g

EXPRESS SHRIMP & SAUSAGE JAMBALAYA

Prep Time: 15mints, Cooking Time: 25mints, Total Time: 40mints; Serving: 4

Ingredients
- 1 teaspoon canola oil
- 8 ounces andouille sausage
- 16-ounce bell pepper and onion
- 14-ounce chicken broth
- 2 cups brown rice

- 8 ounces raw shrimp

Instructions
1. Heat oil in a Dutch Oven over medium-high temperature, adding sausage and pepper-onion mixture; cook, mixing periodically, till the vegetables loosen up, 3 to 5mins. Add stock to the pot and heat until boiling.
2. Add rice, mix once, cover with lid and cook for 5 minutes.
3. Add shrimp and mix again.
4. Remove from the heat and let stand, secured until the shrimp are murky and cooked.
5. Cushion with a fork and serve.

Nutrition Fact: Calories 392; Fat 9g, Carbs 44g, Sugar 6g, Protein 27g

KETO STEAMED CLAMS WITH BASIL GARLIC BUTTER

Prep Time: 3mints, Cook Time: 10mints, Total Time: 13mints; Serving: 4

Ingredients
- 1 pound steamer-sized clams in shell small
- 3 tablespoons unsalted butter
- 1 clove garlic
- 10 fresh basil leaves whole
- 1/2 cup chicken broth

Instructions
1. Soften margarine in an enormous pot, one with a tight-fitting top, over medium heat.
2. Add garlic, basil leaves and chicken broth to the pot and heat to the point of boiling over medium-high heat.
3. Toss in the clams and cover with a tight-fitting cover, leaving the heat on medium-high.
4. While clams are steaming, shake the dish to uniformly cover/cook the shellfish.
5. Remove cover; if the sauce looks watery, leave the skillet to overheat without a top until sauce thickens. Discretionary: Add an extra tablespoon of margarine to the skillet to suit your macros.
6. Remove from heat when sauce reaches expected consistency.
7. Dispose of any shellfishes that have not opened and serve right away.

Nutrition Fact: Calories: 80, Fat 8g, Carbs 5g, Sugar 3g, Protein 14g

OYSTER BROILED WITH SPICY SAUCE

Prep Time: 10mints, Cook Time: 2mints, Total Time: 12mints; Serving: 2

Ingredients
- 12 oysters shucked
- 1 tablespoon Huy Fong's garlic chili paste
- 1 tablespoon olive oil
- 1/8 teaspoon salt
- 7-8 basil leaves fresh

Instructions
1. In a medium-size bowl, mixture garlic chili paste, olive oil, and salt.
2. Add shellfish to the sauce combination and completely coat.
3. Spread the basil leaves on a stove dish to make a mattress for the clams to cook on.
4. Pour the shellfish and the sauce over the basil leaves and unfold the clams out right into a solitary layer.
5. Turn the oven on high.
6. Sear for 2-3 minutes. Remove from the oven and serve promptly.

Nutrition Fact: Calories: 102, Fat 8g, Carbs 2g, Sugar 1g, Protein 4g

GARLIC LEMON BUTTER CRAB LEGS

Prep Time: 10mints, Cook Time: 5mints, Total Time: 15mints; Serving: 2

Ingredients
- 1 lb. king crab legs
- 1/2 stick salted butter
- 3 cloves garlic and lemon
- 1 tablespoon chopped parsley
- 1/2 tablespoon lemon juice

Instructions
1. Preheat stove to 375°F.
2. Defrost the crab legs if frozen. Utilizing a sharp blade or a couple of scissors, cut the crab legs into equal parts to uncover the tissue. Place them equally on a heating sheet or plate.
3. Soften the margarine in a microwave, for around 30 seconds. Add the garlic, parsley and lemon juice to the liquefied spread. Mix to blend well. Spread the margarine blend on the crab. Spare some for dipping.
4. Place the crab legs in the stove for around 5 minutes, or until the crab legs are warmed. Serve quickly with the rest of the garlic lemon margarine and lemon cuts. Press some lemon squeeze on the crab before eating.

Nutrition Facts: Calories 401, Fat 24g, Carbs 2g, Sugar 1g, Protein 42g

LOW CARB SOFT SHELL CRAB

Prep Time: 8mints, Cook Time: 8mints, Total Time: 16mints; Serving: 2

Ingredients
- 8 soft shell crabs
- ½ cup powdered Parmesan
- 2 eggs
- 4 tablespoons Carolina BBQ sauce

Instructions
1. Heat a solid iron skillet with ½ cup of fat with medium-excessive heat and pat the crab dry with a paper towel.
2. Put the powdered parmesan into a big shallow dish. Put the beaten eggs into another massive shallow dish.
3. Dunk the crab into the eggs and tap, simply so the crab has a mild overlaying. Dunk into the parmesan and make use of your fingers to cover the crab well.

4. Drop 3-4 crabs into the heating oil and cook for 2mins, flip and cook an additional 2mins or till crab is cooked thoroughly.
5. Repeat with the rest of the crab pieces.
6. Use Carolina BBQ sauce as a dip when serving.
Nutritional Fact: Calories 388, Fat 14g, Carbs 2g, Sugar 1g, Protein 60g

SALMON ROASTED IN BUTTER

Prep Time: 5mints, Cook Time: 15mints, Total Time: 20mints; Serving: 4
Ingredients
- 1/4 cup unsalted butter
- 3 Tbsp minced fresh dill
- 4 salmon fillets
- Salt and ground black pepper
- 1 tsp garlic and Lemon wedges
- 1 Tbsp minced fresh parsley

Instructions
1. Preheat stove to 475 degrees F.
2. Put spread in a little broiling dish, sprinkle dill, place in stove and heat till the margarine has softened and dill is sizzling, around 4 - 5mins.
3. Remove from stove and put fillets. Come back to the stove and dish 4 minutes.
4. Season with salt and pepper and turn fillets to season reverse side with salt and pepper, sprinkle garlic into the surrounding sauce.
5. Return to stove and cook till it reaches desired level of cooking.
6. Plate salmon and spoon margarine in a dish over salmon, sprinkle with parsley and serve warm with lemon wedges for taste.
Nutrition Facts: Calories 344, Fat 25g, Carbs 12g, Sugar 4g, Protein 28g

SALMON GARLICKY BLACK PEPPER AND EGG FREE LEMON AIOLI

Prep Time: 5mints, Cook Time: 20mints, Total Time: 25mints; Serving: 6
Ingredients
- 4 bundles Bumble Bee Super
- Egg Free Lemon Aioli
- 1/2 cup veggie-lover mayo
- 1/4 cup additional virgin olive oil
- 2 cup of lemon juice
- 2 cloves garlic

Instructions
1. Preheat stove to temperature shown on the bundle.
2. Put each fillet on a heating sheet.
3. Heat 20 minutes
4. Whisk aioli ingredients together in a little bowl and put aside until fish is finished.
5. To serve, cautiously open a material bundle, be cautious about steam.
6. Top each fillet with 1 ounce of sauce and chopped parsley and lemon juice if desire.

7. Any sauce ought to be kept refrigerated.
Nutrition Facts: Calories 427, Fat 35g, Carbs 6.6g, Sugar 1.6g, Protein 25g

KETO BACON WRAPPED SALMON WITH PESTO

Prep Time: 5mints, Cook Time: 15mints, Total Time: 20mints; Serving: 1
Ingredients
- 170g salmon fillet
- 1 slice streaky bacon
- 2 tbsp pesto

Instructions
1. Put the streaky bacon on a chopping board.
2. Put the salmon filet over the bacon.
3. Put 1-2 tbsp pesto inside the center.
4. Put in the skillet, unfold, and fry tenderly for 10 minutes until the salmon and bacon are cooked.
Nutrition Facts: Calories 449, Fat 31g, Carbs 3g, Sugar 1g, Protein 38g

GRILLED SALMON WITH CREAMY PESTO

Prep Time: 15mints, Cook Time: 10mints, Total Time: 25mints; Serving: 4
Ingredients
- 4 - 6 skinless salmon fillets
- Olive oil
- Salt and freshly ground black pepper
- 4 oz. cream cheese
- 1/4 cup milk
- 3 Tbsp homemade

Instructions
1. Preheat a barbecue over medium-high heat to around 425 degrees F. Brush the two sides of salmon with olive oil and season the two sides with salt and pepper. Brush with oil and barbecue salmon around 3 minutes on each side or as much as needed.
2. While salmon is cooking, heat cream cheddar with milk in a pan set over medium heat, blending continually until softened, around 1 - 2 minutes. Remove from heat and mix in pesto.
3. Serve salmon warm with velvety pesto sauce. Spoon around 1 tsp pesto over rich pesto sauce for added flavor
Nutrition Facts: Calories 467, Fat 27g, Carbs 2g, Sugar 2g, Protein 36g

GRILLED SWORDFISH SKEWERS WITH PESTO MAYO

Prep Time: 15mints, Cooking Time: 10mints, Total Time: 25mints; Serving: 4
Ingredients
- 1 lb swordfish
- 16 cherry tomatoes, salt, and pepper
- 1 tsp olive oil to coat
- 1/4 cup pesto
- 1/4 cup mayonnaise

Instructions

1. Gap the swordfish into four equal elements.
2. Place the swordfish with the cherry tomatoes on your sticks.
3. Place the skewers on barbeque and cook for around 1 minute on each side.
4. Serve warm or chilled with a plate of blended greens.
5. Add the pesto and mayonnaise in a bowl and blend well.

Nutrition Fact: Calories 162, Fat 6g, Carbs 2g, Sugar 1.2g, Protein 23g

SCHLEMMERFILET BORDELAISE HERBED ALMOND AND PARMESAN CRUSTED FISH

Prep Time: 20mints, Cooking Time: 35mints, Total Time: 55mints; Serving: 4

Ingredients
- 1 lb Alaska pollock
- 3 oz salted butter
- 2/3 cup almond flour
- 2/3 cup freshly grated Parmesan
- 2 tsp Italian herb seasoning

Instructions
1. Preheat the stove to 350 °F.
2. Put the fish fillets into a glass or fired heating dish.
3. Set up the ingredient: join the margarine, almond flour, Parmesan, herb flavoring and the salt in a medium bowl.
4. Blend in with an electric blender until well-mixed.
5. Pour the blend over the fish fillets.
6. Leave to cook for 35-40 minutes, or till the juices run clear and the garnish is notably darker.

Nutrition Fact: Calories 213, Fat 5g, Carbs 6g, Sugar 2g, Protein 32g

BAKED LEMON BUTTER TILAPIA

Prep Time: 10mints, Cooking Time: 10mints, Total Time: 20mints; Serving: 4

Ingredients:
- 1/4 cup unsalted butter
- 3 cloves garlic
- 2 tablespoons freshly squeezed lemon juice
- 4 tilapia fillets
- Kosher salt, 1 lemon, and pepper
- 2 tablespoons parsley leaves

Instructions
1. Preheat range to 425 ranges F. Delicately oil a preparing dish or coat with a nonstick spray.
2. In a little bowl, whisk collectively margarine, garlic, lemon juice, and lemon, put aside for later use.
3. Season tilapia with salt and pepper for flavor and place onto the prepared heating dish.
4. Put into stove and heat till fish breaks easily with a fork, around 10-12mins.
5. Serve right away, decorated with parsley.

Nutrition Facts: Calories 276.4, Fat 14.5g, Carbs 1.8g, Sugars 0.3g, Protein 35.5g

LOW-CARB FISH CURRY WITH COCONUT AND SPINACH

Prep Time: 5mints, Cook Time: 20mints, Total Time: 25mints; Serving: 6

Ingredients
- 1 kg firm white fish
- 2-4 tbsp curry paste
- 400 ml of coconut cream
- 400 ml of water
- 500g spinach

Instructions
1. Heat the oil in an enormous pan, add the curry paste and fry on moderate heat for 2-3 minutes to bring forth the flavors.
2. Add the coconut cream and water and bring to boil.
3. Cautiously add the fish pieces and lessen the heat. Stew for 10-15 minutes.
4. Add the spinach and cook for another 3-4 minutes, or until the spinach has shriveled.
5. Serve in huge dishes.

Nutrition Facts: Calories 314, Fat 18.5g, Carbs 5.8g, Sugar 2.3g, Protein 33.4g

LOW-CARB ALMOND AND PARMESAN BAKED FISH

Prep Time: 15mints, Cook Time: 20-30mints, Total Time: 35-45mints; Serving: 3-4

Ingredients:
- 3-4 Tilapia
- 1/4 cup melted butter
- 1/3 cup almond meal
- 2 T finely grated Parmesan
- 1/2 tsp. garlic powder and 1/4 tsp. pepper

Instructions
1. Preheat stove to 425°F/220°C.
2. Cover heating dish with a non-stick spray.
3. Liquefy butter together over low heat.
4. In a level bowl huge enough to hold the fish, blend almond meal.
5. Plunge each fish filet in the spread, covering both sides, then place into the almond blend.
6. Attempt to get as a great part of the almond blend to adhere to the fish as you can
7. Cook for 20-30 minutes, or until fish is firm to the touch and darker in color.
8. The preparing time will rely upon the thickness of the fish, so watch it cautiously.

Nutrition Facts: Calories 423, Fat 18g, Carbs 8g, Sugar 3g, Protein 24g

KETO FRIED FISH

Prep Time: 10mints, Cook Time: 15mints; Servings: 4

Ingredients
- 1 lb White Fish cod, tilapia
- 3/4 cup Almond Flour

- Salt, pepper, and Oil
- 2-3 tsp Tony Chachere's Creole
- 2 eggs beaten

Instructions
1. Heat the oil over medium-high heat in a large skillet. On the off chance that you have an electric skillet, set it to 375 degrees F
2. Set up the well-beaten eggs in a rectangular dish. At that point blend the almond flour and Tony Chachere's Creole and put on a plate or shallow dish for plunging the fish.
3. Utilizing paper towels, pat the fish dry and season the two sides with salt and pepper.
4. Dunk in the egg, at that point, coat the two sides in the almond flour blend shaking to remove the abundance.
5. Put the fish into the hot oil in the skillet. Permit cooking for around 2-4 minutes for each side, depending on the thickness of your fish.
6. Present on a platter, permit to cool before serving.

Nutrition Fact: Calories: 344, Fat 25g, Carbs 4g, Sugar 2g, Protein 25g

BAKED WHITE FISH WITH PINE NUT, PARMESAN WITH BASIL PESTO CRUST

Prep Time: 30mints, Cook Time: 10-15mints, Total Time: 40-45mints; Serving: 2

Ingredients
- 2 white fish fillets
- 3 T pine nuts
- 2 T Parmesan Cheese
- 1/4 tsp garlic
- 1 tsp basil pesto and 1 1/2 T mayo

Instructions
1. Preheat stove or toaster stove to 400F/200C. Shower singular goulash dishes with a non-stick spray of olive oil
2. Remove the fish fillets from the cooler and let them come to room temperature while the stove warms.
3. Utilize an enormous culinary specialist's blade to finely cut the pine nuts and mince the garlic. Combine cut pine nuts, Parmesan, minced garlic, basil pesto and mayo.
4. Utilize an elastic scrubber to spread the outside layer blend equally over the outside of each fish fillet. Heap it on so all the outside layer blend is used.
5. Cook fish for 10-15 minutes, until fish is firm to the touch and outside blend is beginning to gently darken in color.
6. Serve hot.

Nutrition Fact: Calories: 213, Fat 15g, Carbs 3g, Sugar 5g, Protein 28g

SMOKY TUNA PICKLE BOATS – LOW CARB & GLUTEN-FREE

Prep Time: 10mints, Cooking Time: 20mints, Total Time: 30mints; Serving: 4

Ingredients
- oz albacore tuna
- 6-oz smoked tuna
- 1/3 cup sugar-free mayonnaise
- 1/4 tsp garlic powder
- 1/4- tsp pepper and 1- Tbsp onion
- 6 large whole dill pickles

Instructions
1. Add all the ingredients aside from the pickles in a medium bowl and blend well.
2. Cut the pickles down the middle and tenderly scoop out the seeds from the center.
3. Spoon around 3 Tbsp of the blend of mixed greens and fish into each pickle half.
4. Chill and serve.

Nutrition Fact: Calories: 118, Fat 7g, Carbs 1.5g, Sugar 0.2g, Protein 11g

EASY KETO FRIED COCONUT SHRIMP

Prep Time: 5mints, Cook Time: 12mints, Total Time: 17mints; Serving: 4

Ingredients
- 1 lb Raw Shrimp
- 1/4 cup Bob's Red Mill Organic Coconut Flour
- 3/4 Cup Organic Unsweetened Coconut Flakes
- 1 Tablespoon Lakanto Monk Fruit Sweetener
- 2 Eggs and Coconut Oil

Instructions
1. In a small bowl combine the salt, Monk Fruit Sweetener and coconut flour
2. Make and a mechanical production system of 3 dishes, one with the flour blend, the second one with the eggs and the third with the unsweetened shredded Coconut
3. Set air fryer to 380°F
4. Cook for round 12 minutes or until shrimp is darkish in color.

Nutrition Fact: Calories: 40, Fat 2.4g, Carbs 1.5g, Sugar 1g, Protein 3.2g

SHRIMP RECIPE WITH GARLIC BUTTER CAULIFLOWER RICE

Prep Time: 10mints, Cook Time: 15mints, Total Time: 25mints; Servings: 4

Ingredients
- 2 lbs Raw large frozen shrimp thawed
- 1 head Cauliflower rice
- 1/2 cup Salted butter
- 1 tbsp minced garlic
- 1/4 tsp fresh ground black pepper

Instructions
1. Preheat stove to 400°F
2. Cut the florets off of the stem of the cauliflower and dispose of the stem. Add the florets

to a nourishment processor and procedure till it looks like the surface of rice. On the other hand, you can purchase ready-made rice cauliflower.

3. On the off risk that your "rice" is solidified and in portions, place in a microwave-secure container and microwave until the lumps can be separated

4. In a big bowl, consisting of defrosted and clean shrimp, season with garlic, parsley and dark pepper.

5. Pour the shrimp and cauliflower mixture onto a sheet field, ensuring the shrimp are in a solitary layer. Prepared within about 15mins.

Nutrition Fact: Calories 423, Fat 24g, Carbs 8g, Sugar 6g, Protein 24g

LOW CARB SPICY SHRIMP HAND ROLLS

Prep Time: 15mints, Cooking Time: 20mints, Total Time: 35mints; Serving: 5

Ingredients
- 2- cups cooked shrimp
- 1/4 - cup mayonnaise and 1 Tbsp Sriracha
- 2- Tbsp cilantro leaves
- 1/4- cucumber
- 5- hand roll nori sheets

Instructions
1. In a medium bowl, mix the cooked shrimp, mayonnaise and Sriracha sauce.
2. Place the hand roll nori sheets in a manner so that the most extensive part is facing you. Put 1/5 of your shrimp blend on the correct side of the wrap, leaving around 2/3 of the wrap vacant. Add cilantro leaves and cucumber strips. Roll the sheets into a cone shape.
3. Use water to seal the edges and serve.

Nutrition Fact: Calories: 130, Fat 10g Carbs 1g, Sugar 2g, Protein 9g

CHIMICHURRI SHRIMP

Prep Time: 15mints, Cooking Time: 20mints, Total Time: 35mints; Serving: 4

Ingredients
- One batch chimichurri sauce
- Pound raw shrimp
- Tbsp olive oil
- Salt
- Fresh cracked black pepper

Instructions
1. Mix the shrimp with the olive oil, salt and pepper.
2. Heat a critical skillet on medium warm temperature, and when it is hot, then place the shrimp.
3. Cook just until the shrimp turn and turn dark red, then flip and cook for one additional minute.
4. Spread the chimichurri sauce in a feast dish, serving dish or skillet, and set the cooked shrimp down into the sauce.
5. Present with evaporated bread for dipping, or serve over rice, couscous, or pasta.

Nutrition Fact: Calories: 231, Fat 4g Carbs 3.1g, Sugar 1.3g, Protein 21g

ZERO CARB FRIED SHRIMP

Prep Time: 20mints, Cook time: 10mints, Total Time: 30mints; Serving: 4

Ingredients
- 1 pound of shrimp
- 2 eggs
- 1/2 teaspoon salt and Olive oil
- 1/2 cup Now Foods Almond Flour
- 1 1/2 cups pork panko

Instruction
1. In a little bowl mix the salt and almond flour
2. Set up 3 dishes, one with the flour blend, the second one with the eggs and the third with the pork panko
3. Dig the shrimp within the almond flour combination, followed then by the egg and lastly by the pork panko.
4. Fill a sauté dish with olive oil and put on medium-high temperature
5. When the oil is warm put shrimp in oil and cook for 1-2 minutes on every surface.
6. Shrimp cook easily so be careful not to over-cook.
7. Present with Spicy Bang Dipping Sauce

Nutrition Fact: Calories: 321, Fat 42g, Carbs 2g, Sugar 3g, Protein 32g

BAKED BUTTER GARLIC SHRIMP

Prep Time: 10mints, Cook Time: 20mints, Total Time: 30mints; Serving: 5-6

Ingredients
- 1 lb raw shrimp
- 5 tbsp softened butter
- 3-4 large cloves garlic
- Salt and fresh ground pepper
- Dried parsley and Lemon wedges

Instructions
1. Preheat stove to 425 degrees F. Smear spread uniformly over the base of the heating dish
2. Sprinkle the squashed garlic over the spread
3. Add the shrimp and sprinkle everything with salt and pepper
4. Heat for 7 minutes and afterward mix/turn the shrimp and prepare for 7-10 additional minutes, or until shrimp is done.
5. Top with parsley, if desired, and crush a lemon wedge over it for the final touch.
6. Fill in as a side with steak or add the cooked shrimp and margarine sauce to pasta. On the off chance that you do this, cook the pasta while the shrimp is preparing for a brisk feast

Nutrition Fact: Calories: 242, Fat 22g, Carbs 2.3g, Sugar 1.7g, Protein 26g

GRILLED SALMON WITH CREAMY PESTO SAUCE

Prep Time: 15mints, Cook Time: 10mints, Total Time: 25mints; Serving: 4

Ingredients
- 4 - 6 skinless salmon fillets
- Olive oil
- Salt and freshly ground black pepper
- 4 oz. cream cheese
- 1/4 cup milk and 3 Tbsp pesto

Instructions
1. Preheat a flame broil over medium-high heat to around 425 degrees F. Brush the two sides of salmon with olive oil and season the two sides with salt and pepper. Brush barbecue grates with oil and flame cook salmon around 3 minutes for each side or to wanted doneness.
2. While salmon is cooking, heat cream cheese with milk in a pan set over medium heat, mixing continually until softened, around 1 - 2 minutes. Remove from heat and mix in pesto.
3. Serve salmon warm with smooth pesto sauce. Spoon around 1 tsp pesto over rich pesto sauce for added flavor

Nutrition Facts: Calories 467, Fat 27g, Carbs 2g, Sugar 2g, Protein 36g

KETO GRILLED LOBSTER TAILS WITH CREOLE BUTTER

Prep Time: 10mints, Cook Time: 8mints, Total Time: 18mints; Serving: 4

Ingredients
- Ounce raw lobster tails
- 1/2 cup salted butter
- 2 teaspoons minced fresh garlic
- 1 tablespoon Creole seasoning
- 2 tablespoons fresh parsley

Instructions
1. Add melted butter, garlic, Creole flavoring, and parsley in a little bowl and blend well with a fork until mixed.
2. Set up the lobster tails for cooking by slicing down the middle or slicing through the base and removing the meat from the shell.
3. Preheat your stove to about 400°F and put the lobster's meat side down over direct heat for around 3 minutes.
4. Turn the tails over and treat the meat liberally with the mollified Creole spread.
5. Cook for an extra 3 to 4 minutes, or until the meat is cooked thoroughly.
6. Serve promptly with extra dissolved Creole margarine if needed.
7. Store extra margarine in the cooler for as long as a week or in the freezer for as long as 3 months

Nutrition Fact: Calories: 213, Fat 13g, Carbs 2g, Sugar 0.3g, Protein 23g

SMOKED SALMON PINWHEELS

Prep Time: 10mints, Cooking Time: 10mints, Total Time: 20mints; Serving: 4

Ingredients
- 8 ounces cold smoked salmon
- 4 ounces 1/3 less fat cream cheese
- 1/4 medium cucumber
- 2 tsp red onion and 2 tsp capers
- 1/2 lemon

Instructions
1. Lay a big piece of dangle wrap on a work floor.
2. Organize the cuts of salmon in a covering fashion to make a square form round 6 inches wide by 12 inches long, with perhaps the longest part facing you.
3. Tenderly spread the creamy cheese over the salmon but not over-doing it.
4. Utilizing the hang wrap, roll salmon up firmly across the cucumber sticks.
5. Utilizing a pointy blade, reduce the fold into 16 1/2-inch thick cuts
6. Sprinkle with crimson onion and with lemon cuts.

Nutrition Fact: Calories: 168, Fat 10g, Carbs 5g, Sugar 1.5g, Protein 13.5g

KETO TUNA SALAD

Prep Time: 10mints, Cooking Time: 15mints, Total Time: 25mints; Serving: 2

Ingredients
- Cup of canned tuna fish
- Tbsp of "real" mayonnaise
- Tsp dried onion flakes
- Salt and pepper

Instructions
1. Add the fish, mayonnaise, and dried onion pieces in a little bowl.
2. Mix and taste
3. Season with salt and pepper according to taste.

Nutrition Fact: Calories: 248, Fat 19g, Carbs 2g, Sugar 2g, Protein 20g

SALMON FLORENTINE

Prep Time: 2mints, Cook Time: 20mints, Total Time: 22mints; Servings: 2

Ingredients
- tbsp ghee
- oz spinach raw and 1 clove garlic
- tbsp apple cider vinegar
- 1/2- tbsp red chili flakes
- 1/2- tsp sea salt, 1/8 tsp black pepper
- 16- oz salmon fillet skinless

Instructions
1. Preheat stove to 350 degrees Fahrenheit.
2. Soften ghee in an enormous skillet over medium heat. Add spinach, vinegar, red chili flakes,

garlic, and 1/2 of the sea salt and dark pepper. Blend to join.
3. Placed spread on the stovetop for 3 minutes.
4. Put salmon fillets in a goulash dish and season with remaining salt and pepper. Partition the cooked spinach between the salmon, covering and molding over the highest point of each fillet.
5. Heat for 15 minutes or until salmon is altogether cooked

Nutrition Fact: Calories: 430, Fat 22g, Carbs 6g, Sugar 3g, Protein 49g

ROASTED SALMON WITH PARMESAN DILL CRUST

Prep Time: 2mints, Cook Time: 10mints, Total Time: 12mints; Serving: 2

Ingredients
- 2- Pieces of salmon
- ¼- cup mayonnaise
- ¼- Cup grated parmesan cheese
- Tbsp dill weed
- Tsp ground mustard

Instructions
1. Preheat stove to 450 degrees F.
2. Combine mayonnaise, parmesan, dill, and mustard.
3. Put salmon on a foil-lined heating sheet.
4. Smear half of the mayonnaise blend over each bit of salmon.
5. Cook in the stove for around 10 minutes, until the outside layer, is darker and the fish roasts.

Nutrition Fact: Calories: 666, Fat 37g, Carbs 10g, Sugar 2g, Protein 76g

PARMESAN CRUSTED COD

Prep Time: 10mints, Cook Time: 15mints, Total Time: 25mints; Serving: 4

Ingredients
- ¾- cup Parmesan cheese 2- Tsp paprika
- Tsp fresh parsley and 1 tsp extra virgin olive oil
- ¼ - Tsp of sea salt
- 4- Cod fillets

Instructions
1. Preheat the stove to 400ºF. Line a heating tray with fabric paper or foil.
2. In a shallow bowl, combine the Parmesan, paprika, parsley, and salt. Sprinkle the cod with olive oil, and immediately dip inside the cheese combo, squeezing it in gently along with your palms. Move to the tray. Top cod with any last cheese combo.
3. Heat until the fish is misty within the thickest phase, 10-15 minutes.
4. Present with the lemon cuts.

Nutrition Fact:: Calories 115, Fat 7.6g, Carbs 1.5g, Sugar 0.3g, Protein 10.7g

BAKED BUTTER GARLIC SHRIMP

Prep Time: 10mints, Cook Time: 20mints, Total Time: 30mints; Serving: 5-6

Ingredients
- lb raw shrimp
- 5- tbsp softened butter
- 3-4- large cloves garlic
- Salt and fresh ground pepper
- Dried parsley and Lemon wedges

Instructions
1. Preheat stove to 425 degrees F.
2. Smear margarine equally over the base of the cooking dish
3. Sprinkle the crushed garlic over the margarine. Add the shrimp and sprinkle everything with salt and pepper
4. Heat for 7 minutes and afterward mix/turn the shrimp and prepare for an additional 7-10 minutes, or until shrimp is done.
5. Enhance taste with parsley and/or squeeze a lemon wedge over it.
6. Fill in as a side with steak or add the cooked shrimp and margarine sauce to pasta. On the off chance that you do this, cook the pasta while the shrimp is being prepared for a brisk feast

Nutrition Fact: Calories 188; Fat 5g, Carbs 10g, Sugar 6g, Protein 24g

BAKED LOBSTER TAILS WITH GARLIC BUTTER

Prep Time: 10mints, Cook Time: 15mints, Total Time: 15mints; Serving: 4

Ingredients
- 4 lobster tails and 5 cloves garlic
- 1/4 c. grated Parmesan
- Juice of 1 lemon
- 1 tsp. Italian seasoning
- 4 tbsp. melted butter

Instructions
1. Preheat stove to 350 degrees F. In a medium bowl, combine garlic, Parmesan, Italian seasoning, and melted butter and season with salt.
2. Utilizing sharp scissors cut the tidy skin up the lobster and brush the lobster tails with the garlic spread flavoring.
3. Put the lobster tails on a heating sheet fixed with material and cook the lobster tails for 15 minutes. The lobster meat inside will be firm and dark. The inward temperature should peruse 140 to 145 degrees.

Nutrition Fact: Calories 266; Fat 11g, Carbs 1g, Sugar 0.1g, Protein 28g

KETO COCONUT SHRIMP RECIPE

Prep Time: 10mints, Cook Time: 5mints, Total Time: 15mints; Serving: 2

Ingredients
- 3- Tablespoons of coconut flour
- Medium egg
- ½ - cup of coconut flakes

- 7-oz raw shrimp, lime, and oil
- Salt and black pepper

Instructions
1. Line a plate with paper towels. Put aside.
2. Plan three dishes. Put the coconut flour in one bowl, the whisked egg in the second and the coconut flakes in the last.
3. Place all the shrimp in the coconut flour. Each shrimp in plunged in the egg, shaking slightly to remove excess flour. At that point plunge the shrimp in the coconut, squeezing the coconut into the shrimp solidly.
4. Heat enough oil to deep fry the shrimp. When hot, fry the shrimp for a moment or two and remove with a spoon and place on the plate with paper towels
5. Season with salt, pepper and lime. Serve warm.

Nutrition Fact: Calories: 267, Fat 15g, Carbs 8g, Sugar 2g, Protein 25g

KETO SHRIMP AND CUCUMBER APPETIZER RECIPE

Prep Time: 10mints, Cook Time: 10mints, Total Time: 20mints; Serving: 6

Ingredients
- 2 cucumbers
- 12 shrimps
- 1 tomato
- Salt and pepper, and 1/4 onion
- 3 Tsp olive oil

Instructions
1. Split the cucumber into eight with the purpose that you can stuff the sauce and shrimp on pinnacle.
2. Make the sauce by way of combining the onion, pepper, tomato, and salt and pepper in a little bowl.
3. Scoop a touch of the sauce onto every cucumber location
4. Then wedge a shrimp on top and sprinkle olive oil on pinnacle.

Nutrition Fact: Calories: 112, Fat 8g, Carbs 3g, Sugar 1g, Protein 8g

PALEO/GF POPCORN SHRIMP RECIPE

Prep Time: 5mints, Cook Time: 20mints, Total Time: 25mints; Serving: 2

Ingredients
- ½ - lb of small shrimp
- 2- eggs
- Tsp Cajun seasoning
- 6- Tablespoons of coconut flour
- Coconut oil for frying

Instructions
1. Liquefy the coconut oil in a pan or profound fryer.
2. Put the beaten eggs into one big bowl and add the coconut flour and seasoning into a separate bowl.
3. Drop the shrimp into the beaten eggs and mix around so each shrimp is blanketed.
4. Then, take the shrimp from the eggs and put them into the flavoring bowl.
5. Toss the battered shrimp into the fryer for a few minutes.
6. Utilizing an opened spoon, remove the shrimp and place on paper towels to remove excessive oil, repeat for the remainder of the shrimp.
7. Cool for 10 minutes and serve and enjoy with/out Paleo ketchup.

Nutrition Fact: Calories: 412, Fat 22g, Carbs 17g, Sugar 4g, Protein 33g

KETO LEMON BAKED SALMON RECIPE

Prep Time: 5mints, Cook Time: 20mints, Total Time: 25mints; Serving: 2

Ingredients
- 2- Lemons
- 2- Fillets of salmon
- 2- Tablespoons of olive oil
- Salt and freshly ground black pepper
- Thyme

Instructions
1. Preheat the stove to 350°F.
2. Put a huge part of the cut lemons on the bottom of a dish.
3. Lay the salmon fillets over the lemons and unfold with the rest of the lemon cuts.
4. Sprinkle olive oil over the salmon and heat inside the stove for 20mins.
5. Season with salt, pepper and thyme

Nutrition Fact: Calories: 571, Fat 44g, Carbs 2g, Sugar 2g, Protein 42g

KETO SMOKED SALMON SALAD WITH POACHED EGG

Prep Time: 5mints, Cook Time: 5mints, Total Time: 10mints; Serving: 1

Ingredients
- 1 large handful of salad greens
- 2 Tbsp olive oil and 1 poached egg
- 1 tsp freshly squeezed lemon juice
- 100 g smoked salmon slices
- 2 Tsp pistachios

Instructions
1. Place greens into a bowl and toss with 1 tablespoon of olive oil and 1 teaspoon of lemon juice
2. Poach an egg.
3. Place the poached egg over the smoked salmon.
4. Sprinkle the squashed pistachios over the egg.
5. Sprinkle with the rest of the olive oil and enjoy.

Nutrition Fact: Calories: 460, Fat 38g, Carbs 3g, Sugar 1g, Protein 27g

QUICK KETO BACON-WRAPPED SALMON

Prep Time: 10mints, Cook Time: 20mints, Total Time: 30mints; Serving: 2;
Ingredients
- 2 fillets of salmon
- 4 slices of bacon
- 1 Tsp of olive oil, 2 Tsp of Basil Pesto
- 2 Tsp of Paleo mayo
- Salt and ground black pepper

Instructions
1. Preheat the stove to 350°F.
2. Pat dry the salmon and wrap it with the bacon. Put onto an oven tray and sprinkle with the olive oil. Heat for 15-20mints
3. In the meantime, mix the pesto and mayonnaise together in a bowl. Season with salt and ground pepper
4. When ready to serve, swab a dab of the pesto and mayo mix on every bacon-wrapped salmon.

Nutrition Fact: Calories: 1175, Fat 109g, Carbs 3g, Sugar 1g, Protein 49g

LOW CARB OATMEAL WITH COCONUT FLOUR

Prep Time: 2mints, Cook Time: 3mints, Total Time: 5mints; Serving: 4
Ingredients
- 2 tablespoons coconut flour
- 4 tsps shredded coconut
- 1 tsp sugar-free crystal sweetener
- 3/4 cup unsweetened almond milk
- 1 tablespoon almond butter

Instructions
1. Put each one of the ingredients into a medium pan.
2. Heat till it begins to stew, until mildly bubbling, at that point reduce the temperature and stew for 2-three minutes, mixing once in a while, until thickened.
3. Remove from heat when it reaches the consistency you want.
4. Serve hot with your preferred ingredients and add extra unsweetened almond milk when desired.

Nutrition Facts: Calories 361, Fat 28.8g, Carbs 14.9g, Sugar 4.1g, Protein 14.6g

BAKED ROSEMARY SALMON

Prep Time: 5mints, Cook Time: 30mints, Total Time: 35mints; Serving: 2
Ingredients
- 2 salmon fillets
- 1 tsp fresh rosemary leaves
- 1/4 cup olive oil
- 1 tsp salt

Instructions
1. Preheat the stove to 350°F (175°C).
2. Blend the olive oil, rosemary, and salt together in a bowl.
3. Rub the blend onto the salmon fillets.
4. Enclose each fillet in a bit of aluminum foil with a portion of the rest of the blend.
5. Cook for 25-30 minutes.

Nutrition Fact: Calories 188; Fat 5g, Carbs 10g, Sugar 6g, Protein 24g

KETO BAKED SALMON WITH LEMON AND BUTTER

Prep Time: 10mints, Cooking Time: 25mints, Total time: 35mints; Serving: 6
Ingredients
- 2 lbs salmon
- 1 tsp sea salt and 1 lemon
- Ground black pepper
- 7 oz. butter
- 1 tbsp olive oil

Instructions
1. Preheat the stove to 400°F
2. Layer a large oven dish with olive oil. Put the salmon, with the skin face down, onto the dish.
3. Cut the lemon and squeeze over the salmon. Spread with half of the butter in dainty cuts.
4. Prepare on the center rack for around 20-30min, or until the salmon is murky and cuts easily with a fork
5. Heat the remainder of the butter in a pot until it starts to bubble. Remove from warm temperature and allow to cool forming a chunk.
6. Delicately add some lemon juice.
7. Serve the fish with the lemon butter and a dish of your selection.

Nutrition Fact: Calories 573, Fat 49g, Carbs1g, Sugar 15g, Protein 31g

KETO FRIED SALMON WITH ASPARAGUS

Prep Time: 5mints, Cooking Time: 10mints, Total Time: 15mints; Serving: 2
Ingredients
- 8 oz. green asparagus
- 3 oz. butter
- 9 oz. salmon
- salt and pepper

nstructions
1. Rinse and trim the asparagus.
2. Heat up a generous bit of butter in a griddle.
3. Fry the asparagus over medium heat for 3-4mins. Season with salt and pepper. Gather the whole thing in one part of the skillet.
4. Add more butter to fry the bits of salmon for numerous minutes on each side.
5. Mix the asparagus every now and again. Lower the warm temperature towards the finish.
6. Season the salmon and add the rest of the butter to it.

Nutrition Fact: Calories 591, Fat 52g, Carbs 2g, Sugar 10g, Protein 28g

PINK PEPPERCORN SMOKED SALMON SALAD RECIPE

Prep Time: 5mints, Total Time: 5mints; Serving: 1;
INGREDIENTS
- 1 handful of arugula salad leaves
- 1 teaspoon of pink peppercorns
- 4 olives
- 50 grams smoked salmon
- 1 slice of lemon

Instructions
1. Put the arugula serving and olives into a shallow bowl or plate.
2. Put the smoked salmon over the serving of mixed greens.
3. Sprinkle the softly squashed pink peppercorns over the smoked salmon.
4. Enhance flavor with a cut of lemon and serve right away

Nutrition Fact: Calories: 80, Fat 8g, Carbs 5g, Sugar 3g, Protein 14g

FIVE-MINUTE KETO CURRIED TUNA SALAD RECIPE

Prep Time: 5mints, Total Time: 5mints; Serving: 1
Ingredients
- 170g of tuna
- 3 Tablespoons mayo
- 2 teaspoons curry powder
- 1 teaspoon dried parsley
- Salt and pepper

Instructions
1. Drain and place the fish in a bowl. Blend in with the mayo, curry powder, and dried parsley. Season with salt and pepper, for taste.
2. Present with a serving of mixed greens or cauliflower rice.

Nutrition Fact: Calories: 520, Fat 41g, Carbs 0.5g, Sugar 0.2g, Protein 41g

FIVE-MINUTE KETO FRIED SARDINES RECIPE WITH OLIVES

Prep Time: 5mints, Cook Time: 5mints, Total Time: 10mints; Serving: 1
Ingredients
- 100g sardines in olive oil
- 5 black olives
- 1 Tablespoon garlic flakes
- 1 teaspoon parsley flakes
- 1 Tablespoon olive oil

Instructions
1. Add the tablespoon of olive oil to the griddle and fry everything together for 5 minutes.

Nutrition Fact: Calories: 416, Fat 33g, Carbs 7g, Sugar 2g, Protein 21g

FIVE-MINUTE KETO SARDINES AND ONIONS RECIPE

Prep Time: 5mints, Total Time: 5mints; Serving: 1
Ingredients
- 100g sardines in olive oil
- 1/4 red onion
- 1 teaspoon apple cider vinegar
- 1 Tablespoon olive oil
- Salt

Instructions
1. Put the cut onions at the base of a bowl. Sprinkle with vinegar and olive oil.
2. Top with sardines.
3. Sprinkle salt.

Nutrition Fact: Calories: 385, Fat 33g, Carbs 3g, Sugar 1g, Protein 20g

EASY SARDINES SALAD RECIPE

Prep Time: 5mints, Total Time: 5mints; Serving: 1
Ingredients
- 120g sardines in olive oil
- 100g salad greens
- 50g deli meat
- 1 Tsp olive oil
- 1 Tsp lemon juice and Salt

Instructions
1. Set up the plate of mixed greens and add olive oil and lemon juice.
2. Add the deli meat in.
3. Top with the drained sardines.
4. Sprinkle with salt for taste.

Nutrition Fact: Calories: 400, Fat 34g, Carbs 2g, Sugar 0.2g, Protein 30g

FRIED MAHI FISH BITES

Prep Time: 15mints, Cooking Time: 20mints, Total Time: 35mints; Serving: 4
Ingredients
- 3 mahi-mahi fillets
- 1/2 cup tapioca flour and 1/3 cup almond flour
- 1 tsp onion powder
- 2 tsp salt and 2 eggs
- 3 tsp coconut oil
- 1 lime

Instructions
1. Utilizing kitchen shears, cut the mahi-mahi fillets into generally 1.5"x1.5" 3D shapes. Put aside
2. Add the custard flour, almond flour, onion powder, and salt in a huge bowl or holder
3. Heat a huge skillet over medium-high and add the coconut oil
4. Place the Mahi fillets into the whisked eggs, at that point into the flour blend, shaking the bowl or holder to cover the fish equally
5. Move the fish into the hot coconut oil and fry for 1 min, then using kitchen tongs, flip the fillets and fry an extra 45 seconds – 1 min the other side.

6. Cut the lime down the middle and squeeze onto the cooked fish before serving
Nutrition Fact:: Calories 113, Fat 6g, Carbs 10g, Sugar 2g, Protein 4g

POACHED COD IN TOMATO SAUCE

Prep Time: 5mints, Cook Time: 20mints, Total Time: 25mints; Serving: 4

Ingredients
- 4 6-ounce boneless cod fillets
- Kosher salt
- 2 cups Paleo-friendly marinara sauce
- Freshly ground black pepper
- ¼ cup chopped fresh herbs

Instructions
1. In case you're utilizing frozen fillets, defrost first. Try not to be disappointed if the fillets aren't totally defrosted by dinnertime; try placing the cod parcels in a bowl and run cool water on them.
2. Blotch the fish with paper towels and sprinkle the two sides with salt.
3. Get a skillet with a top and pour two cups of marinara sauce or salsa. The skillet ought to be enormous enough to fit the fillets cozily in a solitary layer.
4. Wrench the heat up to high to heat the sauce to the point of boiling then cautiously slip in the prepared fillets.
5. Cook for 5 to 8 minutes or until the fish is dark and cooked to your likeness.
6. Top the fish with grounded black pepper and fresh herbs.
7. Serve the saucy fish with a serving of mixed greens, a major platter of broiled vegetables, or cauliflower rice.
Nutrition Fact: Calories: 160, Fat 15g, Carbs 9g, Sugar 1g, Protein 2g

KETO BAKED SALMON WITH LEMON AND BUTTER

Prep Time: 10mints, Cooking Time: 25mints, Total Time: 35mints; Serving: 6

Ingredients
- 1 tbsp olive oil
- 2 lbs salmon
- 1 tsp sea salt and black pepper
- 7 oz. butter
- 1 lemon

Instructions
1. Preheat the stove to 400°F.
2. Oil an extensive heating dish with olive oil. Put the salmon, with the skin-surface down, onto a dish.
3. Liberally season with salt and pepper
4. Cut the lemon and squeeze over the salmon. Spread with 1/2 of the butter in flimsy cuts.
5. Heat at the middle rack for around 20-30minutes, or till the salmon is darkish and can easily be cut with a fork
6. Heat the remainder of the butter in a pan till it starts to bubble. Remove from heat and allow to cool.
7. Serve the fish with the lemon butter and dish of your selection.
Nutrition Fact: Calories 573, Fat 49g, Carbs 1g, Sugar 11g, Protein 31g

PROSCIUTTO-WRAPPED SALMON SKEWERS

Prep Time: 10mints, Cooking Time: 15mints, Total Time: 25mints; Serving: 4

Ingredients
- Salmon fillets and 8 wooden skewers
- ¼ cup fresh basil
- 1 lb salmon and 1 cup mayonnaise
- 1 pinch ground black pepper
- 3½ oz. prosciutto
- 1 tbsp olive oil

Instructions
1. Spray the skewers.
2. Cut the basil finely with a sharp blade.
3. Cut the nearly defrosted fillet pieces lengthwise and mount on the sticks.
4. Roll the sticks in the chopped basil and pepper.
5. Cut the prosciutto into flimsy strips and fold over the salmon.
6. Spread in olive oil and fry in a dish, cook in a stove or on the flame grill.
7. Present with the mayonnaise or a generous plate of mixed greens and a rich aioli.
Nutrition Fact: Calories 680, Fat 62g, Carbs 1g, Sugar 12g, Protein 28g

KETO TUNA PLATE

Prep Time: 5mints, Cooking Time: 10mints, Total Time: 15mints; Serving: 2

Ingredients
- 4 eggs
- 2 oz. baby spinach
- 10 oz. tuna in olive oil
- 1 avocado and ½ cup mayonnaise
- salt and pepper

Instructions
1. Start by cooking the eggs. Lower them cautiously into bubbling water and bubble for 4-8 minutes depending on whether you like them delicate or hard-boiled.
2. Cool the eggs in super cold water for 1-2 minutes when they're set; this will make it simpler to remove the shell.
3. Put eggs, spinach, fish and avocado on a plate. Present with a healthy amount of mayonnaise and maybe a wedge of lemon.
4. Season with salt and pepper
Nutrition Fact: Calories 931, Fat 76g, Carbs 3g, Sugar 21g, Protein 52g

VEGETARIAN RECIPES

KETO SIMPLE VEGAN BOK CHOY SOUP

Prep Time: 1mints, Cook Time: 3minsts, Total Time: 4mints; Serving: 1
INGREDIENTS
- 2 Bok choy stalks
- 1 cup vegetable broth
- 1 tsp nutritional yeast
- 2 dashes garlic powder
- 2 dashes onion powder
- salt and pepper

Instructions
1. Add all fixings in a bowl and mix to blend.
2. Microwave for 3 minutes

Nutrition Facts: Calories 28, Fat 1g, Carbs 4g, Sugar 2g, Protein 7g

ZUCCHINI NOODLES

Prep Time: 15mints, Cooking Time: 10mints, Total Time: 25mints; Serving: 4
INGREDIENTS:
- 3-6 Zucchinis
- Salt

Instructions
1. Wash the zucchini and afterward utilizing a mandolin slicer julienne cut the zucchini.
2. Put zucchini noodles in a colander over an unfilled bowl. Salt zucchini and let represent a few moments. Get dry the noodles.
3. Put noodles in a pot of water on the stove and heat to the point of boiling for around 1-2 minutes.

Nutrition Fact: Calories: 213, Fat 5.3g, Carbs 2.4g, Sugar 2g, Protein 16g

BALSAMIC MARINATED TOMATOES

Prep Time: 5mints, Cooking Time: 10mints, Total Time: 15mints, Serving: 4
Ingredients
- Grape tomatoes
- Balsamic vinegar
- Sea salt and black pepper

Instructions
1. It's so simple. Just cut the tomatoes and pour enough vinegar over to cover them without over-soaking. Sprinkle with a little ocean salt and dark pepper.

Nutrition Fact: Calories 180; Fat 6g, Carbs 9g, Sugar 7g, Protein 24g

PAPRIKA ROASTED RADISHES WITH ONIONS

Prep Time: 20mints, Cooking Time: 20mints, Total Time: 40mints, Serving: 4
Ingredients
- 2- large bunches radishes
- Small onion
- 2- tbsp butter and 2 tbsp olive oil
- tsp fennel seeds
- 1/2- tsp smoked paprika
- Sea salt and black pepper

Instructions
1. Preheat stove to 350° Line a rimmed oven tray with parchment paper.
2. In a blending bowl, add radishes and onion. To the bowl, add spread, olive oil, fennel seeds, paprika, ocean salt, and dark pepper. Remove until radishes and onions are uniformly covered.
3. Pour radishes and onions in a solitary layer onto the parchment paper. Pour any additional spread and flavoring over the top.
4. Prepare for 20 minutes.

Nutrition Fact: Calories: 289, Fat 21.8g, Carbs 14.2g, Sugar 4.2g, Protein 12.3g

SPAGHETTI SQUASH WITH CRISPY SAGE GARLIC SAUCE

Prep Time: 5mints, Cook Time: 15mints, Total Time: 20mints, Serving: 4
INGREDIENTS
- 1 medium spaghetti squash
- 1 cup water and 1 small bunch fresh sage
- 3-5 cloves garlic
- 2 tsp olive oil
- 1 tsp salt
- ⅛ teaspoon nutmeg

INSTRUCTIONS
1. Divide the squash and scoop out the seeds.
2. Add water into the weight cooker and lower the squash parts looking up - stacking them one over the other, if necessary.
3. Close and lock the top of the weight cooker. Cook for 3-4 minutes at high weight.
4. Meanwhile, in a virus sauté dish adds savvy, garlic, and olive oil. Cook the oil blend on low heat, mixing incidentally to cook the savvy leaves. At the point when time is up, open the cooker by discharging the weight.
5. Coax the squash strands out of the shell utilizing a fork and thud them into the sauté' skillet.
6. When the entirety of the squash is there turn off the heat, sprinkle with salt and nutmeg, at that point swoosh everything around to blend well.

Nutritional Fact: Calories: 88.6, Fat 4g, Carbs 13.8g, Sugar 5g, Protein 1.5g

CILANTRO LIME CAULIFLOWER RICE

Prep Time: 15mints, Cooking Time: 10mints, Total Time: 25mints, Serving: 4
Ingredients
- 1 head of cauliflower
- 1 lime
- 2 cloves of garlic
- 1 handful chopped cilantro

Instructions

1. Remove the leaves from the cauliflower and cut the head down the middle. Remove the cauliflower from the center so you just have the florets.
2. Put a large portion of the cauliflower into the processor and procedure until just little pieces remain. Remove from the processor and put it into a container. Procedure the rest of the cauliflower repeating the means
3. Mince the garlic and add to the cauliflower in the dish. Cook over medium heat for around 5 minutes, blending continually.
4. At the point when cauliflower is marginally toasted, and garlic cooked, remove from heat.
5. Remove with cilantro and juice from the entire lime.
Nutrition Fact: Calories: 40, Fat 0.3g, Carbs 9g, Sugar 1g, Protein 3g

OVEN ROASTED CABBAGE WEDGES
Prep Time: 15mints, Cook Time: 45mints, Total Time: 1hr, Serving: 4
Ingredients
- Head Green Cabbage
- ¼- Cup Olive Oil
- 1 ½- tsp garlic salt
- tsp onion powder and 1 tsp fennel seeds
- ¼- tsp black pepper

Instructions
1. Preheat the stove to 400°F. Line a rimmed heating sheet with a silicone preparing mat or parchment paper.
2. Cut the cabbage in 1" cuts through and through.
3. Lines cuts in a solitary layer on an oven tray. Brush each wedge with a liberal covering of olive oil.
4. In a little bowl, add garlic salt, onion powder, fennel seeds, and dark pepper. Sprinkle flavoring over each wedge.
5. Prepare for 45 minutes on the center rack–flipping part of the way through.
Nutrition Fact: Calories 120, Fat 9g, Carbs 9g, Sugar 2g, Protein 2g

BUTTER ROASTED RADISHES
Prep Time: 10mints, Cooking Time: 15mints, Total Time: 25mints, Servings: 4
Ingredients
- 1 lb. Radishes
- 6 Tbs. Butter or Ghee
- 1 tsp. Italian Seasoning
- Garlic Salt

Instructions
1. Preheat stove to 400°
2. Soften spread and blend in Italian flavoring and garlic salt.
3. In an enormous blending bowl, add radishes and spread blend. Remove until radishes are uniformly covered.
4. Line radishes in a solitary layer on a rimmed heating sheet, prepare for 15 minutes.
Nutrition Fact: Calories 173, Fat 17g, Carbs 2.5g, Sugar 2.5g, Protein 1g

PARMESAN-ROASTED CAULIFLOWER
Prep Time: 10mints, Cook Time: 10mints, Total Time: 20mints, Serving: 7
Ingredients
- 1 head cauliflower
- 1 tsp mixed herbs
- 1/2 tsp ground black pepper
- 3 tsp olive oil and 1 tsp salt
- 1/2 cup grated Parmesan cheese

Instructions
1. Preheat range to 450 degrees F. Line a heating sheet with aluminum foil.
2. Organize cauliflower on the readied heating sheet. Sprinkle with salt, combined herbs, and pepper.
3. Sprinkle with olive oil; remove till very a good deal protected. Sprinkle Parmesan cheddar on pinnacle.
4. Broil in the preheated stove until clean, 10 to 15 minutes.
Nutrition Facts: Calories 171, Fat 13.2g, Carb 8.4g, Sugar 6.1g, Protein 6.8g

ROASTED BUFFALO CAULIFLOWER
Prep Time: 10mints, Cook Time: 40mints, Total Time: 50mints, Serving: 7
Ingredients
- 1/3 cup Buffalo wing sauce
- 2 tablespoons extra-virgin olive oil
- 1 tablespoon butter
- 1 head cauliflower, broken into small florets
- 1/4 cup grated Parmesan cheese

Instructions
1. Preheat the stove to 375 tiers F.
2. Put Buffalo sauce, olive oil, and margarine in a massive microwave-safe bowl. Heat until margarine is dissolved, 30 seconds to at least one second.
3. Spread cauliflower on a rimmed oven tray.
4. Prepare within the preheated stove for 30 minutes. Sprinkle Parmesan cheddar on pinnacle.
5. Keep heating till really toasted, round 10mins more.
Nutrition Facts: Calories 164, Fat 11.9g, Carb 11.2g, Sugar 2.4g, Protein 5.5g

LEMON PARMESAN BROCCOLI SOUP
Prep Time: 10mints, Cooking Time: 15mints, Total Time: 25mints, Serving: 4
Ingredients
- 2.5-3 lbs of fresh broccoli florets
- 4 cups of water
- 2 cups unsweetened almond milk
- 3/4 cup parmesan cheese

- 2 tbsp lemon juice

Instructions
1. Put the broccoli and water in an enormous pan. Cover and cook on medium-high until the broccoli are delicate.
2. Hold one cup of the cooking fluid and dispose of the rest.
3. Add half of the broccoli, the held cooking fluid, and almond milk into a blender. Mix until smooth.
4. Come back to the pot with the remainder of the broccoli. Add the parmesan and lemon squeeze and heat until hot.
5. Simply season with pepper or salt for taste

Nutrition Facts: Calories 85, Fat 3.1g, Carbs 10.3g, Sugars 2.5g, Protein 6.8g

COLD SESAME CUCUMBER NOODLE SALAD RECIPE

Prep Time: 20mints, Total Time: 20mints, Servings: 4

Ingredients
- 2 cucumbers
- 1 tsp salt
- 2 tbsp sesame oil
- 2 tbsp rice vinegar
- 2 tbsp sesame seeds white

Instructions
1. Utilize a spiralizer to cut cucumbers into slender noodle-like strands. Spread out on paper towels and sprinkle salt over the cucumber.
2. Let sit down for 15 minutes and pat dry.
3. Taste a piece of cucumber. On the off danger that it's far unreasonably salty in your flavor, wash the cucumber noodles off.
4. Pat dry with paper towels
5. Dress the cucumber noodles with the readied vinaigrette and enhance with taste sesame seeds. Add salt for taste if necessary.

Nutrition Fact: Calories: 107, Fat 9g, Carbs 4g, Sugar 2g, Protein 1g

LOW-CARB CAULIFLOWER HASH BROWNS

Prep Time: 10mints, Cooking Time: 30mints, Total Time: 40mints; Serving: 4

Ingredients
- 1 lb cauliflower
- 3 eggs
- ½ yellow onion
- 2 pinches pepper and 1 tsp salt
- 4 oz. butter

Instructions
1. Wash, trim and mash the cauliflower utilizing a nourishment processor or grater.
2. Place the cauliflower into a huge bowl. Add remaining ingredients and blend. Put aside for 5–10 minutes.
3. Soften a liberal measure of spread or oil on medium heat in a huge skillet. The cooking procedure will go faster on the off chance that you intend to have space for 3–4 flapjacks one after another. Utilize the stove on low heat to keep the main groups of hotcakes warm while you make the others.
4. Put scoops of the ground cauliflower blend in the griddle and allow to spread
5. Fry for 4–5 minutes on each side. Keep in mind that if you flip the pancakes too early they may get destroyed and loose shape.

Nutrition Fact: Calories 282, Fat 26g, Carbs 5g, Sugar 4g, Protein 7g

ROASTED CABBAGE

Prep Time: 20mints, Cooking Time: 35mints, Total Time: 55mints, Serving: 4

Ingredients
- 1 head of green cabbage
- 1 tsp avocado oil
- Salt and pepper to taste

Instructions
1. Preheat stove to 450 tiers
2. Cut the pinnacle of cabbage into 8 wedges and see on a rimmed oven tray.
3. Brush the two aspects with avocado oil and sprinkle salt and new broke pepper to taste on the two aspects.
4. Put cabbage wedges into the range for 25-30 minutes flipping a part of the manner via till you get pleasant company darkish-colored edges.

Nutrition Fact: Calories: 432, Fat 22g, Carbs 8g, Sugar 4g, Protein 34g

NO-COOK REFRESHING MINT AVOCADO CHILLED SOUP

Prep Time: 5mints, Total Time: 5mints, Serving: 2

Ingredients
- 1 medium ripe avocado
- 2 romaine lettuce leaves
- 1 cup of coconut milk
- 1 Tsp lime juice
- 20 fresh mint leaves and salt to taste

Instructions
1. Place every one of the ingredients into a blender and mix well.
2. The soup must be compact but now not as solid as a puree.
3. Chill in the fridge for 5-10 minutes and serve.

Nutrition Fact: Calories: 280, Fat 26g, Carbs 12g, Sugar 2g, Protein 4g

KETO FRIED HALLOUMI CHEESE WITH MUSHROOMS

Prep Time: 5mints, Cooking Time: 10mints, Total Time: 15mints; Serving: 2

Ingredients
- 10 oz. mushrooms
- 10 oz. halloumi cheese
- 3 oz. butter
- 10 green olives

- salt and pepper

Instructions
1. Wash and trim the mushrooms and cut.
2. Heat up a healthy amount of butter in a griddle where you can fit both halloumi and mushrooms
3. Fry the mushrooms on medium heat for 3-5 minutes until they are dark in color. Season with salt and pepper
4. Add more butter and fry the halloumi for a few minutes on each side. Mix the mushrooms from time to time. Lower the heat towards the end.
5. Present with olives.

Nutrition Fact: Calories 830, Fat 74g, Carbs 7g, Sugar 22g, Protein 36g

GOAT CHEESE SALAD WITH BALSAMICO BUTTER

Prep Time: 5mints, Cooking Time: 10mints, Total Time: 15mints; Serving: 2

Ingredients
- 10 oz. goat cheese
- ¼ cup pumpkin seeds
- 2 oz. butter
- 1 tbsp balsamic vinegar
- 3 oz. baby spinach

Instructions
1. Preheat the stove to 400°F (200°C).
2. Put cuts of goat cheese in a lubed dish and heat for 10 minutes.
3. While the goat cheese is in the stove, toast pumpkin seeds in a dry griddle over high temperature till they get a little darker and begin to pop.
4. Lower the heat, add butter and allow to stew till it turns darker in colored and gives out a nutty aroma.
5. Add balsamic vinegar and allow to bubble for a couple of extra minutes.
6. Spread out baby spinach on a plate. Put the cheese on pinnacle and add the balsamic vinegar.

Nutrition Fact: Calories 824, Fat 73g, Carbs 3g, Sugar 25g, Protein 37g

ROASTED GARLIC PARMESAN CAULIFLOWER

Prep Time: 10mints, Cook Time: 40mints, Total Time: 50mints; Serving: 6

Ingredients
- 1 large head cauliflower
- ½ cup grated Parmesan cheese
- 1 tsp Italian Seasoning
- 3 cloves garlic and 3 tsp olive oil
- Sea salt and black pepper

Instructions
1. Preheat the stove to 400°F.
2. In a huge blending bowl, add the cauliflower, Parmesan cheese, Italian flavoring, garlic, olive oil, salt and pepper. Remove until all ingredients are very much joined and the cauliflower is covered.
3. Line in a solitary layer, on a rimmed oven tray and heat on the top rack for 30 to 40 minutes

Nutrition Fact: Calories: 133, Fat 10g, Carbs 4.5, Sugar 3.2g, Protein 6g

CRUNCHY & NUTTY CAULIFLOWER SALAD

Prep Time: 15mints, Cooking Time: 15mints, Total Time: 30mints; Serving: 3

Ingredients
- 3 cups cauliflower
- 1 cup leek
- 1/2 cup organic walnuts
- 1 cup full-fat sour cream
- unrefined sea salt OR Himalayan salt

Instruction
1. Add all ingredients in a huge bowl. Blend until very much blended.
2. Move into a sealed shut compartment.
3. Refrigerate for 3 hours before serving with the goal that the flavors blend further.

Nutrition Fact: Calories: 571, Fat 44g, Carbs 2g, Sugar 2g, Protein 42g

ZUCCHINI NOODLES WITH AVOCADO SAUCE

Prep Time: 10mints, Total Time: 10mints; Serving: 2

Ingredients
- 1 zucchini and 1 avocado
- 1 1/4 cup basil and 1/3 cup water
- 4 tbsp pine nuts
- 2 tbsp lemon juice
- 12 cherry tomatoes

Instructions
1. Make the zucchini noodles utilizing a peeler or the Spiralizer
2. Mix the remainder of the ingredients in a blender until smooth.
3. Add noodles, avocado sauce and cherry tomatoes in a blending bowl.
4. These zucchini noodles with avocado sauce are better eaten fresh; however, you can store them in the cooler for 1 to 2 days.

Nutrition Fact: Calories: 313, Fat 26.8g, Carbs 18.7g, Sugar 6.5g, Protein 6.8g

GRAIN-FREE KETO GRANOLA

Prep Time: 2mints, Cook Time: 20mints, Total Time: 22mints; Serving: 4

Ingredients
- 1 cup nuts and seeds
- 1 tablespoon agave syrup
- 1/2 teaspoon vanilla extract
- 1 teaspoon almond extract
- 1 tablespoon coconut
- 1/4 cup coconut chips

Instructions
1. Preheat stove to 325°F.

2. Blend agave syrup, vanilla concentrate, almond concentrate and coconut oil in a bowl. Heat in microwave 20-30 seconds.
3. Pour blend over nuts and seeds and mix. Heat at 325°F for 10 minutes. Flip and heat again for 5 minutes. Add coconut chips and heat 5 minutes more.
4. Serve

Nutrition Fact: Calories: 299, Fat 8g, Carbs 14g, Sugar 4g, Protein 6g

CHEESY RANCH ROASTED BROCCOLI

Prep Time: 15mints, Cooking Time: 25mints, Total Time: 40mints; Serving: 3

Ingredients
- 4 cups broccoli florets
- 1/4 cup ranch dressing
- 1/2 cup sharp cheddar cheese
- 1/4 cup heavy whipping cream
- kosher salt and pepper to taste

Instructions
1. Place the entirety of the ingredients together in a medium-sized bowl until the broccoli is very much covered.
2. Spread out the broccoli blend in an 8 x 8 ovenproof dish. Heat in a preheated stove at 375 degrees (F) for 30 minutes
3. If not soft enough, place back in the stove for another 5 – 10 minutes, or until satisfied with t's tenderness.
4. Serve warm.

Nutrition Fact: Calories 135, Fat 11g, Carbs 3g, Sugar 2g, Protein 4g

KETO CREAMY AVOCADO PASTA WITH SHIRATAKI

Prep Time: 10mints, Cooking Time: 15mints, Total Time: 25mints; Serving: 4

Ingredients
- packet of shirataki noodles
- avocado ripe
- 1/4- cup heavy cream
- tsp dried basil
- tsp black pepper and 1 tsp salt

Instructions
1. Channel the shirataki noodles in a colander to remove the fluid they come bundled in. Wash completely under running water.
2. Heat up some water and cook the shirataki for 1-2mins to evacuate any waiting aroma. Drain and wash once more.
3. Heat a perfect dry skillet and toss in the shirataki. The noodles contain a lot of water, so this will help dry them out further.
4. Add the rest of the ingredients (you can chose to blend or leave as is) and serve.

Nutrition Fact: Calories: 453, Fat 42g, Carbs 16g, Sugar 3g, Protein 4g

EASY ZUCCHINI NOODLE ALFREDO

Prep Time: 12mints, Cook Time: 10mints, Total Time: 22mints; Servings: 4

Ingredients
- pound zucchini
- 1 Tablespoon olive oil
- ounces cream cheese
- 1 Tablespoon low-fat sour cream
- 1/4 cup Parmesan cheese grated

Instructions
1 Utilize a spiralizer or vegetable peeler to made zucchini noodles.
2 Heat olive oil in a huge skillet over medium heat
3 Add zucchini noodles to the container and sauté for around 5 minutes.
4 Remove noodles to serving dish.
5 Add cream cheese, sour cream, and Parmesan to the skillet and mix to join.
6 Pour sauce over noodles.
7 Top with extra Parmesan cheese if you desire.

Nutrition Fact: Calories: 100, Fat 7g, Carbs 4g, Sugar 3g, Protein 4g

CREAMY MUSHROOM AND CAULIFLOWER RISOTTO RECIPE

Prep Time: 20mints, Cooking Time: 15mints, Total Time: 35mints; Serving: 5

Ingredients
- Cauliflower
- Garlic Cloves
- Sliced Mushrooms
- 1/4 to 1/2 cup Liquid
- Butter/Coconut Oil

Instructions
1 Rice the cauliflower either in a nourishment processor or with a container grater.
2 Heat a little coconut oil or spread in a skillet over medium to high heat
3 When hot, add the garlic and mushrooms.
4 Sauté until diminished.
5 Add the cauliflower and your fluid of decision.
6 Stew delicately, mixing normally until the cauliflower is cooked thoroughly.

Nutrition Fact: Calories: 460, Fat 38g, Carbs 3g, Sugar 1g, Protein 27g

GRILLED HALLOUMI BROCHETTE

Prep Time: 10mints, Cook Time: 10mints, Total Time: 20mints; Servings: 12 slices

Ingredients
- 2 medium tomatoes
- 1/4 cup chopped fresh basil
- 2 to 3 cloves garlic
- 2 tbsp olive oil, Salt, and pepper
- 2 7- ounce packages Halloumi cheese

Instructions
1 In an enormous bowl, add tomatoes, basil, garlic, olive oil, salt, and pepper. Blend well and refrigerate

2 Cut each bit of halloumi once transversely and afterward cut into even 1/2 inch to 1/2-inch slender cuts.
3 You will get around 12 cuts of cheddar. Barbecue over medium heat until marks show up on the cheese, around 2 to 3 minutes on every side. You should relax the cheddar with a metal spatula to turn.
4 Move to a serving plate and top with tomato basil blend.
Nutrition Facts: Calories 134, Fat 11.24g, Carbs 0.96g, Sugar 0.26g, Protein 7.24g

SIMPLE CAULIFLOWER KETO CASSEROLE

Prep Time: 10mints, Cook Time: 35mints, Total Time: 45mints; Serving: 3
Ingredients
- 1/2- head cauliflower florets
- cup shredded Cheddar cheese
- 1/2- cup heavy cream
- Salt and ground black pepper

Instructions
1. Preheat the stove to 400 degrees F.
2. Heat a huge pot of lightly salted water to the point of boiling and cook cauliflower until soft yet firm to the nibble, around 10 minutes. Then drain.
3. Join cheddar, cream, salt and pepper in a huge bowl. Add cauliflower in a dish and cover with cheese blend.
4. Heat in the preheated stove until cheddar is bubbly and turns darker, around 25 minutes.
Nutrition Facts: Calories 469, Fat 40.9g, Carbs 10g, Sugar 13g, Protein 18.1g

STUFFED ZUCCHINI WITH GOAT CHEESE & MARINARA

Prep Time: 15mints, Cooking Time: 25mints, Total Time: 40mints; Serving: 4
Ingredients
- 4 medium-sized zucchinis
- 1 5- ounce log goat cheese
- 1-2 cups marinara sauce
- Chopped parsley

Instructions
1. Preheat oven to 400°F.
2. Cut zucchini down the center the lengthy manner and scoop out the seeds.
3. Season with salt and ground dark pepper and set on a heating sheet
4. Utilizing half of the goat cheese, spread a modest quantity at the base of every zucchini.
5. Spoon marinara sauce on pinnacle.
6. Cook till goat cheese is soft around 10 minutes.
7. Serve right away.
Nutrition Fact: Calories: 412, Fat 22g, Carbs 17g, Sugar 4g, Protein 33g

SIMPLE GREEK SALAD

Prep Time: 20mints, Cooking Time: 15mints, Total Time: 35mints; Serving: 4
Ingredients
- 2 cucumbers
- 1-pint grape tomatoes
- 4 oz feta cheese cubed
- 2 tbsp fresh dill
- 2 tbsp extra virgin olive oil

Instructions
1. Join the initial four ingredients in a medium bowl. Sprinkle with the olive oil.
Nutrition Facts: Calories 118, Fat 9g, Carbs 7g, Sugars 4g, Protein 4.1g

MOROCCAN ROASTED GREEN BEANS

Prep Time: 20mints, Cooking Time: 25mints, Total Time: 45mints; Serving: 4
Ingredients
- cups raw green beans
- 1 tsp kosher salt
- 1/2 tsp ground black pepper
- 1 Tbsp Ras el Hanout seasoning
- 2 Tbsp olive oil

Instructions
1 Remove the green beans, olive oil, and seasonings collectively and spread out on a great parchment sheet.
2 Cook at 400 degrees F for 20 minutes.
3 Remove from the stove and blend.
4 Place back in stove and cook an extra 10 minutes.
5 Remove and serve heated or chilled.
Nutrition Fact: Calories 73, Fat 5g, Carbs 4g, Sugar 2g, Protein 8g

CAPRESE STYLE PORTOBELLO'S

Prep Time: 15mints, Cooking Time: 20mints, Total Time: 35mints; Serving: 4
Ingredients
- Large Portobello mushroom caps
- Cherry tomatoes
- Shredded or fresh mozzarella
- Fresh basil
- Olive oil

Instructions
1 Heat stove to 400degrees F.
2 Line a oven tray with foil for simple cleanup.
3 Brush the tops and edges with olive oil on every mushroom.
4 Cut cherry tomatoes down the middle, place in a bowl, sprinkle with olive oil, and season with chopped basil, salt, and pepper.
5 Put your cheese on the bottom of the mushroom top, spoon at the tomato basil blend and put together until cheese melts and mushrooms are cooked but not overcooked.
Nutrition Fact: Calories: 520, Fat 41g, Carbs 0.5g, Sugar 0.2g, Protein 41g

CHEESY GARLIC ROASTED ASPARAGUS

Prep Time: 10mints, Cook Time: 20mints, Total Time: 30mints; Serving: 4-6
Ingredients
- 1 pound asparagus spears
- 3 tsps olive oil
- 1 tsp minced garlic and 3/4 tsp kosher salt
- 1/4 tsp fresh cracked black pepper
- 1 1/4 cups mozzarella cheese

Instructions
1 Preheat stove to 425°F. Delicately oil an oven tray with nonstick cooking oil spray.
2 Organize asparagus on the prepared sheet. Put aside.
3 In a little bowl combine olive oil, garlic, salt, and pepper
4 Sprinkle the oil blend over the asparagus.
5 Top with mozzarella cheese. Heat for 10-15 minutes until soft, at that point sear until the cheese gets golden.
6 Add salt and pepper, if necessary. Serve right away.
Nutrition Fact: Calories: 440, Fat 48g, Carbs 0.2g Sugar 0.4g, Protein 4g

EASY ROASTED BROCCOLI

Prep Time: 20mints, Cooking Time: 15mints, Total Time: 35mints; Serving: 4
Ingredients:
- 2- Tablespoons olive oil
- ounces broccoli florets
- 1/2- teaspoon salt
- 1/4- teaspoon crushed red chili flakes
- pepper
- juice of half a lemon

Instructions:
1 Preheat the stove to 400 degrees Fahrenheit. Shower a sheet dish with 1 tablespoon olive oil. Put it in the stove while the stove preheats. In an enormous bowl, add the broccoli with the rest of the oil, salt, squashed red chili flakes, and pepper to taste.
2 With a stove glove, remove the sheet dish from the stove and add the broccoli in a solitary layer.
3 Cook for 15 minutes, at that point flip the broccoli and cook for an additional 5 minutes.
4 Remove from the stove. Sprinkle the lemon squeeze over the hot broccoli and taste a piece to check whether you need extra salt or pepper. Serve and enjoy!
Nutrition Fact: Calories: 696, Fat 58g, Carbs 2g, Sugar 0.3g, Protein 42g

THREE-STEP GREEN BEANS RECIPE

Prep Time: 5mints, Cook Time: 10mints, Total Time: 15mints; Serving: 4
Ingredients
- 2 cups heaping green beans
- 1 tablespoon butter
- Salt
- Pepper

Instructions
1. In a big pot, boil salted water. Add green beans, and boil, mixing sometimes, until clean and soft, around 4 to 5mins.
2. Remove beans from heat and throw in a large bowl of ice water till cool, around 3 minutes.
3. Dissolve butter in a big skillet over medium warm temperature. Add beans, season with salt and pepper, and blend till warm and uniformly mixed. Serve right away.
Nutrition Fact: Calories: 117, Fat 10g, Carbs 4g, Sugar 1g, Protein 6g

HASSEL BACK CAPRESE SALADS

Prep Time: 25mints, Cooking Time: 20mints, Total Time: 45mints; Serving: 4
Ingredients:
- 1/2 cup balsamic vinegar
- 6 large, good quality tomatoes
- 1 ball fresh mozzarella cheese
- Few sprigs fresh basil
- Salt and black pepper

Instructions:
1. Start by lessening the balsamic vinegar. Empty it into a little pan and stew over medium-high heat for a few moments, until decreased significantly.
2. Cut thick cuts in the tomatoes, trying not to carve right through. I found that cutting around 4 or 5 cuts for each tomato worked well.
3. Tenderly stuff every tomato with cheese and basil.
4. Sprinkle servings of mixed greens with salt and pepper, and serve showered with the balsamic vinegar.
Nutrition Fact: Calories: 713, Fat 56g, Carbs 0.2g, Sugar 0.3g, Protein 48g

STEAMED ARTICHOKE AND GARLIC BUTTER

Prep Time: 15mints, Cooking Time: 15mints, Total Time: 30mints; Serving: 1
Ingredients:
- 1 artichoke
- 1/2 stick butter
- 1 clove garlic

Instructions
1. Wash the artichoke in cool water. Utilizing a serrated blade, cut off 1/4 of the artichoke
2. Trim the stem with the goal that it is around 1/2-inch lengthy and the artichoke is upstanding.
3. Bring half an inch water to boil in a pot massive enough to keep your artichoke.
4. When boiling add the artichoke and reduce heat to stew.
5. Cover and cook for around 30-40mins.
6. While your artichoke is steaming, heat the butter in a skillet until completely softened. Add the garlic and mix it till aromatic.
7. Serve right away with a variety of napkins and an extra plate to dispose of leaves.

8. To devour an artichoke, pull off a leaf, dunk the bottom into the garlic margarine, and afterward scratch the buttered tissue off together with your teeth.

Nutrition Fact: Calories: 454, Fat 31g, Carbs 26g, Sugars 4.4g, Protein 22g

ACORN SQUASH SLICES

Prep Time: 15mints, Cooking Time: 40mints, Total Time: 55mints; Serving: 6

Ingredients
- 2 medium acorn squash
- 1/2 teaspoon salt
- 3/4 cup maple syrup
- 2 tablespoons butter
- 1/3 cup chopped pecans

Instructions
1. Cut squash down the middle longwise; remove and dispose of seeds. Cut every half widthwise into 1/2-inch cuts; dispose of finishes.
2. Put cuts in a lubed 13-inch. x 9-inch. preparing dish. Sprinkle with salt. Join syrup and spread; pour over squash. Sprinkle with walnuts.
3. Cover and cook at 350°F for 40-45 minutes or until soft.

Nutrition Facts: Calories 170, Fat 7g, Carbs 31g, Sugars 0.2g, Protein 2g

KETO PARSLEY CAULIFLOWER RICE

Prep Time: 10mints, Cook Time: 10mints, Total Time: 20mints; Serving: 2

Ingredients
- 1 head cauliflower washed and dried
- 1 tablespoon olive oil
- 2 cloves garlic and Pinch cayenne
- 1/3 cup parsley
- salt and ground black pepper

Instructions
1. Dispose of the leaves and cut a medium-sized cauliflower head in quarters and mesh each one in every one of them using a container grater with medium openings.
2. Heat a drag of olive oil in a large skillet. Sauté minced garlic.
3. Add cauliflower rice, mix and unfold with a top. Cook for around 10 minutes, blending on more than one occasion.
4. Add chopped parsley, salt, black pepper and a tad of cayenne.
5. Serve and enjoy!

Nutrition Fact: Calories: 141, Fat 7g, Carbs 15g, Sugar 5g, Protein 6g

SAUTÉED RADISHES WITH GREEN BEANS

Prep Time: 10mints, Cooking Time: 10mints, Total Time: 20mints; Serving: 4

Ingredients
- 1 tablespoon butter
- 1/2 pound fresh green
- 1 cup thinly sliced radishes
- 1/2 teaspoon sugar and 1/4 tsp salt
- 2 tsps pine nuts

Instructions
1. In an enormous skillet, heat butter over medium-high heat.
2. Add beans; cook and mix 3-4 minutes or until soft.
3. Add radishes; cook 2-3 minutes longer or until vegetables are soft, mixing once in a while. Mix in sugar and salt; then sprinkle with nuts.

Nutrition Facts: Calories 75, Fat 6g, Carbs 5g, Sugars 2g, Protein 2g

SWEET POTATO & BEAN QUESADILLAS

Prep Time: 15mints, Cooking Time: 15mints, Total Time: 30mints; Serving: 4

Ingredients
- 2 medium sweet potatoes
- 4 whole-wheat tortillas
- 3/4 cup canned black beans
- 1/2 cup shredded pepper jack cheese
- 3/4 cup salsa

Instructions
1. Clean sweet potatoes; penetrate a few times with a fork. Put on a microwave-safe plate. Microwave on high until soft, 7-9mints
2. At the point when cool enough to handle, cut every potato the long way down the middle. Scoop out the mash. Spread onto half of every tortilla; top with beans and cheese
3. Heat a cast-iron skillet or frying pan over medium heat, cook tortillas until golden and cheese has dissolved, 2-3 minutes on each side.
4. Present with salsa.

Nutrition Facts: Calories 306, Fat 8g, Carb 46g, Sugars 9g, Protein 11g

TOASTED RAVIOLI PUFFS

Prep Time: 15mints, Cooking Time: 15mints, Total Time: 30mints; Serving: 2 dozen

Ingredients
- 24 refrigerated cheese ravioli
- 1 tsp reduced-fat Italian salad dressing
- 1 tsp Italian-style panko bread
- 1 tsp grated Parmesan cheese
- Warm marinara sauce

Instructions
1. Preheat stove to 400°F. Cook ravioli as indicated on packet then drain. Move to a lubed parchment sheet.
2. Brush with serving of mixed greens dressing. In a little bowl, blend bread morsels and cheese; sprinkle over ravioli.
3. Heat 12-15 minutes or until golden dark-colored.
4. Present with marinara sauce.

Nutrition Facts: Calories 21, Fat 1g, Carbs 3g, Sugars 0.2g, Protein 1g

TOMATO & AVOCADO SANDWICHES

Prep Time: 5mints, Cooking Time: 5mints, Total Time: 10mints; Serving: 2

Ingredients
- 1/2 medium ripe avocado
- 4 slices whole-wheat bread
- 1 medium tomato
- 2 tsps shallot
- 1/4 cup hummus

Instructions
1. Spread avocado on two cuts of toast. Top with tomato and shallot.
2. Spread hummus and serve.

Nutrition Facts: Calories 278, Fat 11g, Carbs 35g, Sugars 6g, Protein 11g

APPLE, WHITE CHEDDAR & ARUGULA TARTS

Prep Time: 15mints, Cooking Time: 15mints, Total Time: 30mints; Serving: 4

Ingredients
- 1 sheet frozen puff pastry
- 1 cup shredded white cheddar cheese
- 2 medium apples
- 2 tsps olive oil and 1 tsp lemon juice
- 3 cups fresh arugula

Instructions
1. Preheat stove to 400°F. On a floured surface, lay puff pastry, fold into a 12-in. square. Cut baked goods into four squares; place on a parchment paper-lined tray.
2. Sprinkle half of each square with cheese on the inside, 1/4 in. from the edges; top with apples. Crease baked good packing.
3. Press edges with a fork to seal.
4. Heat 16-18 minutes or until golden.
5. In a bowl, whisk oil and lemon juice until mixed; add arugula and remove to cover.
6. Present with cooked pastries.

Nutrition Facts: Calories 518, Fat 33g, Carbs 46g, Sugars 8g, Protein 12g

RISOTTO CAKES

Prep Time: 15mints, Cooking Time: 15mints, Total Time: 30mints; Serving: 4

Ingredients
- 1 large egg
- 2 cups cold leftover risotto
- 1 cup coarse -wheat breadcrumbs
- 2 teaspoons extra-virgin olive oil

Instructions
1. Beat egg in an enormous bowl; mix in leftover risotto and ½ cup breadcrumbs. Put the remaining ½ cup breadcrumbs in a shallow dish. Structure the risotto blend into eight 2½-inch cakes and dig in the breadcrumbs.
2. Coat an enormous nonstick skillet with 1 teaspoon oil and heat over medium heat. Add the cakes and cook until caramelized on the main site, 2 to 4 minutes.
3. To make your very own breadcrumbs, trim the outsides of the wheat bread.
4. Spread on a heating sheet and prepare at 250°F until dry, around 10 to 15 minutes.
5. For locally acquired coarse dry breadcrumbs, we like Ian's image, marked "Panko breadcrumbs." Find them at well-supplied grocery stores.

Nutrition Fact: Calories 303, Fat 9g, Carb 40g, Sugar 0.2g, Protein 11g

APPENDIX : RECIPES INDEX

10-Minute Keto Toast Recipe 24
2 Ingredient Paleo Crockpot Chicken 38
3 Ingredient Flourless Sugar Free Cookies 99
3 Ingredient Keto Almond Butter Cups 99
3 Ingredient Keto Chocolate Coconut Cups 102
3-Ingredient Bacon And Egg Breakfast Muffins 23
3-Ingredient Keto No-Bake Coconut Cookies Recipe 97
3-Ingredient Keto Peanut Butter Fudge 98
3-Ingredient Keto Raspberry Lemon Popsicles 101
4 Ingredient Chocolate Peanut Butter No-Bake Cookies 97
4 Ingredient Keto Vegan Chocolate Coconut Cookies 99
4 Ingredient Keto Vegan Chocolate Snowball Cookies 100
4 Ingredient Low Carb Hot Chocolate Ice Cream 97
4-Ingredient No-Bake Chocolate Coconut Crack Bars 98
4-Ingredient Pancakes 22
5 Ingredient Bacon Wrapped Chicken Breast 46
90-Second Keto Bread In a Mug 90

A

Acorn Squash Slices 133
Almond Coconut Milk Creamer 113
Almond Joy Fruit And Nut Bars 106
Apple Martini 109
Apple, White Cheddar & Arugula Tarts 134
Asparagus + Goat Cheese Frittata 87
Avocado Baked Eggs 75
Avocado Chicken Salad 39

B

Bacon & Egg Fat Bombs 79
Bacon Avocado Ranch Chicken Burger And Tabasco Sauce 44
Bacon Onion Butter 78
Bacon, Braunschweiger, & Pistachio Truffles 85
Bacon-Wrapped Avocado Fries 74
Bacon-Wrapped Chicken Tenders With Ranch Dip 45
Bacon-Wrapped Meatloaf 12
Bacon-Wrapped Mozzarella Sticks 78
Bacon-Wrapped Pork Chops 59
Bacon-Wrapped Scallops 89
Bacon-Wrapped Tahini And Sun-Dried Tomato Stuffed Chicken Breasts 39
Baked Butter Garlic Shrimp 119
Baked Butter Garlic Shrimp 121
Baked Chicken Meatballs - Habanero & Green Chili 43
Baked Eggs And Asparagus With Parmesan 76
Baked Lemon Butter Tilapia 117
Baked Lobster Tails With Garlic Butter 121
Baked Pesto Chicken 34
Baked Rosemary Salmon 123
Baked Sausage With Creamy Basil Sauce 13
Baked White Fish With Pine Nut, Parmesan With Basil Pesto Crust 118
Balsamic Marinated Tomatoes 126
Balsamic, Garlic, And Basil Marinated Chicken Breasts 43
Basic Keto Cheese Crisps 77
Basil Stuffed Chicken Breasts 49
Bbq Chicken Livers And Heart 36
Bbq Chicken Livers And Hearts 38
Beef (Heart) Steak 56
Beef Tongue Into Delicious Crispy Beef 35
Best Keto Popcorn Cheese Puffs 74
Better Than Fat Head Pizza – Pizza Crust 85
Black Beauty – Low Carb Vodka Drink 109
Blackened Dijon Chicken 48
Blackened Ranch Pan-Fried Chicken Thighs 48
Blueberry Coconut Yogurt Smoothie Recipe 25
Blueberry Martini 109
Boiled Eggs With Butter And Thyme 34
Boiled Eggs With Butter And Thyme 70
Boneless Pork Chops Recipe 63
Breakfast Egg Crepes With Avocados 9
Broccoli & Cheddar Keto Bread 69
Broiled Chicken Thighs With Artichokes And Garlic 47
Brussels Sprouts Chips 81
Butter Coffee Rubbed Tri-Tip Steak 54
Butter Roasted Radishes 127
Buttery Coconut Flour Waffles 29

C

Cacao Coffee Recipe 110
Caesar Egg Salad Lettuce Wraps 71
Caesar Egg Salad Lettuce Wraps 88
Caesar Salad Deviled Eggs 71
Caprese Grilled Eggplant Roll-Ups 89
Caprese Style Portobello's 131
Caramelized Onion And Bacon Pork Chops 63
Carrot Chips 81
Cauliflower Fried Rice With Bacon Recipe 68
Cauliflower Mac And Cheese In 4 Minutes 83
Cauliflower-Spinach Side Dish 77
Chamomile Mint Tea Recipe 110
Cheddar And Everything Seasoning Fat Bombs 74
Cheese Meatloaf 20
Cheesy Egg White Veggie Breakfast Muffins 32
Cheesy Garlic Roasted Asparagus 131
Cheesy Keto Biscuits 77
Cheesy Ranch Roasted Broccoli 130
Chicken Al Forno With Vodka Sauce & Two Kinds Of Cheese 46
Chicken Bacon Ranch Casserole 46
Chicken Breast With Olive Tapenade 35
Chicken Caesar 41
Chicken Liver With Raw Garlic And Thyme 39
Chicken Pepper Poppers For Bbqs And Potlucks 40

Chicken, Bacon, And Apple Mini Meatloaves Recipe 41
Chili Roasted Chicken Thighs 45
Chimichurri Shrimp 119
Chipotle Steak Bowl 59
Chocolate Chip Ice Cream 94
Chocolate Coconut Gummies 102
Chocolate Peanut Butter Balls 107
Chocolate Protein Pancakes 105
Chocolate Protein Waffles 27
Cilantro Lime Cauliflower Rice 126
Cinnamon "Rice" Breakfast Pudding 33
Cinnamon Bun Fat Bomb Bars 95
Cinnamon Chocolate Breakfast Smoothie Recipe 28
Cinnamon Faux-St Crunch Cereal 30
Cloud Eggs 88
Coconut Fat Bombs 19
Coconut Flour Crepes 30
Coconut Flour Pizza Crust Recipe 85
Coconut Macadamia Bars – Breakfast In Five 24
Coconut Milk Latte 110
Coconut Milk Strawberry Smoothie 25
Coco-Nutty Grain-Free Granola 31
Coffee Barbecue Pork Belly 60
Cold Brew Protein Shake Smoothie 31
Cold Sesame Cucumber Noodle Salad Recipe 128
Corned Beef And Cauliflower Hash 58
Corned Beef Hash 52
Cosmopolitan Cocktail Recipe 112
Cowboy Burgers (Keto) 52
Cranberry Ginger Mulled Wine 109
Cream Cheese Pancakes – Low Carb & Keto 105
Cream Of Celery Soup 10
Creamy Mexican Slow Cooker Keto Chicken 49
Creamy Mushroom And Cauliflower Risotto Recipe 130
Creamy Triple Chocolate Keto Shake 24
Crispy Cheddar Crisps 80
Crispy Green Bean Chips 81
Crispy Keto Chicken Thighs Recipe 17
Crispy Pork Chops Keto 63
Crispy Sweet Potato Fries 75
Crock Pot Chicken Stock 37
Crockpot Chicken Stock 38
Crockpot Green Chile Chicken 47
Crunchy & Nutty Cauliflower Salad 129
Cube Steak 55
Cucumber Basil Ice Cubes Recipe 111
Cucumber Lime Water 111
Curry-Roasted Shrimp With Oranges 114

D

Dairy-Free Boosted Keto Coffee 109
Dairy-Free Peanut Butter And Jelly Smoothie 26
Dirty Chai 111

E

Easy 5 Ingredient Paleo Roast Chicken 42
Easy Broiled Table Seasoned Mini Beef Patties 52
Easy Crockpot Bone Broth 86
Easy Keto Avocado Toast Recipe 27
Easy Keto Broccoli Beef Recipe 64
Easy Keto Fried Coconut Shrimp 118
Easy Keto Fudge Recipe With Cocoa Powder 107
Easy Keto Garlic Roasted Bok Choy 99
Easy Keto Ham And Cheese Rolls Recipe 104
Easy Keto Instant Pot Chile Verde 61
Easy Keto Pepperoni Meatballs 9
Easy Low Carb Cauliflower Pizza Crust Recipe 83
Easy Low Carb Keto Breakfast Casserole 32
Easy Marinated Grilled Steak Tacos 54
Easy Mexican Chicken Casserole With Chipotle 46
Easy Mozzarella & Pesto Chicken Casserole 45
Easy Paleo Broccoli Beef Recipe 58
Easy Paleo Chicken Pepper Stir-Fry 44
Easy Pan-Fried Lemon Chicken 11
Easy Roasted Broccoli 132
Easy Sardines Salad Recipe 124
Easy Slow Cooker Keto Pot Roast 50
Easy Stovetop Sugar-Free Candied Almonds 98
Easy Taco Casserole Recipe 70
Easy Zucchini Beef Saute, Garlic, And Cilantro 58
Easy Zucchini Beef Saute, Garlic, And Cilantro 64
Easy Zucchini Noodle Alfredo 130
Egg & Chorizo Muffins 76
Egg Fast Fried Boiled Eggs With Yum Yum Sauce 72
Egg Fast Recipe: Egg Puffs 72
Egg Muffins With Sausage, Spinach, And Cheese 76
Egg Nest Recipe With Braised Cabbage 87
Eggplant French Toast 79
Eggs En Cocotte Recipe 87
Energizing Keto Smoothie 27
English Toffee Fat Bombs 95
Everything But The Bagel 33
Express Shrimp & Sausage Jambalaya 114

F

Fancy Af Egg Clouds Recipe 87
Farmhouse Beans & Sausage 22
Fat Bombs 96
Fat Head Pizza - The Holy Grail 86
Fathead Pizza Dough- Keto 85
Five-Minute Keto Curried Tuna Salad Recipe 124
Five-Minute Keto Fried Sardines Recipe With Olives 124
Five-Minute Keto Sardines And Onions Recipe 124
Five-Spice Tilapia 114
Fluffy Microwave Scrambled Eggs 71
Fresh Strawberry Lime Popsicles 100
Fresh Tomato Basil Soup 12
Fried Mahi Fish Bites 124
Frozen Blueberry Fat Bombs 18
Frozen Keto Berry Shake 25
Fudgy Macadamia Chocolate Fat Bomb 101

G

Garlic & Rosemary Lamb Chops 65

Garlic Bacon Wrapped Chicken Bites Recipe 10
Garlic Butter Baked Pork Chops 61
Garlic Dill Baked Cucumber Chips 75
Garlic Ghee Baked Chicken Breast 42
Garlic Lemon Butter Crab Legs 115
Garlic Lemon Chicken Breast 41
Garlic Parmesan Baked Tortilla Chips 80
Ghee Aka Clarified Butter 77
Goat Cheese Salad With Balsamico Butter 129
Grain-Free "Whole Grain" Crackers 80
Grain-Free Butter Bread 90
Grain-Free Keto Granola 129
Greek Lamb Chop Marinade 66
Grilled Beef Liver 22
Grilled Chicken Drumsticks With Garlic Marinade 43
Grilled Chicken With Chimichurri Sauce 43
Grilled Halloumi Brochette 130
Grilled Lamb Chops With Dijon-Basil Butter 65
Grilled Lamb In Paleo Mint Cream Sauce 65
Grilled Salmon With Creamy Pesto 116
Grilled Salmon With Creamy Pesto Sauce 120
Grilled Swordfish Skewers With Pesto Mayo 116
Guilt-Free Slow Cooked Shoulder Of Lamb 66

H

Halloumi Cheese With Butter-Fried Eggplant 69
Happy Almond Bombs – Keto Fat Bombs 96
Hassel Back Caprese Salads 132
Healthy 3 Ingredients No Bake Paleo Vegan Coconut Crack Bars 98
Healthy Buffalo Chicken Dip 38
Healthy Chocolate Peanut Butter Low Carb Smoothie 11
Healthy Chocolate Peanut Butter Low Carb Smoothie 25
Healthy No Churn Workout Protein Ice Cream 98
Herb Roasted Bone Marrow 21
Hidden Liver Meatballs 53
High Protein Low Carb Breakfast Casserole 33
Holley's Ham And Swiss Breakfast Muffins 32
Homemade Baked Banana Chips 83
Homemade Thai Chicken Broth 42
Honeysuckle Tea 111
Huevos Pericos Colombian Scrambled Eggs 88

I

Instant Pot Keto Crack Chicken 48
Italian Keto Plate 84

J

Jalapeno Popper Deviled Eggs With Bacon 79
Jello Cream Cheese Fat Bomb 101
Juicy Ranch Chicken 39

K

Kale And Chives Egg Muffins 23
Kale Keto Tofu Stir Fry 11
Kalua Pork 60
Kamikaze Shot Sugar-Free 111
Kathleen's Cottage Pancakes 105
Keto "Everything" Avocado Breakfast 13
Keto "Peanut Butter" Cookies 19

Keto 2 Minute Avocado Oil Mayo 88
Keto 3-Ingredient Muffins Recipe 16
Keto 4-Ingredient Almond Flour Cookies 17
Keto 5-Ingredient Coconut Flour Cookies 15
Keto Almond Butter Chicken Saute 42
Keto Almond Butter Cookie Dough 14
Keto Almond Butter Fat Bomb Sandwiches Recipe 103
Keto Avocado Dessert 104
Keto Bacon Asparagus Mini Frittata Recipe 30
Keto Bacon Wrapped Asparagus With a Secret Sauce 91
Keto Bacon Wrapped Salmon With Pesto 116
Keto Bagels Recipe With Fathead Dough 105
Keto Baked Bacon Omelet 14
Keto Baked Salmon With Lemon And Butter 123
Keto Baked Salmon With Lemon And Butter 125
Keto Barbecue Dry Rub Ribs 61
Keto Beef Liver With Asian Dip 56
Keto Beetroot Shake For Athletes 25
Keto Blueberry Ginger Smoothie 27
Keto Blueberry Mojito 113
Keto Boosted Coffee Recipe 108
Keto Boosted Coffee Recipe 14
Keto Breakfast Pizza 19
Keto Broccoli Beef Stir-Fry 55
Keto Broccoli Beef Stir-Fry Recipe 10
Keto Broccoli Soup Recipe 11
Keto Brunch Spread 15
Keto Brunch Spread 69
Keto Buffalo Cauliflower Wings 36
Keto Cheese Omelet 68
Keto Cheesecake Cupcakes 107
Keto Chicken Hearts Recipe 12
Keto Chili Dog Pot Pie Casserole 60
Keto Chocolate Coconut Cups 16
Keto Chocolate Mason Jar Ice Cream 106
Keto Chocolate Nut Clusters 96
Keto Chocolate Peanut Butter Cookies 100
Keto Chocolate Peppermint Smoothie Recipe 27
Keto Chocolate Raspberry Spinach Green Smoothie 29
Keto Chocolate Smoothie 26
Keto Cinnamon Chocolate Chia Pudding 73
Keto Cloud Bread 10
Keto Coconut Coffee Recipe 108
Keto Coconut Fat Bomb Sandwiches Recipe 103
Keto Coconut Shrimp Recipe 121
Keto Collagen Boosted Coffee 108
Keto Cookie Dough (With Chocolate Chips) 70
Keto Corned Beef And Hash Recipe 56
Keto Creamy Avocado Pasta With Shirataki 130
Keto Crème Brule 94
Keto Crispy Rosemary Chicken Drumsticks 35
Keto Crockpot Garlic Chicken 37
Keto Crockpot Garlic Chicken 44
Keto Crockpot Shredded Chicken 35
Keto Curried Tomato Soup 9
Keto Curry Candied Bacon Recipe 82
Keto Deviled Eggs 84

Keto Dijon Smothered Chicken Drumsticks 34
Keto Electrolyte Drink 14
Keto Fat Bombs | Cookies And Cream 104
Keto Four-Ingredient Pancake With Almond Flour Recipe 30
Keto Fried Cabbage With Crispy Bacon 18
Keto Fried Chicken With Broccoli 15
Keto Fried Fish 117
Keto Fried Halloumi Cheese With Mushrooms 128
Keto Fried Salmon With Asparagus 123
Keto Fried Salmon With Green Beans 22
Keto Frothy Coffee Recipe 108
Keto Garlic Cheese 'Bread' 78
Keto Ginger Cilantro Smoothie 29
Keto Golden Chicken Bacon Fritter Balls Recipe 44
Keto Grilled Lobster Tails With Creole Butter 120
Keto Guacamole Burgers 9
Keto Hollandaise 91
Keto Honey Mustard Chicken 47
Keto Honey Mustard Chicken 49
Keto Honey Mustard Dressing 91
Keto Iced Apple Green Tea 110
Keto Iced Lemon Coffee Recipe 108
Keto Instant Pot Roasted Bone Broth Recipe 51
Keto Jalapeno Poppers 68
Keto Lemon Baked Salmon Recipe 122
Keto Lemon Baked Salmon Recipe 20
Keto Lemon Ginger Green Juice Shots Recipe 28
Keto Lemon Pepper Roast Chicken 41
Keto Low Carb Tortilla Chips 74
Keto Macadamia Crusted Chicken Breast 44
Keto Madeleine Cookies 16
Keto Muffins 107
Keto Mushroom Omelet 23
Keto Oatmeal: 5-Minute Low-Carb Oatmeal 31
Keto Organic Peanut Smoothie 26
Keto Oven-Baked Steak With Garlic Thyme Portabella Mushrooms 51
Keto Oven-Baked Steak With Garlic Thyme Portabella Mushrooms 57
Keto Parsley Cauliflower Rice 133
Keto Peanut Butter Cookies 102
Keto Peanut Butter Fudge Fat Bomb 94
Keto Pecan Crisps Recipe 20
Keto Pizza Casserole 21
Keto Pizza Chips 75
Keto Pork Belly 63
Keto Raspberry Avocado Smoothie 27
Keto Red Velvet Smoothie Recipe 28
Keto Roasted Bone Marrow Recipe 50
Keto Roasted Brussels Sprouts With Garlic 12
Keto Rosemary Roast Beef And White Radishes 55
Keto Salmon-Filled Avocados 21
Keto Salt And Pepper Crackers 82
Keto Sausage And Egg Breakfast Sandwich 32
Keto Sausage Balls 76
Keto Shortbread Cookies 18
Keto Shrimp And Cucumber Appetizer Recipe 122
Keto Simple Vegan Bok Choy Soup 126
Keto Skirt Steak 54
Keto Slow Cooker Greek Chicken 48
Keto Slow Cooker Onions 64
Keto Smoked Salmon And Avocado Plate 17
Keto Smoked Salmon And Avocado Plate 20
Keto Smoked Salmon Plate 16
Keto Smoked Salmon Plate 19
Keto Smoked Salmon Salad With Poached Egg 122
Keto Smoothie - Blueberry 24
Keto Smoothie Recipe {With Chocolate & Chia Seeds} 29
Keto Sous-Vide Fillet Steak Recipe 56
Keto Sous-Vide Fillet Steak Recipe 57
Keto Spicy Beef Avocado Cups 53
Keto Spicy Beef Avocado Cups 55
Keto Spinach Avocado Green Smoothie 28
Keto Steak Au Poivre 53
Keto Steak Au Poivre 57
Keto Steamed Clams With Basil Garlic Butter 115
Keto Stove-Top Bone Broth 74
Keto Traditional Coffee Recipe 108
Keto Tuna Plate 125
Keto Tuna Salad 120
Keto Turmeric Bone Broth 111
Keto Vanilla Almond Fat Bomb 103
Keto Vegan Chocolates 100
Keto-Friendly Baked Cheese Crisps 73

L

Lamb & Leek Burgers 52
Lamb & Leek Burgers With Lemon Cream 66
Lamb Lollipops With Garlic And Rosemary Recipe 65
Lamb, Red Onion And Herb Koftas 66
Lemon Cheesecake Fat Bombs With Cream Cheese 96
Lemon Fruit And Nut Bars 68
Lemon Parmesan Broccoli Soup 127
Lemon Parsley Chicken 36
Lemon Pepper Chicken 38
Lemon Pepper Pork Chops 63
Lemon Turmeric Roasted Cauliflower Keto 70
Low Carb Bacon & Eggs 73
Low Carb Blueberry Mojitos 108
Low Carb Blueberry Protein Power Smoothie 26
Low Carb Cheese Enchiladas 88
Low Carb Chicken Nuggets Keto 49
Low Carb Chocolate Bark 102
Low Carb Chocolate Coconut Fat Bombs 101
Low Carb Chocolate Mason Jar Ice Cream 93
Low Carb Fried Mac & Cheese 89
Low Carb Jello Pops 94
Low Carb Keto Banana Nut Protein Pancakes 106
Low Carb Keto Chocolate Bar 17

Low Carb Keto Egg Noodles 72
Low Carb Margarita 112
Low Carb Margaritas 112
Low Carb Mojito 112
Low Carb Oatmeal With Coconut Flour 123
Low Carb Onion Rings 21
Low Carb Orange Dreamlike Smoothie 32
Low Carb Pina Colada 111
Low Carb Pork Medallions 58
Low Carb Pumpkin Cheesecake Mousse 104
Low Carb Rolls 95
Low Carb Soft Shell Crab 115
Low Carb Spicy Shrimp Hand Rolls 119
Low Carb Strawberry Margarita Gummy Worms 109
Low Carb Tortilla Pork Rind Wraps 60
Low-Carb 5 Minute Mocha Smoothie 29
Low-Carb Almond And Parmesan Baked Fish 117
Low-Carb Blueberry Vanilla Smoothie 26
Low-Carb Cauliflower Hash Browns 128
Low-Carb Fish Curry With Coconut And Spinach 117
Low-Carb Keto Cheese Taco Shells 78
Low-Carb Keto Tuna Pickle Boats 72
Low-Carb Stuffed Poblano Peppers 51
Low-Carb Waffles 106

M
Macadamia Nut Fat Bomb 93
Malted Milk Ice Cream 93
Mckee Strawberry Keto Milkshake 25
Meat-Lover Pizza Cups 31
Meat-Lover Pizza Cups 84
Microwave Paleo Bread 72
Mini Zucchini Avocado Burgers 51
Minty Green Protein Smoothie Shake 25
Mock French Toast 79
Moroccan Roasted Green Beans 131

N
No-Bake Keto Butter Cookies 97
No-Bake Keto Vegan Peanut Butter Cookies 100
No-Cook Refreshing Mint Avocado Chilled Soup 128
Nutella Fat Bombs 103

O
One-Minute Keto Mug Bread 73
One-Pot Braised Lamb With Caramelized Onions And Rosemary 67
Oven Roasted Cabbage Wedges 127
Oven-Baked Bacon 77
Oyster Broiled With Spicy Sauce 115

P
Paleo Crispy Garlic Curry Chicken Drumsticks Recipe 40
Paleo Crock Pot Oxtail With Mustard Gravy 52
Paleo Egg Frittata Muffins Recipe [Keto, Dairy-Free] 31
Paleo Garlic Chicken Nuggets 40
Paleo Guacamole Burger Recipe 13
Paleo Rib Eye Steak 55
Paleo Slow Cooker Pork Recipe 50
Paleo Vegan Coconut Cranberry Crack Bars 97
Paleo/Gf Popcorn Shrimp Recipe 122
Paleo-Italian Carpaccio 54
Pan Seared Duck Breast 57
Pan-Seared Beef Tongue 35
Paprika Roasted Radishes With Onions 126
Parmesan Chicken Tenders 47
Parmesan Chive And Garlic Keto Crackers 91
Parmesan Crisps Baked With Zucchini And Carrots 82
Parmesan Crusted Cod 121
Parmesan-Roasted Cauliflower 127
Peanut Butter Chocolate Cookies 101
Pecan Crusted Pork Chops 62
Perfect Keto Avocado Breakfast Bowl 23
Perfect Keto Peaches And Cream Fat Bombs 24
Pink Peppercorn Smoked Salmon Salad Recipe 124
Pizza Eggs Keto 71
Poached Cod In Tomato Sauce 125
Pomegranate Chicken Salad Recipe 40
Portobello Mushroom Mini Keto Pizzas 73
Pot Pork Chops Dinner 62
Prosciutto-Wrapped Salmon Skewers 125
Protein Pudding - Chocolate Or Vanilla 105
Pumpkin Pie Fruit And Nut Bars 106
Pumpkin Seed Bark And Dark Chocolate & Sea Salt 102
Pumpkin Spice Apple Chips 82
Pumpkin Spice Boosted Keto Coffee 113
Pumpkin Spice Roasted Pecans 90

Q
Quick Keto Bacon-Wrapped Salmon 123

R
Ranch Chicken 46
Raspberry Fat Bombs - Cream Heart Jellies 103
Refreshing Cucumber Celery Lime Smoothie 27
Risotto Cakes 134
Roasted Buffalo Cauliflower 127
Roasted Butternut Squash Cubes 90
Roasted Cabbage 128
Roasted Garlic Parmesan Cauliflower 129
Roasted Salmon With Parmesan Dill Crust 121
Roasted Squash, Pomegranate Seeds And Spiced Walnut Salad 89
Rosemary & Sea Salt Flax Crackers 83
Rosemary And Sea Salt Crackers 83
Rosemary Garlic Butter Pork Chops 62
Rosemary Garlic Chicken Kabobs 47
Rosemary Liver Burgers 50
Rosemary Mint Soda 15

S
Salmon Florentine 120
Salmon Garlicky Black Pepper And Egg Free Lemon Aioli 116
Salmon Roasted In Butter 116
Salt And Vinegar Zucchini Chips 80
Salted Caramel Keto Smoothie 29
Sausage Kale Soup With Mushroom 66

Sautéed Radishes With Green Beans 133
Savory Salmon Fat Bombs 78
Schlemmerfilet Bordelaise Herbed Almond And Parmesan Crusted Fish 117
Seared Salmon With Green Peppercorn Sauce 114
Sesame Mirin Kale Chips 81
Sheet Pan Brussels Sprouts With Bacon 23
Shredded Taco Pork 60
Shrimp Recipe With Garlic Butter Cauliflower Rice 118
Shrimp Stacks 114
Simple Beef Tenderloin Filet Mignon 53
Simple Bone Broth 34
Simple Cauliflower Keto Casserole 131
Simple Greek Salad 131
Simple Marinated Chicken Hearts 42
Sleep In" Smoothie 27
Slow Cook Chicken Curry 37
Slow Cooker Chicken Adobo Keto 37
Slow Cooker Keto Corned Beef Cabbage 59
Slow Cooker Keto Meatballs 64
Slow Cooker Paleo Chicken Broth 36
Slow Cooker Pork 50
Slow-Cooked Keto Corned Beef Brisket 53
Smoked Paprika Chicken 36
Smoked Salmon Pinwheels 120
Smoky Tuna Pickle Boats – Low Carb & Gluten-Free 118
Sour Cream And Chive Crackers 80
Sour Cream And Chive Egg Clouds 71
Spaghetti Squash With Crispy Sage Garlic Sauce 126
Spicy Cheddar Crisps 81
Spicy Keto Cheese Chips 70
Spicy Keto Deviled Eggs 68
Spicy Keto Deviled Eggs 84
Spicy Sausage, Cheese, And Egg Muffins 77
Spiked Root Beer Float 112
Spinach Pizza Crust 86
Spinach-Mozzarella Stuffed Burgers 92
Split Chicken Breast With Onions And Mushrooms 37
Spring Soup With Poached Egg 34
Steamed Artichoke 86
Steamed Artichoke And Garlic Butter 132
Strawberry & Mint Smoothie 28
Strawberry Avocado Coconut Smoothie 28
Strawberry Avocado Keto Smoothie With Almond Milk 26

Strawberry Cheesecake Fat Bombs 95
Strawberry Dole Whip Recipe 104
Strawberry Ice Cream 93
Strawberry Low Carb Popsicles Freezer Pops 101
Strawberry Protein Smoothie 26
Stuffed Chicken With Asparagus & Bacon 45
Stuffed Pork Chops – 5 Ingredients 59
Stuffed Pork Chops – 5 Ingredients 62
Stuffed Pork Chops With Bacon And Gouda 61
Stuffed Zucchini With Goat Cheese & Marinara 131
Sugar-Free Coconut Ice Cream 94
Sugar-Free Low Carb Dried Cranberries 93
Super Easy Spicy Baked Chicken 45
Sweet Potato & Bean Quesadillas 133

T

Taco Sauce – Low Carb, Gluten-Free 85
Taco Sauce 89
The Best Bunless Burger Recipe Burgers 64
The Garden Surprise – Keto Gin Cocktail 113
The Splendido 112
The Ultimate Keto Buns 74
Three Ingredient Keto Steak Sauté 18
Three Ingredient Keto Steak Sauté 54
Three-Step Green Beans Recipe 132
Toasted Ravioli Puffs 133
Tomato & Avocado Sandwiches 134
Tomato Chips 82
Traditional Lime Mojito Recipe With Honey 113
Turkey And Cheese Rolls 73
Turkey Meatloaf 13
Turmeric Ginger Lime Tea Recipe 110
Tuscan-Style Grilled Rib Eye Steak 58

V

Vanilla Latte Martini 108
Vegan Keto Porridge 30
Vegged Up Paleo Beef Burgers 50

W

White Chocolate Fat Bombs 103
White Lasagna Stuffed Peppers 69
Wilted Organic Kale & Bacon 90
World's Moistest Chicken 39
World's Easiest Crockpot Pork Roast 50

Z

Zero Carb Fried Shrimp 119
Zingy Salted Lime Soda 110
Zucchini Noodles 126
Zucchini Noodles With Avocado Sauce 129

www.ingramcontent.com/pod-product-compliance
Lightning Source LLC
Chambersburg PA
CBHW081114080526
44587CB00021B/3588